hormone
intelligence

Also by Aviva Romm, MD

The Adrenal Thyroid Revolution

Botanical Medicine for Women's Health

The Natural Pregnancy Book

Natural Health After Birth

Vaccinations: A Thoughtful Parent's Guide

Naturally Healthy Babies and Children

AVIVA ROMM

hormone intelligence

THE COMPLETE GUIDE TO
CALMING HORMONE CHAOS AND
RESTORING YOUR BODY'S NATURAL
BLUEPRINT FOR WELL-BEING

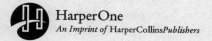

HarperOne
An Imprint of HarperCollinsPublishers

FIRST EDITION

Designed by SBI Book Arts, LLC

Library of Congress Cataloging-in-Publication Data

Names: Romm, Aviva Jill, author.
Title: Hormone intelligence : the complete guide to calming hormone chaos and restoring your body's natural blueprint for well-being / Aviva Romm.
Description: First edition. | San Francisco : HarperOne, [2021] | Includes bibliographical references.
Identifiers: LCCN 2020051682 (print) | LCCN 2020051683 (ebook) | ISBN 9780062796219 (hardcover) | ISBN 9780062796271 (paperback) | ISBN 9780062796240 (ebook)
Subjects: LCSH: Hormone therapy.
Classification: LCC RM286 .R66 2021 (print) | LCC RM286 (ebook) | DDC 615.3/6—dc23
LC record available at https://lccn.loc.gov/2020051682
LC ebook record available at https://lccn.loc.gov/2020051683

21 22 23 24 25 LSC 10 9 8 7 6 5 4 3

For those who have been told you are too sensitive, too outspoken, too emotional, too *hormonal*. Own it. It's your inner guidance system. It's a superpower.

For all who have put your confidence in me as a doctor, healer, teacher, and who have shared your struggles and healing stories. Thank you. I am always listening.

For the girls now—the women of tomorrow—may you inherit a world in which you can thrive and that honors your agency over your body.

And for my daughters, goddaughter, and granddaughters to come.

CONTENTS

WHAT'S IN A NAME

Gender and Language in This Book

My intention is for this book to be inclusive of all people who need help with their hormones or gynecologic concerns. The focus of this book is the health concerns of those born with and/or possessing "women's tack." While I use the words *woman/women/she/her*, as you read, please insert the words that you relate to.

I also want to acknowledge my privilege. I cannot speak from lived experience of the impact of systemic racism on a woman's health but want to acknowledge that there are unacceptable disparities in how most conditions I discuss in this book affect BIWOC.

I use medically defined anatomic terms so that we have a common language that enables us to decipher health information and also speak authoritatively with health care providers. However, I want to note that many of these terms are named by and for men (i.e., *vagina* means "a sheath" for a sword), and that language has played a part in co-opting women's bodies. In my personal life, I use the Sanskrit term *yoni* instead of *vulva*, because it connotes the sacred feminine, and sometimes I might let that fly in the book.

I generally avoid terms like *reproductive* (unless relevant) and *sexual organs* because not all people with these parts want to reproduce, and some might not have those body parts and may be highly sexual. My goal is to help illuminate a new and inclusive approach to women's health in which we all feel whole and safe, including in discussing everything we need to stay healthy.

I sincerely hope that you're able to connect with these words and stories; I take full responsibility for my language shortcomings and appreciate your patience.

introduction

YOU ARE NOT BROKEN

I am no longer accepting the things I cannot change.
I am changing the things I cannot accept.

—Angela Y. Davis

Wouldn't it be incredible if you could look forward to your period—or at least not hate it anymore—knowing you won't be struggling with cramps, crazy-ass mood swings, swollen breasts, and bloating? If you could wake up knowing that endometriosis pain won't make you pop Motrin, Advil, or something stronger just to make it through the day? How fantastic would it be to not have to take "the Pill" to suppress period pain, acne, endometriosis, or polycystic ovary syndrome (PCOS) symptoms? What if you knew you could get pregnant easily, when you're ready to, without spending tens of thousands of dollars and months of physical and mental stress on fertility treatments—or you knew how to make those treatments more effective? What if we all knew we could look forward to a healthy menopause, free of hormone replacement therapy (HRT) to manage hot flashes, vaginal dryness, poor sleep, or a hysterectomy for fibroids? What if you could wake up each morning ready to face the day with energy and vitality, body confidence, and even (dare I say) feeling a bit sexy?

You've probably already been searching online for answers, perhaps even changing your diet, taking supplements, doing yoga, or seeing an acupuncturist, naturopath, therapist, health coach, or all of the above. Brava! But sorting through the morass of options and "expert" guidance out there is overwhelming and even anxiety provoking. There's so much information, it's often conflicting, and it's hard to know who and what to trust. You may have already spent a lot of time and money trying various approaches that just haven't worked. It would make anyone want to throw their hands up, say F-It, and reach for the Motrin!

Welcome to a whole new medicine for women! I invite you to exhale, because all this is possible. I'm Dr. Aviva Romm. The goal of this book is to change all that for you: to share practical, actionable, affordable guidelines that you know you can trust because they've been clinically proven, and that really work to help you reclaim your hormonal, gynecologic, and whole health. You've now got me on this journey with you, and I've spent a combined thirty-six years practicing as a midwife and Yale-trained MD (yes, both!) specializing in women's health. I know a thing or two about why it's time for a major paradigm shift from the old way of doing things with a pill for every ill and dismissive attitudes, to one that respects women, honors our capacity to heal, and doesn't turn to medications and surgery as the first or only solution for everything that ails us. I also know you need answers; I will bring you those that really make a difference.

Undoubtedly, you've picked this book up because you're experiencing a hormone imbalance or gynecologic condition that's somewhere along the spectrum of annoying and troublesome to severe or debilitating. Perhaps you know something is up, can't seem to get a diagnosis, and want to know what's going on. Perhaps you've had a diagnosis but are completely confused about what it means and what you can do. And perhaps you want more natural solutions than the pharmaceutical or surgical treatment you've been told is your only option.

If you're wondering what on earth is going on with your periods, if you're sick and tired of feeling hijacked by your hormones (lately or for as long as you can remember!), or simply uncomfortable, month after month, or day after day; if you're interested in natural alternatives but have no idea what's safe and effective, or if your questions have been dismissed by a doctor for what you were pretty sure were hormone conditions and haven't been able to get a real answer about what's going on, you're not alone, and finally, you're in the right place.

Regardless of whether you're struggling with the specific symptoms or one of the seven major conditions I help you with in this book, you're curious to know more about your hormones and body, or you're not quite sure if a hormone imbalance is at the heart of what you're experiencing—or it's something else—this book finally answers the questions: *What does hormone health look like and how do you get it?*

A Hidden Hormone Epidemic

Why am I so passionate about supporting you on this journey? Because I believe you deserve to live your most powerful life and our hormones significantly influence pretty much everything. Simply put: if your hormones aren't happy, neither are you! Also, as a woman, midwife + physician, and mom of three daughters, I know you need better answers than most women get at their doctor's office.

As you'll soon learn, we're in the midst of a hidden epidemic in which an extraordinary number of women of all ages and life stages—at least 80% of us—will struggle with a hormone or gynecologic problem in our lifetime, significant enough to cause disruption in our life quality, career, or overall health. And though women's hormonal and gynecologic condition, from our teens through menopause, have surged to epic numbers over the past decade, too many in the medical establishment are willing to simply chalk this up to a "new normal," and shrug and say "take the Pill," with women being told in so many different ways that it's no big deal.

But it is a big deal. There have been *far* too many women enduring *far* too much discomfort for *far* too long.

The Many Faces of Hormone-Related Conditions

Hormone-related conditions show up in many ways, including those that commonly bring women to my office and that can be improved with this book:

- PMS
- Polycystic ovary syndrome (PCOS)
- Infertility
- Endometriosis
- Fatigue, low energy
- Hormonal migraines and headaches
- Menstrual cramps
- Miscarriages
- Monthly breast tenderness and lumps
- Sleep problems
- Thyroid problems
- Weight gain
- Anxiety or depression
- Fibroids
- Acne

- Cervical dysplasia (abnormal cellular changes)
- Chronic vaginal infections
- Cravings (sugar, carbs, salt)
- Irritability, mood swings, depression
- Family or personal history of breast, endometrial, or other gynecologic cancer
- Hair loss
- Irregular, skipped, or painful periods
- Low (or no) sex drive
- Perimenopausal symptoms (hot flashes, vaginal dryness, low libido)
- Osteopenia or osteoporosis
- Prenatal or postpartum depression
- Menstrual problems

Enough Medical Mistreatment

Though hormonal health is central to our total well-being—even our economic health is affected by workdays missed for pain, depression, and other symptoms—it's been viewed through a myopic, cracked medical lens.

This isn't new. Women have been told for decades that feeling miserable around our periods is normal, that pain during sex is normal,

that taking the Pill for fifteen years to suppress symptoms is normal. I've worked with countless women who were dismissed—or dissed—by their doctor, or who received a prescription—a birth control pill, something for sleep, something for pain—rather than any explanation of what's really going on "down there." And too many have been left feeling it's all in their heads.

Some women have been shamed or chastised

by physicians, told that what's happening is the result of bad genes, bad luck, their weight, or their own bad habits. Medicine has a history of blaming our conditions on us: endometriosis was blamed on women for working outside the home, low sex drive on "frigid women" who refused their "wifely duties," migraines on those trying to get out of housework, for example. Or we may be told "it's just aging." I've had patients told this even in their twenties!

What's truly frightening is how often we're pushed to rely on drugs and surgery for problems that can be resolved with dietary changes, mind-body support, and natural medicines including targeted nutrients and herbs. But medications and surgeries can have unintended side effects that women may then have to live with for decades. We've been over-medicalized at our own expense, our natural cycles pathologized from puberty through menopause. And it's not equal for all women; if you're white and seeking medical care, you might be labeled as "difficult," though you're still likely to receive treatment—albeit you're at risk of overtreatment. If you're Black or brown, you're more likely to be told to grin and bear it, and are less likely to be given proper treatment, or treatment at all.

As harsh as this sounds, I have to call it what it is: *medical mis/maltreatment*. As a midwife, physician, mother, and grandmother, I'm not okay with any woman being made to feel she's broken or flawed, or any woman being medically mistreated. As a lifelong women's health activist and women's medical doctor, I'm saying enough. Enough blaming us and our bodies. Enough medical mistreatment.

We need a *healthy* new normal. We shouldn't simply accept that one in three women struggling with a hormone problem is an acceptable new normal. Nor should we accept overmedicalization and mistreatment. You deserve more. You deserve better. You deserve to be heard, believed, and respected. You deserve to feel your best. And you deserve to believe in your phenomenal body again. I hope that this starts here, with this book, and that as you feel more body-empowered, it ripples throughout your life.

Your Inner Guidance System

While the medical model treats us otherwise, you are not a bunch of unrelated parts stuck together. You're a whole person, and every aspect of your life influences your hormonal health—from your genetics to your diet to your job to your marriage to your body products to your neighborhood. This is not a romantic notion; yes, the interconnectedness of everything is a spiritual belief, a way of seeing the world, but the concept of internal and external ecosystems shaping our physiology is also hard science.

In fact, a field of science called *exposome science* shows us how this interconnectedness shapes our neurobiology, endocrinology, immunology, microbiology, and more. I'm going to teach you how this relates to your hormone and gynecologic health. This is an important approach that allows for deeply personalized medicine, but that conventional medicine just hasn't caught up with yet. As a result, most doctors fail to address the *root causes of imbalance*, sometimes thus also failing to prevent the potential long-term consequences of improperly treated health imbalances.

In this book, we'll look at what's happened to our hormones and why. I've learned from decades of experience that there's a core set of root cause imbalances that lead to most hormonal imbalances, symptoms, and gynecologic conditions. Though each of us is unique, we all live in a common environment, exposed to a similar set of forces at work tilting our hormones out of balance. We're going to connect the dots between what's going on in your environment, your body, and your hormones. Then, you'll get busy resetting your hormones. No matter how hormonal imbalances show up in your life, addressing the root causes corrects the symptoms and conditions that result from these often hidden causes. I'm going to show you what happens when you get aligned with the natural blueprint meant to guide your cycles, hormones, and gynecological health.

Along the way, we're going to look at why we've come to accept the belief that it's normal to suffer "because you're a woman," or that your symptoms or imbalances are due to something that's wrong with you. I'm going to help you reinterpret your hormones as an inner code, your own unique inner guidance system—your *Hormone Intelligence*—and I'm going to give you tools to help you interpret their messages and tap into your body's innate wisdom. I'm going to show you how to let go of the negative cultural attitudes about our bodies, menstruation, and sex, and more—the insidious norms that stereotype us as "hormonal," a.k.a. unpredictable and irrational, and that shame us into feeling like there's something fundamentally inferior or "gross" about being a woman. Seeing how these archaic yet entrenched patriarchal messages that also abound in medicine have created a warped viewpoint about our hormones will help you claim power over your body and health in a whole new way. And I'm officially asking you to press pause, right now, on any self-blaming you might be doing.

A Bold Promise

I want you to feel at home in your body, in sync with the power of your hormones, and in the driver's seat of your gynecologic health. While doctor after doctor might tell you they have no idea what's causing your symptoms, there's much more to the story than we've been told,

or that most doctors have learned in their medical training. And the science *does* give us clear answers.

I'm making a bold promise: things are going to get better for you. But unlike so many books and programs that promise a miracle overnight or seven-day fast solution, I'm offering steady, lasting changes based on cultivating deeper balance, which happens with small daily shifts, scientifically shown to lead to big changes, day by day, cycle by cycle, season by season in your life. Health is what happens the 98% of the time you're not in the doctor's office. The roller-coaster ride can stop when you're empowered with the knowledge about the multiple influences that disrupt your hormone balance. You'll realize you *don't* just have to grin and bear it anymore. I'm also going to show you why it's so important that you don't—because your hormonal health is a critical vital sign of your total health.

But first, I want to dispel some preconceived notions about holistic health. There's a lot of BS out there that gives integrative medicine a bad name; we're going to leave that behind. Holistic health, the way I practice it, is not about unsubstantiated practices, fistfuls of supplements, or ignoring conventional medicine when it can help you. It's about a whole-woman approach to health.

Unlike some authors, I'm not going to tell you that you have to go off your medication, not take hormones, or quit seeing your conventional doctor if that's what's needed or simply your preference. I don't suggest you throw the medical baby out with the medical industry bathwater. There's a time and place for hormone therapy and even surgery. But I want you to understand why medications and surgeries often aren't the only, the best, the safest, or even the most effective solutions—and that there is another way that respects the effectiveness of dietary, herbal, and other natural remedies, and self-care approaches to healing, which are almost always better to try first.

My approach is holistic in that it looks at how your whole life influences your wellness—including hidden exposures, missing nutrients, and other important factors you'll learn about and can shift. I will guide you through my favorite and most effective hormone-friendly practices, techniques, and tools, the same ones that my patients have used to transform their lives, that I share with my friends and family, and that I live by and use for myself. It's the perfect blend of ancient ways and modern medicine, grounded in common sense—which is what you get when a midwife/MD writes a book for you.

This book will help you find YOUR comfort zone of treatments, and will show you how to understand and work with, not against, your hormones, so they can work for, and not against, *you*. When you see your body as an ally, not an enemy, and your hormones as a guidance system or compass guided by a deep inner intelligence, rather than the source of distress, dysfunction, or disease, you can achieve a level of health, energy, well-being, and vitality you may never have known before. I invite you into an entirely new relationship with the most important person in your hormone life: YOU.

Don't Shoot the Messenger

Your body isn't your enemy, and hormone imbalances aren't just random. They also don't mean you're broken or crazy. They are your body's sane response to a crazy world that demands you live in ways that are absolutely contrary to your natural, innate hormonal blueprint. Your hormones, and your symptoms, are vital signs offering you powerful information that act as a compass, a complete *inner guidance system* and, as such, sometimes a *warning* system, too, alerting you when you're not getting what you need for hormone health—which also means for your best total health. Like the canaries historically sent into the coal mine ahead of the miners to warn them of the presence of dangerous, toxic elements that could harm the miners, hormone imbalances are sensitive, early warning signs of possible greater threats to our well-being.

Hormones exist as the background music of your life. They do their work quietly without calling much attention to themselves, a host of individual notes working in harmony together to set the tone for how you feel, your energy levels, focus, and motivation, to name just a few ways that they subtly impact us. When they're at their optimal levels, your body works with a nice even rhythm that keeps you humming along with no major interference with your life—no static on your physical, emotional, and mental channels. Think smooth jazz or R&B, a powerful steady beat that you're always dancing to.

Hormones exist in *constant* relationship with one another and with the cells, tissues, systems, and organs in your body, connecting various parts of you via pathways or axes of signaling, such as the brain, ovaries, and uterus. They're in constant communication with one another and constantly responding to conditions around them. To do this extraordinary orchestration, they depend on having the right inputs in the right amounts from the larger ecosystem that surrounds them, and not too many of the wrong ones.

Genetics can definitely predispose us to certain conditions, but it's estimated that, at most, genes account for only about 15% of the cause of chronic conditions. So what makes up that other 85%? Well, environmental exposures. But when I say that, I don't simply mean the toxins in our world. I'm referring to the two major ecosystems that determine our health: an inner ecosystem and an outer ecosystem that add up to your *exposome*. This includes what you eat and how your digestive system works, your stress triggers and your nervous system resilience, your toxin exposure and the robustness of your inherent detoxification system, your levels of inflammation and daily lifestyle choices, your level of cellular damage and ability to repair it, the health of your microbiome, and more. The exposome is a constellation of the exposures we have daily, and over the course of our lifetime, from conception on.

Here's where another radical paradigm shift appears. The symptoms you're experiencing, while certainly disruptive and upsetting, are not the core problem. Your hormones give you real-time feedback on how all these factors are impacting you. They're your Siri—but instead of artificial intelligence, it's your innate intelligence or, as I'll show you, your Hormone Intelligence, talking to you, giving you information on your health. Our hormones act as a highly sensitive "radar," alerting us to when there's something creating interference on our signaling pathways. Confused signaling, caused by exposome imbalances, causes hormone symptoms and conditions, sometimes small ones that we might write off as normal discomforts and inconveniences, like menstrual cramps or premenstrual headaches, and sometimes big, loud, disruptive ones that demand our attention, like fertility problems, PCOS, endometriosis, debilitating pelvic pain, menopausal symptoms, and more. Instead of a smooth-groove beat playing, you may feel as if you're living with constant static, aggravating noise, or all-out pandemonium!

Your skin and your hair, your menstrual cycles, the regularity of your bowel movements, the quality of your sleep, your sex drive, your moods, your fertility, how much pelvic pain you experience with your periods—or in general—these, and other signs I'll show you, are all barometers of how well your inner and outer ecosystems are supporting your health. What few of us are taught is that we can use this information to "read" our hormonal health, interpret the messages, and make the changes that restore a steady, healthy hum.

For a long time now, the medical and pharmaceutical industries have sold us on the belief that our bodies are defective, we have no control over our hormones or our health, and basically, our gynecologic organs are a disaster waiting to happen. But this is far from the truth. Thirty years of research and clinical practice has taught me that what's going on in our bodies is absolutely not our fault. Your body is not a lemon. It is *far from broken*. Your body is a gorgeous home for YOU. What *is* broken is our food system, our

On Her Terms

If you're looking for the definitions of a term I use in these pages, for example, anatomical terms, or more information about a term, visit the "On Her Terms" glossary on page 385. For simplicity's sake, going forward in this book I use the terms *hormone imbalance* and *hormone conditions* interchangeably, to encompass common hormonally related symptoms, as well as gynecologic or "reproductive health" problems including PMS, endometriosis, PCOS, uterine fibroids, fertility challenges, and all the additional women's symptoms and conditions addressed in this book.

"environment, a culture that demands we give up healthy sleep schedules . . . and our health care system. What's broken is how we see our hormones—so we "shoot the messenger," suppressing them and blaming ourselves, rather than looking more closely at what's causing hormonal mayhem. This miseducation has come with a cost: it's created an atmosphere of anxiety and mistrust of our bodies and caused us to lose our connection to one of the most powerful and integral sources of information we have—our hormonal intelligence. Your body, via your hormones, is trying to tell you something important. And it never lies. This book is here to introduce you to a revolutionary approach and to help you see your hormones and symptoms as a vital sign, an innate inner guidance system.

What We Don't Know Can Hurt Us

Many common symptoms and hormone problems have potentially serious implications—there are not only immediate issues, but there are increased lifetime risks of obesity, diabetes, and reproductive and other forms of cancer due to the higher levels of estrogen that lead to this condition. Hormone imbalances have been shown to have a serious impact on not only women's health, but also our self-confidence, quality of life, the ease of our relationships, and even financial and career achievement due to days of missed work or just less energy to reach for that next rung of the ladder.

When we just chalk hormone imbalances and gynecologic conditions up as normal or inconvenient, we're also relegated to lives filled with treatments that can have serious consequences. The Pill is so commonly prescribed that most women don't even consider it a medication, and most doctors forget that it can have serious side effects. Don't freak out! It's why you're here—and I'm going to tell you the other half of the story: the one with the safe, effective, affordable solutions to the hormone problems that brought you to this book.

The Hormone Intelligence Solution

It makes sense that you might be wondering, "But okay, Dr. Aviva, how can your one plan reverse all these seemingly separate hormonal problems like infertility AND anxiety AND heavy bleeding?" My answer: "Because they are all connected—and I am going to show you how!"

Hormone Intelligence is the plan I've developed over thirty-five years of helping women to reclaim their hormones and feel like themselves again. Based on solid research, it gets the brain-ovary-uterus connection back online so there's clear communication and hormone signaling between those circuits—the very circuits that control your mood, mind, cycles, weight, sleep, and also your brain, bone, and heart health now and in the long run. It does this by providing your body with the specific elements women need for healthy hormone production, while removing the obstacles that get in the way: the chronic inflammation, toxins, stress, poor foods, and more that are the fires sounding your hormone alarm system. Hormone Intelligence is based on solid research into what makes our hormones "tick" and what gets in their way; it's brought real results to real women, some of whom you'll meet throughout this book (out of respect to my patients, names have been changed and stories have been amalgamated).

These lifestyle changes are the essential, foundational first steps for every woman experiencing hormonal imbalance. But for every "outer" change I encourage you to make, such as in the foods you eat and rhythms of your day, I offer you "inner" shifts as well, like how to have a healthier conversation with your body. This inner/outer balance is powerful and necessary; once you understand what your hormones are telling you, you can respond with healthy inputs—and trust that your body will respond, too.

This book takes you on a profoundly healing journey.

In Part One, I'll show you why hormone problems are so common today, what hormone balance looks like, how to begin to recognize symptoms and gynecologic problems as vital signs, and how to interpret what they are telling you.

In Part Two, I'll teach you all about the six root causes that are at the heart of the hormone epidemic we're currently facing and show you how to implement the six-week Hormone Intelligence Plan solutions that will help you transform your lifestyle into one that resets and optimizes your hormone health and reverses common gynecologic symptoms.

In Part Three, I give you the same advanced, targeted symptom- and condition-specific plans I use in my medical practice to enhance and supplement the core six-week Hormone Intelligence Plan. The Advanced Protocols allow you to further personalize the program to your goals and symptom severity.

In Part Four, I bring it all into your kitchen with recipes that take the work out of figuring out what to eat while keeping the plan filling and delicious, hopefully inspiring you to eat for hormone health for your lifetime.

What to Expect

Let's get clear from the outset: if you're seeking a "wham-bam miracle solution" built on exaggerated promises and claims, this is not it. We've been taught to take a pill and expect a result in an hour. Healing works differently. We're reframing the outdated medical mindset of quick fixes and silver bullets here, rejecting the belief that we always have to be in a rush for everything to happen, and that results have to be immediate and dramatic for us to believe something is making a difference.

Hormone Intelligence is about creating a nourishing, sustainable pathway to lifelong hormonal and gynecologic health. The underlying issues that led to your hormone imbalances are complex and multifactorial. They didn't happen overnight, and they won't likely get turned around overnight. This is a restorative plan; it's important to give your body ample time to repair, reset, and rebalance, and that also means patience with the process. It can take weeks, and sometimes even months for changes in bigger symptoms and conditions to resolve. But they can!

PCOS can be reversed, women with endometriosis can experience lesion and symptom remission, and there are at least a few babies out there named Avi or Aviva—named by women who reversed an infertility diagnosis using the very same protocols in this book. I truly believe that your diagnosis does not have to be your destiny! But some conditions are complex; therefore, it's okay if you need a combination of conventional and alternative approaches. That's the beauty of a truly integrative, holistic plan, and everything in this book can be used as a stand-alone plan, or in conjunction with conventional medicine if needed.

That said, this doesn't mean you won't notice improvements quickly—even just a week or so into the program. Microchanges can happen in a very short time, including significant improvements in energy (woot!), digestion (no more bloating!), sleep (ahhh . . .), mental clarity and outlook (as one patient said to me, "The lights are back on!"), and relief from sugar cravings, anxiety and depression, low self-esteem, and sluggish metabolism. You might notice more vibrant skin and shinier hair—or your friends asking you what you're doing to look so good so they can do it, too. That's how beautifully your body responds when you give yourself what you need to be nourished.

Ready to hit the reset button and finally get off the hormone roller coaster? Pour a cup of tea, cozy up in your favorite chair, and keep reading while I get real about women's health and hormones. Let's journey into your personal Hormone Intelligence and find solutions to your hormonal conditions—even the tough ones. No more suffering. Your body is simply waiting for you to say, "Yes!"

know yourself

UNDERSTANDING HORMONE INTELLIGENCE

Stepping onto a brand-new path is difficult,
but not more difficult than remaining in a situation
which is not nurturing to the whole woman.

—Maya Angelou

the hidden hormone epidemic

There's a saying: "Stories are data with a soul." In my career as a midwife and physician specializing in women's health, I've had the privilege of hearing tens of thousands of women's stories about the challenges they've experienced with their hormonal health and how this has impacted their lives. Some have minor but chronic discomforts that they "just deal with" or use medications like ibuprofen or "the Pill" to manage; many experience cyclic or daily anxiety-provoking or embarrassing symptoms; and a surprising number of women are living with worrisome, painful, or distracting symptoms or conditions affecting their daily well-being and plans for their future.

Their stories share a theme: medical appointments in which they've been made to feel invisible, their concerns were ignored, dismissed, or not taken seriously, or at which they were treated disrespectfully. A startling number of women have been belittled, told they're being "dramatic." So many have faced difficulty finding a provider they trust, or have been met by a surprising lack of care and respect from a medical provider, and most report little guidance beyond what could be written on a prescription pad.

Too many women have been to multiple practitioners only to hear the same thing: "It's stress, you need to relax more"; "It's normal for women to have hormone imbalances—why don't you try taking the Pill"; "Take pain medication, try an antidepressant / anxiety pill / sleeping pill"; or "You should really just have that surgery." Many have left medical appointments so confused that they wondered if their symptoms were "all in their heads" as medical providers have insinuated—or said! Many have spent years struggling alone, not sure whether their symptoms were normal or a sign that something seriously wrong was being missed. Too many find themselves on medications they don't want to be on, facing decisions about surgeries they feel too young to have, and are feeling the tremendous impact of hormone imbalances on their personal and professional lives.

The power and strength of women who cope with all these varying challenges, and still face the day, never cease to amaze me.

Women Unseen and Unheard

The women who reach out to me are mothers, teachers, students, executives, actors, doctors, nurses, wives, yoga teachers, bartenders, writers, pilots, lawyers, salespeople, entrepreneurs, architects, organic farmers, nutritionists, and more. They're part of an alarming trend: a growing frequency and intensity of women's hormone-related conditions. "Hormonal roller coaster" and "hormonal hell" are just a couple of the phrases women have used when talking to me about their periods, moods, sleep, fertility challenges, sex lives, and other "women's problems."

Some have been dealing with these symptoms for as long as they can remember—at least since their teens—others have symptoms that began as they entered a new decade or phase in life—when trying to conceive, after having a baby in their forties, or after a major life stress. Many have spent years on the Pill, many are confused, discouraged, or exhausted by what's going on in their bodies, and frustrated by the difficulty they're having finding answers. They wonder if they can have children, if they will always suffer with pain, if they will need surgery or will develop cancer. Some come with totally normal "symptoms" that they fear are abnormal because, as women, we've been taught so little about how our bodies work, what's normal, and what's not. The quantity and poignancy of their stories of turbulence, bewilderment, and secret, unspoken fears, often completely at odds with the successful public face of the women sharing them, strikes a powerful chord.

When I'm able to confirm or provide a diagnosis for a patient, her relief fills the whole room. As one woman said to me, "If just one doctor had listened to me, I wouldn't have lost years of my life to this." When I'm able to show a woman that her body or symptoms are normal, her relief is palpable. Why, in an age of so much female empowerment, so much claiming of our voices and our rights, are so many women harboring the anxiety—or downright fear—that they are going to spend their lives feeling so out of balance, never truly embodying their best selves and never truly feeling at home in their bodies? And why do they feel so "unseen and unheard"?

The Best of Times, the Worst of Times

We live in an amazing time. Women are owning their power, learning to speak out, and standing up for their rights in ways that would make our foremothers proud. We're breaking down long-standing taboos about our bodies and sexuality. National Public Radio called 2015 "the year of the period," and *Cosmopolitan* magazine declared it "the year the period went public." Poet Rupi Kaur posted a picture of herself on Instagram with a period stain on her sweatpants, the kind that any of us might wake up with on period day 1, and a picture of Harvard Business School graduate, musician, and activist Kiran Gandhi appeared in newspapers around the world running the London Marathon in bloodstained joggers, because she preferred to free-bleed (go *sans* pad or tampon) while running rather than wear an uncomfortable menstrual product. Both went viral to the almost audible exhale of women everywhere. The secret was out, the taboo broken.

We don't have to be embarrassed, mortified, or filled with shame anymore. Women bloody well have periods.

In 2016, after a presidential candidate said it on live television, the word *vagina* went public. Around the same time, actress Lena Dunham opened up publicly about choosing a hysterectomy at the age of thirty after suffering with debilitating pain for over a decade, enduring surgery after surgery that didn't help. Celebrity chef Padma Lakshmi went public about suffering with endometriosis and its impact on her life and fertility. Whoopi Goldberg is among a number of other public figures educating women about this condition. These women began to normalize talking about gynecologic pain, freeing women from living with it in silence.

Similarly, celebrities including fitness coach Jillian Michaels and actress Emma Thompson have become more outspoken about living with PCOS, while performers Kerry Washington, Katy Perry, and Cameron Diaz are among those who have revealed their challenges with severe acne and acne scarring. Menopause isn't so hush-hush anymore, either; actresses Kim Cattrall and Helen Mirren have proclaimed the power of the "pause," while Jane Fonda and Lily Tomlin starred in a sitcom in which they create a vibrator company for older women because, as growing research shows, older women want pleasure, too.

In 2018, the #metoo movement created a tidal wave in sexual politics. Tired of keeping quiet about workplace sexual abuse, women started making noise and with it headlines and magazine covers, including the cover of *Time*. More women are currently in elected office than ever, and young women today are the first to start their work lives close to financial parity to men. And in 2019, like a pièce de résistance, *Period: End of Sentence*, a documentary about the impact of an endemic lack of access to period products on poor women around the world, won an Academy Award, and the word *period* was said, loud and proud, onstage at the Academy Awards. Mic drop.

With the power of social media, women's magazines, and podcasts, for example, we're claiming our power with a new fierceness and freedom, and we're hearing one another and elevating our collective voices. What our feminist foremothers hoped for is happening: a new wave of young women is talking about the power and beauty of their menstrual cycles, bodies, sex, and more. A new kind of conversation has begun. Amen.

Yet, while all this woman-rising has been happening, a hidden hormone epidemic has unfolded, with more women suffering from hormone problems and reproductive health conditions than ever in modern history. Digging into the medical literature, I found that the data confirmed exactly what women's stories were telling me, and the statistics are staggering:

- **Premenstrual Syndrome (PMS):** 85% of women experience troublesome premenstrual symptoms including irritability, sugar or carb binges, bloating, depression, migraines, acne, and more. For 15% of women, symptoms are severe enough to seriously affect their quality of life.

- **Painful or Heavy Periods:** At least three-quarters of us have painful or heavy periods. For one in six women they're severe enough to impact their functioning. As just one example, anemia due to chronic heavy blood loss reduces girls' scores in school enough so that it can reduce career opportunities in math and the sciences later on. Heavy periods can be scary, uncomfortable, and challenging to manage; cramps lead to using medications such as Motrin or Advil to power through, but as you'll learn, regular use can cause short- and long-term consequences.

- **Pelvic Pain / Pain During Sex:** Up to one in five women has chronic pelvic pain lasting more than a year at a time. Chronic pain and burning in the vulva affect approximately six million women in the US. Thirty percent of women report pain during sex. Many just put up with it; some forgo sex, living with the fear that this will damage their relationship. This isn't just "older women" stuff: it's affecting women between the ages of eighteen and fifty.

- **Endometriosis:** Once a relatively uncommon condition, endometriosis, a complex hormone-mediated immunological condition that can cause severe chronic pain, digestive symptoms, depression, and fertility challenges, and is associated with a higher rate of autoimmune disease, affects at least 10% of women in total, with rates probably higher since teenagers are vastly underdiagnosed. It takes nine years on average, and multiple doctors, for a woman to get a proper diagnosis. Endometriosis is a common reason for missed school, missed work, and emergency room visits. It's often not until a woman's fertility is jeopardized that she receives the attention she deserves to explain the pain she's been living with, typically for years.

- **Polycystic Ovary Syndrome:** Between 5 and 10% of women of childbearing age in the United States have polycystic ovary syndrome (PCOS), a complex metabolic and hormonal condition that can lead to frustrating weight gain, distressing hair loss, hair growing in unwanted places

(your chin, breasts, or lower belly, for example), depression, irregular or absent periods, or the emotionally challenging acne that comes with this condition. PCOS is responsible for 70% of infertility issues in women who have difficulty ovulating, as well as increased risks for prenatal problems including miscarriage and gestational diabetes in women who do become pregnant with this condition. For a subset of women, there is also an increased risk of diabetes and heart disease. Yet over 50% of cases of PCOS go unnoticed and untreated, and if women have been diagnosed, most tell me they've received nothing more than a brochure and prescriptions for the Pill to control their hormones and metformin to control their blood sugar.

- **Challenged Conceptions:** According to the CDC (Centers for Disease Control and Prevention), about 10% of women in the United States now have difficulty getting or staying pregnant because their fertility or that of their partner is compromised. One in six of us now seeks a consultation for fertility problems during our reproductive years. A recent study found that miscarriage affected 28% of couples planning a pregnancy, a 42% increase since the 1980s. Not only can the diagnosis be anguishing, there are the ups and downs of treatment, as well as the financial costs that can get as high as $50,000, or more.

- **Acne:** Acne affects at least 15% of adult women and can cause emotional, psychological, and social suffering, with studies showing that its impact on health-related quality of life (HrQOL) is as dramatic as severe debilitating conditions including psoriasis, arthritis, and epilepsy. It can lead to missing school and work, decreased focus, reduced confidence and productivity, and sometimes disabling self-consciousness that interferes with relationships and can cause anxiety and depression. The acne can also drive women to use potentially harmful and excessive amounts of cosmetics to cover it, and chronic antibiotic treatment can affect gut health, worsening hormone balance.

- **Hysterectomy:** Half of all women in the US aged 60 and over will have had a hysterectomy, which is bad enough, but surprisingly, millions are done on women in their twenties, thirties, and forties, usually for benign reasons that could be treated in nonsurgical ways. Fully 20% are considered medically unnecessary, yet only 30% of women who have been advised to have one are informed of nonsurgical alternatives by their doctor.

- **Hypothyroidism:** An estimated 30 million women have hypothyroidism, which not only affects metabolism and weight, but also interferes with the production of other hormones, including estrogen and progesterone, and can cause infertility, miscarriage, irregular cycles, skipped periods, heavy periods, cognitive problems, and much more.

- **Premature Puberty:** Perhaps most striking is the rise in premature puberty. The Kotex "Tween" line brings this point home profoundly. Emblazoned with hearts and stars, the brand has menstrual pads and products for the increasing number of girls getting their periods by the time they're eight years old. In the United States, 15 to 23% of girls are now beginning puberty—experiencing noticeable breast development and even having their first period—by age seven, compared to age

twelve in our mothers' and grandmothers' day. The implications of early puberty are serious; not just the emotional issues, but increased lifetime risks of obesity, diabetes, and reproductive and other forms of cancer due to the early onset of exposure to higher levels of estrogen.

Eighty percent of us will have a hormonal imbalance in our lifetime that gets our attention or raises our level of concern. Ominously, the trend is skewing younger and younger: PCOS, PMS, and endometriosis are presenting in girls as young as twelve. Hormone conditions are leading tens of millions of women in the US alone to miss out on the pleasure of their lives as a result of days of discomfort—suffering serious immediate and long-term health consequences—and are causing hundreds of millions of women to be in confusion about their bodies.

This data may not even capture the full scope of the epidemic. Because our hormones orchestrate so many functions in our bodies, not just our cycles and reproduction, but weight and metabolism, immunity, brain health, and more, the list of symptoms and medical conditions that stem from hormonal imbalances is extensive. Some of the "hidden" or unexpected problems stemming from women's hormone imbalances can include: sleep problems, fatigue, brain fog, weight gain, food cravings, digestive symptoms, hair loss, anxiety or depression, loss of creativity, bone loss (osteopenia, osteoporosis), autoimmune diseases (Hashimoto's thyroiditis, rheumatoid arthritis, and others), breast and endometrial cancer, diabetes, and high cholesterol, to name a few.

And here's one more important statistic: 96% of the symptoms and conditions we face, including most of those in this book, will take the form of what is called "invisible illness." To the world you look fine, while you silently deal with symptoms that steal your energy, sap your joy, make you feel self-conscious, and keep you from living your big beautiful life to its fullest.

There's a hidden hormone epidemic going on and it's made up of a lot of silent suffering. But how can these two realities—liberating empowerment and chronic, silent suffering—coexist in such dramatic fashion?

A Biased Medical System

The fact that a veritable tsunami of hormone conditions has remained hidden cannot be separated from the medical establishment's systemic failure to adequately study, understand, and take women's health concerns seriously. The medical conditions that uniquely affect more than half of all humans (women) are consistently the least-prioritized, least-funded (if funded at all) areas of research, every single year. A 2014 report, *Sex-Specific Medical Research: Why Women's Health Can't Wait*, on bias in medical research stated, "Medical research that is either sex- or gender-neutral or skewed to male physiology puts women at risk for missed opportunities for prevention, incorrect diagnoses, misinformed treatments, sickness, and even death."

Consequently, lack of adequate training in women's health also continues to be a problem in medical education. Most doctors aren't taught to recognize, diagnose, or treat even the most common women's conditions. One study found, for example, that 63% of general practitioners said they felt ill at ease in the diagnosis and follow-up of patients with endometriosis. One-half could not cite three main symptoms of the disease outside of menstrual pain, pain during sex, chronic pelvic pain, and infertility. Only 38% of general practitioners indicated that they perform a clinical gyneco-logic examination for suspected endometriosis, and 28% recommended MRI to confirm the diagnosis—which is the incorrect test. This is a big deal when it comes to our health and safety. At least half of all women with PCOS remain undiagnosed, and in one survey of primary care doctors, 70% said they neither recognized the symptoms of endometriosis nor knew how to treat patients for this condition. A recent study found that one in three women who were later diagnosed with endometriosis were told by their medical providers that their pain was normal, and that they did not have a medical problem. Some are misdiagnosed as having "gas" or irritable bowel syndrome.

Even when they do have patients in their practice with this diagnosis, doctors often miss the forest for the trees—meaning that they just aren't aware of the scope of the statistics, so they see it as an individual problem rather than as the bigger public health problem that it is.

Inherent biases against women, which are endemic in medical care, more often than not make matters worse, reinforcing negative or inaccurate medical and cultural beliefs about hormonal and gynecologic health. That's why, when we express concerns about menstrual pain to our doctors, for example, we are likely to be told that they are a normal part of being a woman, even if they cause us to be doubled over every month, unable to go to work, or are serious enough to bring us to the emergency department. A 2001 study, "The Girl Who Cried Pain," found that when both men and women present the same symptoms, health care providers are more likely to give pain-relieving medications to men, while women are more likely to receive sedatives, suggesting that medical experts perceive women as "hysterical," with psychogenic or emotional symptoms, and not "real" pain or a medical problem.

Silencing and Blaming Ourselves—and Our Hormones

Most of us have inherited centuries of negative, dismissive, and confusing beliefs and misinformation about our bodies, cycles, and hormones. We enter womanhood unprepared for the hormone roller coaster. Few of us experienced our teens feeling like our bodies were our besties or that becoming a woman was all that it was hyped up to be. We all did our best to figure out how to navigate body, mood, and life changes, often with some level of sucking up discomfort, embarrassment, and uncertainty along the way.

We're taught so little about how our bodies work, what's normal, and what's not, that we often just keep discomforts to ourselves, living with quiet, chronic concerns about our reproductive and sexual health, unclear what's normal, what's not. Inherited cultural (and family) shame, embarrassment, and squeamishness may keep us from asking.

And so this culture of shame leads us to think we're alone, broken, the only ones going through this body battle. We're tacitly taught that it's normal to suffer, so we assume that our monthly pain, digestive problems, headaches, cravings, bloating, and heavy bleeding are to be expected. Heck, it's normal to have menstrual cramps, to bleed like crazy each month, for our breasts to hurt during our periods, for sex to hurt, to get headaches, even to struggle to get pregnant—after all, so many women do, right? We've been encouraged to ignore or suppress the physical and emotional symptoms we experience with medications, to replace our natural scents with "garden fresh" ones, and, in order to succeed in a male-dominated work environment, pretend we weren't "hormonal."

Further, we don't want to be "complainers,"

so we tend to "stuff it down and soldier on." For most women, perhaps you, too, these feelings persist until we get fed up and fill a prescription or end up with a hysterectomy we're not sure we truly needed. Along the way, we were told to put our trust in the medical model, and to be polite. It's easy to see why so many of us disengage from the system altogether and seek alternatives.

We're also told that our hormones make us unreliable and irrational. Or that our problems aren't real. In one study, one in ten women with endometriosis was overtly told "it's all in your head" (or as Abby Norman, author of *Ask Me About My Uterus*, described, being treated as a "Freudian hysteric with an iPhone"), 20% saw as many as five health care providers over as many as ten years before receiving a proper diagnosis. This story repeats itself thousands of times a day, in doctor's offices around the country. A woman is told that her pain is normal when it's due to an ovarian cyst, told her PCOS is caused by being "too fat," and the list goes on. A 2010 study reported that "Health care professionals are more likely to dismiss women's pain reports as emotional, psychogenic, hysterical or oversensitive, and therefore not real, leading to more frequent mental health diagnoses." So we start blaming our hormones, we begrudge our monthly cycles, and we do our best to ignore them as much as possible.

The result? Not only missed diagnoses, but women starting to wonder if they are "gaslighting" themselves—convincing themselves of symptoms that aren't there—even severe pain! As one woman said to me, "Surely all these doctors couldn't be wrong; after all, they were the experts."

Too many women feel invisible *even in front of their own doctor.* And when women try to press for deeper answers, ask for alternative solutions, or mention something they've read on the internet that might be helpful, they're often met with skepticism or downright disrespect (many women have had a doctor ask, "Where did you get your degree, Google University?") or made to feel like they have two heads for considering possible alternatives to pharmaceuticals and surgery as their first-line treatments. Until, that is, they bring a man with them—which many women report they've had to do in order to have their symptoms taken seriously.

Women are routinely told that they're overreacting when they know that they've gained fifteen pounds but haven't changed their diet or exercise routine, that their depression is not just overwhelm or being a new mom, or due to menopause, that they're not just lying awake at night, staring at the ceiling, unable to sleep because they're under stress. Women's hormone conditions have become so common that even we as women have made the mistake of assuming it's just normal for us to experience hemorrhagic-level periods, monthly cramps, or fifty soaking hot flashes a day.

Common and *normal* are different. Just because so many women experience something doesn't mean it's inherent to our biology—being a woman is not a diagnosis! We learn to ignore our inner compass when we're told that uncomfortable, painful, or unpleasant symptoms are normal. I'm here to help you reclaim what is truly normal—a life in which your hormones aren't whipping you around, where you're not in pain, where you feel comfortable in your own skin, where you can achieve your goals. Taboos about talking about our vaginas, clits, discharge, menstrual cycles and vaginal bleeding, sex, fertility, and menopause have been endangering women's health for too long and in measurable ways. This book will help you put an end to any embarrassment you have about talking about your body and cycles and will empower you with the language to help you do this.

Being a Woman Is Not a Disease

I can't shed light on the ways that women's hormonal symptoms and gynecologic conditions are *underrecognized* and dismissed without also revealing the flip side of this behavior: the rampant *medicalization* of women's bodies (and emotions!) by the medical and pharmaceutical industries.

Medicalization, the social and economic control of women's bodies, begins at the first sign of period problems, and if not then, with a first prescription for a contraceptive or a first Pap smear at age twenty-one or so. The medical profession has led us to believe that our bodies are "lemons"—machines that chronically break down; that disease is inevitable; that the only "real solutions" and "right answers" are pharmaceuticals, surgery, and other invasive interventions; and that science always trumps nature.

The pharmaceutical and medical device industries exert a shocking amount of influence over medical practice—even creating diagnoses so that specific treatments can be targeted at us—and as women, we're the biggest target.

Premenstrual dysphoric disorder (PMDD) and female sexual dysfunction are two examples of pharmaceutical companies inventing new diseases to sell medications. Look, I've performed thousands of procedures and I've seen the lifesaving powers of Western medicine and have truly been in awe. I'm grateful to have the training and skills I do. But there's a saying aptly applied to medical doctors: "If all you have is a hammer, you tend to see everything as a nail." Medicine is the hammer. But women are not nails. We need—and deserve—more lasting, effective, and safe solutions than conventional medicine currently has to offer.

Here are just a few ways that this medicalization perpetuates the hidden epidemic (and lines a lot of deep pockets):

- Fifty percent of all birth control pills are not prescribed for contraception, but for menstrual pain and problems, as a first-line option.

- Eighty percent of women now self-diagnose PMS, labeling even normal mood shifts before their periods as a medical condition. One in four women is now on an antidepressant, one of the most common treatments for PMS. Yet only about half of all women benefit from this treatment, and few are warned about side effects.

- Fertility medicine is projected to be a $41 billion industry by 2026, and no wonder—if you don't get pregnant within a few months of trying you're sent for a fertility evaluation. Yet fertility medications and procedures carry risks, while efficacy is currently only about 50%. Companies like Facebook and Apple offer egg freezing as a perk to their employees—selling the idea that your fertility might not be something you can bank on.

- Pregnant women are particularly subjected to "sickification"; 90% receive a medication prescription in pregnancy (50% of which have not been proven safe to the fetus). Pregnant women receive multiple unnecessary ultrasounds and dozens of lab tests, and one in three gives birth by cesarean section, an estimated 50% of which are considered unnecessary, and which increase a woman's risks of injury, infection, and mortality.

- Menopause has been medically manipulated and treated like a disease since the 1950s when the book *Forever Feminine* touted the use of estrogen as a female fountain of youth. Not long after, normally declining estrogen was described as a deficiency, and hormone replacement therapy (HRT) was prescribed to tens of millions of women to prevent the "ravages" of aging, despite known serious risks. Most purported benefits have now been disproven and risks have come to light including increased risks of certain cancers.

- One in three women having a hysterectomy in her lifetime in the US, much higher than any European country, is another example of gross overmedicalization. They are largely done for benign conditions for which there are nonsurgical alternatives. It's now thought that there are direct connections between the uterus and the brain through the autonomic nervous system, which may protective women against dementia. If the ovaries are removed, a woman may experience primary ovarian insufficiency (POI), which also has risks.

(continued)

No wonder we think that being a woman is itself a disease, that we all have some screwed-up genes, and that we couldn't live without constant medical surveillance. We've been the subjects of medical misapplication for over a century now—and we're not the ones profiting from it. We're sold sickification—and with it fear for our health—by a direct-to-consumer pharmaceutical industry making us believe there's a disease lurking around every corner. New diseases are even created by Pharma to support sales of medications. Pfizer creating the disease "female sexual dysfunction" to sell "pink Viagra" is just one of many notorious examples of off-label marketing without any proof of effectiveness and safety. Our bodies are big business.

And get this: While 70% of all pharmaceuticals are prescribed to women (half of all women over fifty are on at least two), most have never been tested in women! Differences in how we metabolize medications put us at major risk for adverse events compared to men. Even medications we rely on for common symptoms, ibuprofen for example, has been associated with unintended consequences, which I'll explain. Yet pharmaceutical advertising downplays the risks while exaggerating the benefits—to consumer and practitioners alike.

Then there are the episodes of sheer ignorance and greed:

- DES, a synthetic form of estrogen doctors prescribed to women from 1938 until 1971 to prevent miscarriages and premature delivery, which not only was discovered to be ineffective but also led to reproductive tract cancers in the offspring of mothers who took it

- The Dalkon Shield, an IUD sold from 1970 to 1985, was released without any clinical trials and almost immediate knowledge by the manufacturer and FDA to have serious risks, which ultimately led to over 300,000 lawsuits from women who had been severely damaged. The device was removed from the market in the late 1970s, though it was still used in developing countries into the early 1980s.

- Two decades of overtreatment of women under twenty-one for cervical changes found on Pap smears, leading to cervical damage that prevented conception and led to higher rates of pregnancy and birth interventions.

- Use of the Essure "permanent birth control" though hundreds of women's symptoms of hemorrhaging and pain were denied by doctors. The device was removed from the market in 2019; it was found to be terribly dangerous and the source of irreparable pelvic organ damage in tens of thousands of women.

I could list many more Western medical "whoopsies"—gynecologic treatments that, even just in the past decade, were found to cause more harm than good.

What's Going On?
Many Branches, a Few Roots

So why *are* increasing numbers of women struggling with hormone conditions? Why are seven-year-olds getting their periods? Why are women having so much trouble getting pregnant? Why are so many women in pain so much of the time? Should we just accept this as "the new normal?"

The answer is a straight-up *no*.

The fact that hormone-related conditions have now reached epidemic proportions should be a big flashing red light telling us that something concerning is happening.

But what (the heck!!!) is it?

To answer that question we have to put on a new set of lenses that are different from the broken ones we've been taught to see our bodies through. This is the lens—and heart—of *holistic gynecology*, which is way more than pink bathrobes and fuzzy stirrups! It's founded on a deep understanding of the factors affecting women's whole lives and our hormones: it's based on seeing your hormone-related symptoms as more than discomforts and diagnoses, but as clues to underlying imbalances asking to be addressed.

Hormones Are Messengers, Symptoms Are Messages

Do you remember the game "Telephone"—the one where you pick a word or phrase, and "pass it on," each person whispering it to the person next to them, until it reaches the last person in a circle? This person then announces the message to the group. The goal of the game is to pass the message on down the line without it becoming garbled along the way, but the fun is that the final message is usually totally different than how it started, and the result is often hilarious.

Hormone imbalances happen a lot like those scrambled messages. Our hormones are messengers, to be specific, chemical messengers, which carry signals from their point of origin—a gland in one part of your body that secretes it (i.e., your ovaries, thyroid, pancreas, or adrenals)—to its targets—the cells that are its final destination.

The message is meant to be delivered clearly, and when it is, the hormone's actions are carried out with ease and we feel the results: easy periods, good sleep, clear skin, healthy weight, sharp thinking—among the thousands of functions our hormones do to keep us in a state of dynamic balance. Hormones take their cues from internal signals (i.e., our blood sugar status, other hormone levels), and also the world around us. For example, when it's dark at night, the hormone *melatonin* helps us feel sleepy; as the sun comes up, *cortisol* makes us feel awake. This is part of our circadian rhythm, which you'll learn about in Chapter 8.

Throughout human history this has occurred every millisecond with remarkably few errors. While women have always experienced some mild hormonal disruptions here or there, we haven't been plagued by severe hormone problems en masse. Over the past few decades something has changed. Our hormonal messaging has become muddled, but unlike words in a party game, when these messages get scrambled, the results aren't funny—they're the problems that brought you to this book.

So what is it that's gotten this ancient, hard-wired system so confused?

There's a guiding principle in this book: your body is an incredible organism with a tremendous desire for dynamic balance. When symptoms and conditions arise, they're a warning that something needs attention. Hormone conditions aren't the root of the problem—they're the symptom trying to tell you something. But what are they trying to say? Understanding exactly this will help you take the reins back on your hormone health.

Putting the *Ecology* Back into Gynecology

If you look in medical textbooks (or ask most doctors), you'll find the phrase "we just don't know" a whole lot. "We just don't know" what causes endometriosis, "we just don't know" what causes PCOS, "we just don't know" why women get PMS, "we just don't know" what causes menstrual migraines, "we just don't know" why so many women are experiencing fertility problems. The list of what "we just don't know" is staggering.

But I believe we do know. In fact, there's a whole field of research that can help us to answer these very questions—and that gives us the direction we need to start to take our health back as women.

Over the past decade, a major field of science has emerged that illuminates how a specific set of influences we're all exposed to, to a greater or lesser extent depending on personal and social factors, are impacting our health. It's called *exposome science.* I call it our *total health ecology.* Exposome science divides our total ecology into two overlapping realms, inner and outer ecosystems. Our exposome plays an even greater role in determining our health than our genes, but does influence whether our "health promoting" or "disease triggering" predispositions are activated. It weaves a variety of medical disciplines into a holistic model: environmental medicine, toxicology, chronobiology (the branch of biology concerned with natural physiological rhythms and other cyclical phenomena such as sleep and menstrual cycles), the latest on microbiome research, trauma psychiatry, and more—research that rarely reaches the desks of primary care doctors, internists, gynecologists, and fertility doctors.

Your **internal ecosystem** includes your nutritional status, stress resilience, sleep quality and quantity, microbiome and digestive system, environmental "body burden" (lifetime toxin accumulation), inflammation, and something called *oxidative stress,* the amount of cellular damage you have as a result of all these factors cumulatively.

Your **external ecosystem** includes the quality and types of foods you eat, the level and type of stress you're under (including economic and cultural stressors like sexism, racism, threat of violence, history of trauma), the toxins and medications you're regularly exposed to, and interestingly, your health beliefs, as you'll learn more about in Chapter 5.

Exposome medicine takes a 360-degree view of your health terrain—the variables that conventional medicine overlooks, largely because physicians aren't taught to explore them, or are so busy seeing 35 patients a day, with an average of only 17 minutes per patient, that they don't have time even when they know better.

Gynecology has in it the roots *gyn,* which means woman, and *ecology,* which means our relationship to our total environment—making exposome science the perfect medicine for us. Exposome medicine also reveals the importance of what ancient philosophers, ecofeminists, and indigenous cultures believe: that women's bodies are a microcosm of the greater environment we all live in. We can't separate what's happening in our culture, our lives, our diets, our environment, our microbiome, or our minds and moods from what's going on in our health. The diseases we're seeing are diseases of our modern living and of a planet in distress, reflected in women's bodies. We're all interconnected, and our individual problems are also a collective one.

Exposome medicine validates the importance of a holistic approach to gynecology, one that puts YOU at the center of your care and that explores your experience as a whole woman; it takes a full-circle look at all the factors influencing your health—what's causing or contributing to your symptoms.

A Perfect Storm: Overwhelmed and Undernourished

How do I apply this in the Hormone Intelligence Plan? Many years ago I began asking myself two questions as I sat with my patients:

- What's overwhelming this woman's innate healing potential that we can reduce or remove?
- What's missing that her body needs to activate innate healing that we can add?

Think of it this way: When you don't adequately water or fertilize a plant, its roots don't receive the nourishment the plant needs for growth. However, if you overfeed or overwater a plant, it becomes overloaded and can't handle the burden. Not unlike a plant, though much more complex, our health depends on receiving the right amount of the right kind of inputs, but not too much or the wrong kind. Lack of one or too much of the other can throw our hormone-producing (endocrine) system for a loop—and that's exactly what's happening for most women.

These questions—and their answers—form the basis of my entire medical practice, and Hormone Intelligence.

Over the past seventy years there have been massive changes in countless aspects of our lives, from our modern diets, stress levels, sleep cycles, to the sheer volume of hormone-mimicking chemicals found in our environment (air, soil, and water), the very same factors associated with every hormonal and gyneco-logic condition in this book. Most of us are experiencing a perfect storm—multiple and interrelated factors affecting us—at any given time, and we're simultaneously experiencing multisystem overwhelm and undernourishment in our inner and outer ecosystems. The problem isn't that our hormones are faulty, nor are our genetic predispositions simply setting us up for disaster. And generally, we can easily rebound from a small single impact to our exposome, but most of us are experiencing a tsunami of them, daily.

These "hits" to our exposome create static in our hormone-signaling pathways, the delicate networks of hormonal, neurologic, and immunologic messengers, nerves, cells, and more, that are supposed to allow our hormones to ebb and flow with relative ease, daily and throughout the seasons of our lives. These hits accumulate, eventually tipping the scale away from balance and overwhelming our innate capacity to reset. I call these factors the *root causes*. Our hormone imbalances and gynecologic conditions are themselves the symptoms of deeper root cause imbalances. We've been blaming these messengers when they've just been trying to warn us.

Getting to the underlying factors that are causing interference on your hormone-signaling pathways helps you eliminate or drastically lessen the static on your hormone pathways, allowing you to once again sync up with your own natural hormonal rhythms and balance. In healing the imbalances in each of your root causes, you'll simultaneously be taking care of not just your hormones, but your lifetime health.

A New Medicine for Women

As you can see, it's not enough to just name a condition and treat it with medication, surgery, or even a sprinkling of the supposedly natural bioidentical hormones offered by many alternative practitioners. They might help in the short run, but they're a Band-Aid on deeper, hidden root causes. Conventional medicine misses the complexity of most of the symptoms and conditions we're experiencing, treating the surface but not the roots, so problems keep coming back, and we eventually turn to more drastic solutions.

Each of the root causes you're going to learn about are interconnected; as when you touch one part of a spider's web and the whole web moves, a disruption in one root impacts the others. When you begin to heal the roots in one or several areas, you experience whole-system improvements. A whole-woman approach that integrates your "total ecology" is vital. This new approach to medicine for women is the heart of holistic gynecology—our *hormone ecology*—and the Hormone Intelligence Plan you find in this book.

It's never too late to embrace the incredible power of your hormones, to see them as your allies, and to start celebrating the wonder of your body. I've taught thousands of women to become body-wise, to use diet, natural medicines, and lifestyle changes to shift their hormones into balance, and how to easily course-correct when "life happens." I've watched women gain confidence and agency over their well-being. I'm not saying it's fast and easy; it may be more challenging for some of you than others. But time and experience have shown me that every woman can experience greater ease and confidence in her body—and with it joy in her life. And I know you can, too.

When you learn just how many influences are affecting your hormones you'll see that your personal symptoms are not something you've been doing wrong. It's not you or your hormones that are broken. It's that twenty-first-century living is creating mixed messages and interference on our hormone channels. It's that the medical system is broken. My hope is that as you understand that there are big systemic, cultural, and economic forces at play, you'll feel kinder to and more patient with yourself, and more fired up to reclaim your role as CEO of your health. You've already taken the first step by picking up this book. Let's take the next step together, as I teach you to understand and recognize what's normal and what's not. Body knowledge is power.

the language of your cycles

A dame that knows the ropes isn't likely to get tied up.
—Mae West

Within us is an ancient blueprint meant to guide our hormones, monthly cycles, and life cycles. This isn't a romantic notion, nor is it biological reductionism; it's human physiology. Our hormones are guided by our *neuroendocrine system*, an information superhighway that's hardwired between our brain, ovaries, uterus, and vagina, with pathways interconnecting our thyroid gland, adrenals, heart, bones, and digestive and immune systems. This blueprint determines the arc of your hormonal journey from before you're born (when your ovarian cells are formed in your mother's womb), through your menstrual cycles and motherhood (if that's part of your journey), and into your mid-fifties, after which, with good health, a gentle pilot light of hormones keeps the flame alive for another forty years. This blueprint guides predictable changes over the course of our lives, most obviously, physical and emotional qualities unique to each phase of our life cycle.

I call this blueprint *Hormone Intelligence*. My aim is to teach you to become fluent in and able to decode your body's own Hormone Intelligence. Being *body-wise*, literate in and attuned to your personal cycles and the specific signs each hormone gives you, will help you to identify and get help when things *aren't* going according to the blueprint, recognize symptoms, detect changes early, and take action on simmering problems. Knowing what's normal (and normal for YOU) will dispel worries and misconceptions you may be harboring about your body and help you stop stressing over symptoms day after day, month after month, or year after year.

Your hormones and cycles not only give you physical signals as to what's going on, but you've got a whole under-the-radar navigation system of subtle cues you'll learn about, which can, if you listen to them, give you greater self-awareness and help you live a more harmonious and empowered life. You'll understand your hormones—how they're affecting not only your brain, uterus, ovaries, vulva, and vagina, but also your digestive system, moods, sleep, cravings, attractions, shopping habits, creative flow, focus, and more—and you'll be able to use this information to your advantage.

Welcome to your messy, mysterious, miraculous body. Let's start at the beginning.

The Arc of Our Life Cycles

Women have a powerful capacity for transformation—we change monthly and throughout our life's seasons—sometimes subtly, sometimes obviously. We shift through our life cycles like a vinyasa (yoga) flow, our hormones quietly instructing our moves. Knowing where you are on your hormone arc can help you understand what you might be experiencing—and why. Here are the phases:

Puberty: The is the new moon of the arc. Ideally between ages eleven and fourteen (as early as age ten and up to age sixteen are still considered normal) the ride of your life begins. Your brain's naturally scheduled programming, combined with your genetics and environmental exposures, tell your body when it's time to—presto chango—make you taller, solidify your bones, and sprout armpit and pubic hair. You menstruate for the first time, your breasts bloom, and you start to experience sexual interests.

Twenties and Thirties: Concerns about your monthly cycles, questions and concerns about sex, contraception, avoiding sexually transmitted infections, and getting pregnant (if that's on your life to-do list) are at the forefront. If you're having a smooth hormone ride, you can expect monthly periods, approximately 26 to 34 days apart, with midcycle fertility occurring when you ovulate between days 14 and 18. But as you've learned from your own personal experience, and in Chapter 1, most women aren't having a smooth ride. Hence, this book.

Late Thirties and Early Forties: For women with robust hormone health, these years are typically a continuation of regular cycles and midcycle ovulation and are often smoother than all the years until now. Then somewhere in our late thirties or early forties we begin to notice some degree of irregularity in period frequency, length, and amount of blood loss because of a natural decline in ovarian function as we get closer to perimenopause, the transitional phase to menopause. Fertility also might still be big on your mind, even into your mid-forties.

Mid- to Late Forties and Early Fifties: We enter the perimenopause phase now, which can last as long as eight years before menopause (complete cessation of ovulation and menstruation; international average age is 52 years old). As a result of a natural decline in estrogen and eventual cessation of ovulation, our periods typically become irregular, initially often more frequent, and then much less so; our flow may at first become heavier, then lightens; and as you get closer to menopause, you may notice hot flashes, sleep changes, changes in your urinary frequency, and changes in your sex drive along with some vaginal dryness.

This book is meant to be a lifelong companion—one you can return to in the various seasons of your life—as a touchstone of hormone support.

Hormones 101

In modern terms, your hormones are wireless signaling messengers circulating throughout every part of your body. The word *hormone* comes from the Greek "to arouse" or "to set in motion"—and do they ever! Our endocrine system, the biological system that produces all our hormones, is composed of glands (small secretory organs) including the hypothalamus, pituitary, thyroid, and adrenal glands, and ovaries (and to a lesser degree include your fat cells, skin, and even your brain). Over fifty hormones are continually produced daily. Manufactured in one location, they travel to a cell somewhere else in your body, bind to a receptor, sort of like "docking ports" with a shape that matches a specific hormone, and initiate a chain reaction that gets an action done—like maturing an egg in your ovary or telling your hair to grow or your period to start. You have hormone receptors in the more obvious places like your breasts, uterus, and ovaries, and also in your brain, your heart, your bones, to name a few locations.

Hormones regulate millions of functions including metabolism (the rate at which you burn calories, thus determining your energy levels and weight, for example), growth, development, tissue function, sexual function, reproduction, sleep, mood, and more. They must be present in specific amounts to do their jobs properly—as in Goldilocks's case, there can't be too little or too much, the levels have to be juuuuust right, so your body is constantly adjusting hormone production through *feedback loops*.

Brain to Body and Back Again: Your Hormones Really Are "Loopy"

Feedback loops work similarly to a thermostat in your house: When the temperature reaches the set point, say 68°F, the thermostat slows heat production to keep your home at the desired temperature. When your house cools to below that, the heater kicks back on. When your bloodstream reaches a required level of a specific hormone, a message relays to the brain (or ovary, or thyroid, etc.) to slow production of that hormone; this is called a *negative feedback loop*. When hormone levels get below optimal, your brain (or ovary, or thyroid, etc.) sends out signals that ramp up production—a *positive feedback loop*. This happens every millisecond with each hormone being constantly calibrated to meet your needs. External clues also drive hormone production; light and dark

The Hormone Superhighways

These 3 major information pathways, or *feedback loops*, are the holy trinity of women's hormones; I refer to them throughout the book.

- **The Hypothalamic-Pituitary-Ovarian (HPO) Axis:** the main brain-ovary signaling loop, stimulating and regulating female hormone production and your monthly cycles.
- **The Hypothalamic-Pituitary-Adrenal (HPA) Axis:** the signaling loop between your brain and adrenal glands, controlling cortisol production and adrenaline release regulating your stress response, sleep, inflammation, blood sugar, and much more.
- **The Hypothalamic-Pituitary-Thyroid (HPT) Axis:** the signaling loop between your brain and thyroid, which also has a strong say in your menstrual cycles, energy levels, metabolism, and cognitive function.

exposure affect melatonin production; connecting with a loved one ramps up oxytocin; and stress increases cortisol. Seeing someone you think is hot gets you "turned on," hearing a baby cry may cause milk letdown if you're breastfeeding, smelling your favorite food activates digestive hormones. Hormones are thus a bridge between our inner and outer ecosystems.

It Takes a Symphony

Hormone health requires a well-tuned symphony. Your hypothalamus serves as the conductor; your pituitary gland is the baton conveying the conductor's messages to key sections of the orchestra, which includes your ovaries, thyroid, and adrenals.

Within each of these organs are the musicians, your hormones—estrogen, progesterone; testosterone, cortisol, thyroid hormones, and others—translating the conductor's instructions into actions: menstruation, ovulation, fertility, conception, breast health, and more. A missed beat might go unnoticed, but if the conductor isn't leading, if an instrument isn't tuned, if a musician is off tempo, or someone has the wrong sheet music, there's disharmony—or chaos! Hormone Intelligence is designed to tune this orchestra, giving your endocrine system everything it needs to make beautiful music for you each month and over your life cycles.

Meet Your Leading Ladies and Supporting Cast

I'd like to introduce you to a small but powerful set of the most influential hormones involved in women's health—and in the conditions that brought you to this book.

The Leading Ladies

The three leading ladies of women's health are estrogen, progesterone, and testosterone—collectively known as "sex hormones."

Estrogen is the "Queen Bee." We produce three types of estrogen in our ovaries, fat cells, and to lesser amounts, our skin. The one I'd like you to get to know best is *estradiol* (E2), the diva who influences your puberty, your menstrual cycles, pregnancy, and menopause. At puberty she causes us to develop breasts and hips, and all our female sex characteristics. Made in your ovarian follicles, estradiol drives the activity of the first half of your menstrual cycle, making another appearance after ovulation. Her reach is extraordinary. While preparing the uterus for implantation should you become pregnant, she makes your features more symmetrical and your skin glow, while boosting your confidence around ovulation.

Endocrine System

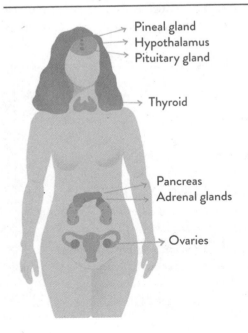

Pineal gland
Hypothalamus
Pituitary gland

Thyroid

Pancreas
Adrenal glands

Ovaries

Estrogen is also more than a reproductive hormone. It stimulates cell growth and is involved in the production of neurotransmitters, chemicals like dopamine and serotonin, that influence your mood. Estrogen receptors are found not only in the ovaries and uterus, but in the heart, brain, bones, and immune system and are known to play a role in maintaining your cognitive function (preventing Alzheimer's disease), building bone density; controlling inflammation (and helping to develop and prevent autoimmune disease), controlling cholesterol, maintaining skin and hair vibrancy, as well as maintaining weight, healthy metabolism, urinary tract health, and vaginal health. Estrogen helps you connect with others through empathy and facial expression recognition, while supporting healthy stress response.

Progesterone, the "calming" hormone, which is produced in the ovary after ovulation, plays a role in early breast development, stabilizes the endometrium for pregnancy, and if fertilization occurs, helps to maintain pregnancy. It may act as a "homing signal," drawing sperm toward the egg at ovulation. Progesterone levels have important implications for brain function and mood; a breakdown product called *allopregnanolone* creates calm, as well as deep, restful sleep. It also protects brain tissue from inflammation and injury; it's involved in serotonin production and calms the nervous system so much it protects against and may help treat addiction. Progesterone also enhances your skin elasticity and vitality, keeps your immune function working well, and even plays a role in blood sugar balance and healthy insulin signaling.

Androgens, like the estrogens, are a group of hormones, **testosterone** being the one we're most familiar with. While we think of these as male hormones, we've got them too. I think of them as the huntress hormones; they inspire drive and strength—emotionally and physically. Produced in the adrenal glands and ovaries, androgens are key players in regulating your menstrual cycle. They are also builders, helping to increase bone and muscle strength, enhance your sex drive (especially just before ovulation), and strengthen your confidence and assertiveness.

The Supporting Cast

Cortisol is our "healer" hormone, more commonly known as the "stress" hormone because of its central role in the fight-flight-freeze response. Produced in the adrenal glands, cortisol is released when the brain detects a threat; it initiates a cascade of changes in your nervous system that activate the primary stress response. Cortisol also regulates sleep (or lack thereof), immunity and inflammation, hormone production, and our menstrual cycles and ovulation. Both acute and chronic stress play a major role in sex hormone, thyroid hormone, and melatonin production.

The **thyroid** hormones are your "energizer" hormones. Produced in your thyroid gland, a butterfly-shaped organ at the front of your neck, thyroid hormones regulate energy, metabolism, and cognitive function, and play a significant role in ovarian hormone production, cycle regularity, fertility, menopause, and more.

Melatonin, a neurohormone produced in your brain's pineal gland, is referred to as the "sleep" hormone. It not only helps you settle into needed rest at night, but helps your body with important detoxification functions. Your ovarian follicles are rich in melatonin, providing your eggs with protection against something called *oxidative stress*, addressed in Chapter 11, which is part of melatonin's role in detoxification.

Insulin, made by the pancreas, allows your body to use sugar (glucose) from carbohydrates in the foods you eat for energy, or to store glucose for future use. It keeps your blood sugar level from getting too high (hyperglycemia) or too low (hypoglycemia). Insulin resistance, a significant contributing factor to PCOS and to inflammation, is involved in many gynecologic symptoms, including pain, PMS, and endometriosis. We reverse this in Part Two.

Behind the Scenes

Numerous other important hormones also influence our cyclic, reproductive, and sexual health. Those that are going to get honorable mention throughout the book, and therefore you'll want to be familiar with, are:

Follicle-stimulating hormone (FSH): produced in the pituitary gland, it stimulates the growth of ovarian follicles prior to ovulation and also increases estradiol production.

Luteinizing hormone (LH): also a pituitary hormone, it's a driving force in ovulation, stimulating the ovarian follicles to produce estradiol, which causes the ovarian follicle to release the mature egg. In the second half of the menstrual cycle, LH stimulates the corpus luteum to produce progesterone.

Prolactin: plays a role in the complex feedback loop that tells your brain when to produce more or less of the hormones I've introduced you to. It also plays a major role in breastfeeding.

Which Symptoms, Which Hormones?

Now that you know a thing or two about the main players and supporting hormones affecting your gynecologic health, you may be curious to know which hormones are related to the symptoms you might be experiencing. The Hormones and Their Symptoms chart (pages 33–37) will help you connect those

dots, and the Hormone Blueprint Questionnaire (pages 38–40) will help to personalize this information.

Should I Get My Hormones Tested?

I don't run routine hormone testing on every patient who sees me for hormonal or gynecologic symptoms. If their symptoms obviously point to a diagnosis, it's usually unnecessary. For example, if a woman has mild PMS or menstrual cramps, I'd be unlikely to order lab tests. If she has obvious symptoms of PCOS (see Chapter 4), then I wouldn't run blood tests to confirm PCOS, though I'd run labs to check for problems that can accompany PCOS, like insulin resistance or high cholesterol.

However, a basic **Women's Hormone Panel** can be helpful in confirming a diagnosis or illuminating root causes, for example, why periods may have gone AWOL, whether you're experiencing primary ovarian insufficiency (POI), if low progesterone or a slow thyroid is contributing to fertility problems, whether you have insulin resistance associated with PCOS, or whether your hot flashes, night sweats, and vaginal dryness are due to perimenopause. A basic **Women's Hormone Panel** can also help identify a diagnosis when symptoms aren't fully adding up to a condition. It can also tell you whether your hormones are in the appropriate ranges for your age.

The Hormone Intelligence Basic Hormone Panel includes:

- Estradiol

- FSH and LH (best tested on day 3 of your menstrual cycle)

- Progesterone (best tested on day 19–22 of your menstrual cycle)

- Sex-hormone-binding globulin
- Free testosterone
- Thyroid panel: TSH, free T4, free T3, reverse T3, anti-TPO, and antithyroglobulin antibodies
- 24-hour salivary cortisol
- Prolactin

In Part Three, I discuss when testing is recommended for specific conditions.

Now that you're understanding your hormonal landscape, it's time to dive deeper into the most informative vital sign we have: the menstrual cycle. Even if you think you know everything about cycles and periods, please have a read because you're going to have a whole new appreciation for your cycle—and you're going to learn to use it to your advantage in ways that will become a game changer for how you live your life.

Hormones and Their Symptoms

High Estrogen (particularly estradiol)

Common Symptoms

- Cyclic breast tenderness, breast cysts
- Endometriosis
- Heavy periods
- Menstrual migraines
- Mood swings
- Short menstrual cycles (<21 days)
- Fibroids
- Bloating, water retention

Common Causes

- Estrogen-containing birth control
- Endocrine-disrupting chemicals
- Impaired liver detoxification
- Low-fiber diet
- Obesity
- Intestinal dysbiosis, sluggish elimination

Potential Risks

- Autoimmune disease
- Breast, ovarian, and endometrial cancers
- Hypothyroidism

Low Estrogen (particularly estradiol)

Common Symptoms

- Bone loss (osteopenia, osteoporosis)
- Brain fog, memory problems
- Depression
- Headaches
- Hot flashes, night sweats
- Irritability, anxiety

Hormones and Their Symptoms *(continued)*

- Joint pain
- Decreased skin tone
- Low libido
- Low thyroid function
- Sagging breasts, loss of breast size
- Sleep problems
- Scant or skipped periods
- Thinning hair
- Vaginal dryness
- Urinary tract infection (UTI)
- Weight gain

Common Causes

- Low body fat / energy, malnutrition
- Menopause
- Overexercise
- Primary ovarian insufficiency (POI)
- Stress

Potential Risks

- Alzheimer's disease / dementia
- UTIs
- Heart disease
- Osteoporosis

Low Progesterone

Common Symptoms

- Anovulation
- Anxiety
- Constipation
- Cyclic breast pain
- Depression
- Endometriosis
- Fertility problems
- Insomnia
- Irregular menstrual cycles
- Irritability, anxiety
- Long menstrual cycles (>35 days)
- Low libido
- Miscarriage
- Short luteal phase
- Spotting between periods
- Water retention

Common Causes

- Not ovulating / luteal phase deficiency
- PCOS

Potential Risks

- Abnormal uterine bleeding
- Breast cancer
- Endometrial cancer
- Recurrent miscarriage
- Reduced bone density

Hormones and Their Symptoms *(continued)*

High Testosterone

Common Symptoms

- Acne
- Anxiety
- Blood sugar problems
- Depression
- Fertility problems
- Hair loss, thinning hair
- Hirsutism (hair in unwanted places)
- Irritability
- Oily skin/hair
- Reactivity, irritability, aggression

Common Causes

- Chronic stress
- High-sugar or high-carbohydrate diet
- Insulin resistance
- Polycystic ovary syndrome (PCOS)

Potential Risks

- Depression
- Diabetes
- Heart disease
- High cholesterol
- Infertility
- PCOS

Low Testosterone

Common Symptoms

- "Bat wings" (fat on the back of your arms)
- Decreased sense of well-being
- Depression
- Fatigue
- Low confidence
- Low libido
- Low motivation
- Muscle loss, muscle weakness
- Weight gain

Common Causes

- Low adrenal function
- Naturally decline in menopause
- Stress

Potential Risks

- Not well studied in women

Hormones and Their Symptoms (continued)

High Cortisol

Common Symptoms

- Anxiety/panic attacks
- Frequent illness
- Irregular periods
- Low stress resilience
- Increased abdominal fat ("muffin tops")
- Sleep problems
- Sugar, salt, fat cravings
- (See pages 39–40 for a complete list)

Common Causes

- Chronic stress
- Natural decline in menopause

Potential Risks

- Anxiety
- Bone loss (osteopenia, osteoporosis)
- Fatigue
- High blood pressure
- High blood sugar / insulin resistance
- Hypothyroidism
- Low libido
- Metabolic syndrome

Low Thyroid Hormone

Common Symptoms

- Cold hands and feet
- Constipation
- Depression
- Dry skin
- Enlarged thyroid gland (goiter)
- Fatigue
- Feel "chilly" a lot
- Hoarse voice
- Irregular periods
- Joint pain
- Low energy
- Low libido
- Puffiness
- Skipped, irregular, or heavy periods
- Slow metabolism (weight gain)
- Slower mental function / impaired memory
- Thinning hair / missing outer third of eyebrows
- Weight gain

Common Causes

- Autoimmunity
- Certain medications
- Iodine deficiency
- Pituitary gland problem

Hormones and Their Symptoms (continued)

- Pregnancy
- Radiation or surgery to the neck/thyroid

- Thyroid cancer

Potential Risks

- Depression
- Goiter
- Heart disease
- Infertility
- Miscarriage

- Pregnancy problems, postpartum depression
- Obesity and its associated risks
- Peripheral neuropathy

High Insulin / Insulin Resistance

Common Symptoms

- Blood pressure >130/80
- BMI >25
- Darkened skin of the neck, groin, or armpits
- High blood pressure
- High LDL and low HDL cholesterol

- Increased abdominal fat
- PCOS
- Shakiness between meals
- Skin tags
- Waist circumference >30 inches
- Weight gain

Common Causes

- Chronic stress
- Diet high in sugar or refined carbohydrates

- Inadequate sleep
- Underactive thyroid

Potential Risks

- Dementia
- Fatty liver disease (NAFLD)
- Gestational diabetes
- Heart disease

- High cholesterol
- Obesity
- PCOS
- Type 2 diabetes

Your Hormone Blueprint Questionnaire

Now let's add a self-assessment to help you connect the dots. At avivaromm.com/hormone
-intelligence-resources you'll find a printable version you can use to track improvement as you
go through the plan and beyond. Scoring >4 points in any of the 8 patterns suggests that you
have some measure of the associated imbalance. Scoring >8 points in any section suggests a
more significant imbalance. It's common—in fact likely—to have more than one imbalance. The
Hormone Intelligence Plan is all about addressing these symptoms and imbalances!

Check all boxes that relate to you in each section.

Pattern 1: High Estrogen

- ☐ Heavy periods
- ☐ Painful periods
- ☐ Short menstrual cycles (<21 days)
- ☐ Bloating, fluid retention
- ☐ Breast tenderness, cysts
- ☐ Mood swings
- ☐ Menstrual migraines
- ☐ Uterine fibroids
- ☐ Endometriosis
- ☐ Varicose veins
- ☐ Gallbladder problems
- ☐ History of using estrogen-containing birth control or medication (in the last three months)
- ☐ A pear-shaped body

Pattern 2: Low Estrogen

- ☐ Irregular or absent periods
- ☐ Trouble falling asleep, waking in the middle of the night
- ☐ Anxiety, depression
- ☐ Hot flashes, night sweats
- ☐ Vaginal dryness
- ☐ Urinary frequency or frequent UTIs
- ☐ Low libido
- ☐ Weight gain
- ☐ Brain fog, memory problems, poor focus
- ☐ Long menstrual cycles or scant periods
- ☐ Migraines
- ☐ Joint aches or pains
- ☐ Loss of bone density (osteopenia, osteoporosis, loss of height)
- ☐ Autoimmune disease

Pattern 3: Low Progesterone

- ☐ Irregular menstrual cycles
- ☐ Heavy periods
- ☐ Insomnia, sleep problems
- ☐ Headaches or migraines
- ☐ Anxiety, depression
- ☐ PMS

Your Hormone Blueprint Questionnaire *(continued)*

- ☐ Short luteal phase (ovulation to menstruation less than 12 days)
- ☐ Spotting in the second half of your cycle
- ☐ Low or no signs of ovulation
- ☐ Low basal body temp in the luteal phase
- ☐ Fertility problems

- ☐ Recurrent miscarriage
- ☐ Symptoms of excess estrogen (weight gain, depression, heavy periods, low libido, breast tenderness, fibrocystic breasts, fibroids, gallbladder problems)
- ☐ Endometriosis

Pattern 4: High Testosterone

- ☐ Irregular periods
- ☐ Skipped periods
- ☐ Fertility challenges
- ☐ Hair in unwanted places
- ☐ Hair loss (head)

- ☐ Acne
- ☐ Weight gain
- ☐ Aggression, irritability
- ☐ Polycystic ovary syndrome (PCOS)
- ☐ High LDL cholesterol

Pattern 5: Low Testosterone

- ☐ Fatigue, sluggishness
- ☐ Low motivation
- ☐ Depression
- ☐ Muscle weakness or loss of muscle
- ☐ Hair loss
- ☐ Sleep disturbances

- ☐ Low sex drive
- ☐ Decreased sexual satisfaction, difficulty achieving orgasm
- ☐ Weight gain
- ☐ Irregular menstrual cycles

Pattern 6: High Cortisol

- ☐ Chronic stress, overwhelm
- ☐ Low motivation or drive
- ☐ Often feeling burnout
- ☐ Trouble falling asleep, feeling "tired and wired"
- ☐ Tired during the day, hit a slump around 3–4 p.m.
- ☐ Waking up tired even after a good night's sleep

- ☐ Insomnia, trouble falling asleep or staying asleep
- ☐ Needing coffee to start the day, or a cup in the afternoon
- ☐ Craving sweets, chocolate, or salty foods
- ☐ Bloating, puffiness, or fluid retention
- ☐ Mood swings, PMS, irritability, weepiness, mini breakdowns, or anxiety

Your Hormone Blueprint Questionnaire *(continued)*

- ☐ Low (or no) sex drive
- ☐ Overweight, especially around my middle ("muffin top")
- ☐ Blue or even depressed
- ☐ Increased skin wrinkling for your age
- ☐ Reduced memory or focus
- ☐ Irregular menstrual cycles
- ☐ Miserable menopausal symptoms

- ☐ Trouble getting pregnant, history of miscarriage
- ☐ PCOS
- ☐ High cholesterol
- ☐ Bone loss (osteopenia or osteoporosis)
- ☐ Autoimmune disease
- ☐ Frequent colds or illnesses

Pattern 7: Low Thyroid Hormone

- ☐ Sluggishness, fatigue, zero energy
- ☐ Weight gain without changing eating or exercise habits
- ☐ Trouble losing weight, despite dieting and exercise
- ☐ My memory and concentration aren't what they were
- ☐ Low mood, depression, anxiety
- ☐ Sluggish bowels, constipation
- ☐ Feeling cold all the time, have to wear a sweater even if nobody else is, low body temperature

- ☐ Dry, itchy, or rough skin
- ☐ Brittle or coarse hair or nails
- ☐ Hair loss, hair thinning
- ☐ High cholesterol
- ☐ Puffiness around eyes, face gets puffy
- ☐ Loss or thinning of outer third of eyebrows
- ☐ PMS, heavy periods, or skipped periods
- ☐ Trouble getting pregnant, history of miscarriage
- ☐ History of postpartum depression or trouble producing breast milk

Pattern 8: High Insulin / Insulin Resistance

- ☐ High blood sugar
- ☐ Metabolic syndrome, insulin resistance, or diabetes
- ☐ Shakiness or agitation between meals
- ☐ Skin tags
- ☐ Brown, velvety skin discoloration in my armpits, groin, or neck
- ☐ Tired a lot
- ☐ Overweight, with weight especially around my waist and belly

- ☐ Frequent thirst, frequent urination
- ☐ Waist circumference >30 inches
- ☐ High blood pressure (>130/80)
- ☐ History of gestational diabetes or had a baby who weighed more than 9 pounds
- ☐ PCOS
- ☐ Hair in unwanted places
- ☐ Hair thinning or loss
- ☐ Acne, especially cystic acne

your sixth vital sign

I was twelve, spending the night at my grandparents' when I saw blood in my underwear. I told my grandma, who, red-cheeked, congratulated me and made a quick trip to the grocery store, returning with a box of maxi pads that she hastily handed to me in a paper bag. No fanfare, but no biggie, right?

Then a few months later, it happened: a junior high schooler's worst nightmare! I was leaving sixth-grade English class when a classmate threw her sweatshirt around my waist. (Sound of audience gasping.) "You have blood on the back of your jeans," she whispered. Her armed hooked in mine, she ushered me to the bathroom and whipped a maxi pad out of her backpack, Mary-Fucking-Poppins style, and handed it to me with a smile. To this day I'm grateful for that goddess who covered my ass!

Many of us begin menstruating as I did, more or less in the dark, no thanks to those useless fourth-, fifth-, or sixth-grade "health classes," and we spend a good deal of the rest of our menstrual lives feeling that way—not knowing what's normal, when to be concerned, or how to get the information we need—let alone how to feel "cool" about having periods. Is everyone else having menstrual cramps? Mood swings? Sugar cravings? Heavy bleeding? Should my period hurt this much? What if I bleed through my white jeans on this date?

Statistically, nearly half of all girls don't know what's happening to them when they have their period; teens and women report that the sex education classes they had were useless (or worse, useless *and* scary!), and a 2006 study of Ivy League college students revealed that only 27.5% were able to correctly identify when a woman is fertile during her menstrual cycle. From my interactions with thousands of women each year, from those in their teens to those in their seventies, I've found that most women don't know, beyond a vague sense, what hormones are and do, and how their body works. But it's never too late to get body-wise and body-literate. I hope this chapter is finally the health class you wished you had, taught by the cool auntie who let you in on the juicy secrets. And I hope by the end of the chapter you find yourself a little in love with the amazingness of your hormones and how cool you really are.

Your Sixth Vital Sign

The correlation between our menstrual cycles and our lifelong health is so intertwined and significant that in 2006 the American Academy of Pediatrics (AAP) and the American College of Obstetricians and Gynecologists (ACOG) published a report called "Menstruation in Girls and Adolescents: Using the Menstrual Cycle as a Vital Sign," a position reaffirmed by both organizations in 2015—making women's health symptoms our sixth vital sign, after temperature, blood pressure, heart rate, respiratory rate, and pain.

Paula Hillard, MD, of Stanford University School of Medicine, stated it beautifully, "The menstrual cycle is a window into the general health and well-being of women, and not just a reproductive event"; changes in your menstrual cycle are "the first sign that something else could be going on." Given that most women menstruate about four hundred times in our lives, it's a crying shame not to learn the skill of tapping into what is truly the secret language of our body—our hormone whisperings. Becoming familiar with the dance of your cycle helps you start to "check your own vital sign" and understand how it's affecting your moods, energy, sleep, appetite, weight, focus, sex drive, hair, skin, even your digestion. You get a sense of what your "optimal" and normal cycles are like and discern when symptoms of imbalance are creeping in. You even start to understand those symptoms not as body betrayal, but as an innately intelligent response to changing conditions within. If we don't, when these little whispers are trying to alert us to a problem, they get louder and louder in the form of worsening symptoms or the onset of actual medical conditions, until we're forced to pay attention to them.

We'll talk all about the hormone imbalances you need to know about in the next chapter. First, let's take a journey through what an optimal menstrual cycle looks like. Not cycling anymore? Read on anyway—our menstrual cycle history remains an important vital sign throughout our lives, predictive of the severity of symptoms we might experience in menopause, and you'll find yourself having plenty of "aha" moments.

What Is a Healthy Menstrual Cycle?

First, there's no such thing as a perfect period. You don't have to menstruate every 28 days

On Her Terms: Signs vs. Symptoms

As women, we have shifts in discharge, odors, desire, energy, mood, and all kinds of physical sensations throughout our monthly cycles and life cycles. Going forward, when I refer to normal body functions, I use the word *sign* instead of the usual word *symptom* because it's normal stuff. When I mean that something is in fact a symptom of a condition, I use the word *symptom* or *condition* to differentiate.

like clockwork to be normal, you don't have to bleed at the full moon to be spiritually aligned, and even mild, occasional cramps or other mild symptoms can be perfectly normal. There's a range of normal, varying woman-to-woman, by life cycle, and by age. If you're cycle is generally within the parameters set out in this chapter, then normal is what's normal for YOU. The big thing to look for is major deviations from what I lay out in this chapter, big or persistent shifts from your own typical normal, and anything affecting your quality of life (work, fertility, sex, play, etc.), as I'll explain.

Here are the signs that tell you whether your hormones and cycles are happily in balance, and if they're not right now, where you're aiming for them to be over the next 6 weeks to 6 months from following the plan in this book.

Menstrual Cycle Length

Although some women describe their periods coming "like clockwork" every 28 days, this is the exception. Based on several long-term studies of thousands of women around the world, most women's menstrual cycles are between 26 to 34 days.

Menstrual cycles' lengths also vary with the seasons of our life. In our *teens*, it's normal for our periods to be anywhere from 23 to 90 days apart, in our reproductive years (twenties to mid-forties) for them to be anywhere from 24 to 38 days apart (the average length is 29 days), and as we edge toward menopause, for our cycles to be as short as 24 days apart or to go AWOL for 3 to 4 months at a time. That's of course as long as there are no Red Flag symptoms that indicate a problem like PCOS or endometriosis (more in the next chapter).

In addition, it's normal for your cycle to change pattern over the course of a year, and to vary by as much as 6 days from month to month. This is important to keep in mind as

you read through the four phases of the menstrual cycle below, which, for convenience in presenting the information, is based on a typical 28-day cycle. If your cycle length, time of ovulation, or hormonal signs occur within a few days either way of the suggested weekly time frame, and you're not having problems with your cycle or gynecologic health, then no sweat—that's just *your* normal.

Period Length

3 to 7 days

Amount of Bleeding

No more than six pads or tampons/day. Heaviest flow day is period day two, but this varies.

Pain

No more than occasional mild cramps or pelvic tension; no need for medications, hot water bottles, or other comfort measures; no more than mild breast "fullness"—but no breast pain, cysts, or cyclic lumps; no headaches or migraines.

Mood

Mild shifts in mood, level of desire for social connection, energy, sleep, and cravings are normal; these should not, however, feel extreme, disruptive, or out of control to *you*.

Meet the Four Phases of Your Menstrual Cycle

The menstrual cycle is divided into four phases, each with its own unique hormonal shifts, physical signs, and qualities, though as you'll soon learn, some phases overlap. This cycle repeats every month for, give or take, forty years of most women's lives, except when we're

What's Your Period Code Word?

It's the 21st century and a lotta' women are still so embarrassed about having a period they hide tampons up their sleeves on the way to the restroom (no shame, I've done it, too) and have code words for that time of the month (or TOM if you're texting). Period code words can be funny—a relaxed way to talk about being on the rag (ha, did it again!). There are over 5,000 euphemisms for Aunt Flo in the English language. Here are a few—that I haven't already just dropped:

- Auntie
- Code Red
- Crimson wave, crimson tide
- Lady time, Lady friend, Lady days
- Monthly visitor

- Mother Nature
- Ragging
- Red tide
- Shark Week

In my (hippie) household "moon time" is my homage to an ancient way of honoring our cycles. Do you have a period code word? Is it to avoid awkwardness? Or just for fun? Let's normalize periods by talking about them! Including saying *period* with pride. Period.

pregnant. Let's explore these phases together. To clarify an incredibly common misconception, your menstrual cycle is not just your period; it encompasses the first day of your period through to the last day before your next period starts, and with it, the hormonal, physical, and emotional shifts that occur during this time.

Phase One: Menstruation a.k.a. Your Period (Days 1 to 7)

It seems logical that we'd think of our periods as the end of our cycles, but technically, the first day of your period is **day 1** of the entire cycle. During your period, you're **shedding the old (as in uterine lining) and starting fresh (new cycle of hormone ebbs and flows)**. If you're trying to get pregnant—and haven't—your period can feel like the end. So I like to remind my fertility patients that, technically, it's a chance to start anew. Think of it like Marie Kondo for the uterus.

When you have your period, the uterine lining that "proliferated" (got thicker and lusher) during the preceding cycle, sheds. This is the result of the cyclic drop in **estrogen and progesterone** to their lowest point. This hormone plummet, with an accompanying drop in serotonin and a peak in inflammatory chemicals (i.e., prostaglandins), is responsible for the signs—and symptoms—we experience in the days before and on the first couple of days of bleeding.

How Much Flow Is Normal?

Normal blood loss over the course of a period is **30 to 80 mL**. Think of it this way: a shot glass and a half is about 60 mL, or from 1 to 6 tablespoons. It seems like a lot more blood that than, doesn't it? That's because it gets diluted with vaginal mucus.

A period is considered "heavy" when:

- It lasts 8 or more days.

- It interferes with your ability to do day-to-day tasks.

- You're soaking through maxi pads / tampons on the regular.

- You have to change your tampon or pad more than every 2 hours.

- You need a pad plus a tampon to contain the flow.

- You have to change your pads or tampons during the night.

- You pass blood clots the size of a quarter or larger.

- You experience fatigue, low energy, shortness of breath, or you've been diagnosed with anemia.

How Much Period Pain Is Normal?

You're going to be shocked, but the answer is *None*. I'm serious. You shouldn't ever be in *pain* because of your period. Mild cramps, a bit of heaviness in your pelvis or cooch, mild low-back ache—these are all sensations that tell you your period is about to start—and are normal. But being a woman shouldn't *hurt* every month, all the time, when you're having sex, peeing, pooping, or any other time.

Remember, common is not the same as normal! We've become so indoctrinated to believe that period pain is "normal" that even an emergency room doctor or nurse might ask you "Are you sure it's not just that time of the month?" when you're actually doubled up in pain from a kidney stone, ovarian cyst, or appendicitis! This happens all the time. Really!

While you may never celebrate having your period (unless it was late and you didn't want it to be!), your period should never be

Does Period Blood Color Mean Something Important?

You may have read on the internet that period blood color has all kinds of meanings about your health. Myth busting time! Here's the real deal:

Period blood color changes when it's exposed to air—that's called *oxidation*. The more it oxidizes, the darker the color gets.

Very dark blood is usually old blood being shed from your uterus—possibly some lining remaining from your last cycle, and is not medically significant.

Bright red blood is fresh blood. If your period blood is very pale or light pink and watery, that could be a sign that you have low iron (anemia) so it's worth having a simple blood test to check.

Contrary to another internet myth, it's also perfectly normal to have small clots mixed in with your blood. As your uterine lining sheds, clotting factors kick in to control how much you bleed so every period isn't a life-threating event! Clots smaller than the size of a quarter, happening occasionally, are not medically relevant. Bigger clots? Could be due to heavy periods, endometriosis, or fibroids. We'll talk about this in Chapter 4.

Menstrual Cycle at a Glance

Phase	Happens on These (Approximate) Days of a (28-Day) Menstrual Cycle	What's Happening	What Your Hormones Are Doing
Menstruation	1–6	On the first 1–6 days, the endometrial lining sheds.	Estrogen and progesterone are at their lowest at the start of menstruation; estrogen begins to rise.
Follicular	1–13 (includes the menstrual phase)	The uterine lining is proliferating, the ovary is ripening follicles to induce one egg to release, and the glands in the cervix start to produce fertile mucus.	Estrogen continues to rise, as does FSH, heading toward a midcycle peak; testosterone increases.
Ovulation	14–18	An egg is released from the ovary.	Estrogen begins to peak, stimulating an LH surge. This leads the dominant ovarian follicle to rupture and release an egg.
Luteal	14–28 (includes ovulation)	The time between ovulation and the start of menstruation; implantation occurs if you become pregnant; your body prepares for menstruation if you don't.	Progesterone is produced by the empty follicle, dominating the second half of the menstrual cycle. Estrogen has a second lesser peak. After midluteal phase, progesterone and estrogen levels drop, causing the endometrium to shed, and the cycle begins again with your next period.

more than a mild inconvenience. Period pain is a signal that something is amiss—which we'll talk about in the next chapter.

Phase Two: The Follicular Phase (Days 1 to 13)

The start of your period marks the start of the **follicular phase**, named for the tiny ovum-containing follicles on your ovaries—one of which becomes the diva, the dominant follicle with an ova destined for release.

Estrogen is dominant during this phase, and testosterone starts to rise, making us feel energized, sexier, bolder, and more vibrant and mentally clear. You are on fire! Under the influence of estrogen, your uterine lining proliferates, getting lusher, ready for implantation should the released egg get fertilized after ovulation. Toward the end of the follicular phase,

your pituitary produces a burst of luteinizing hormone, preparing the follicle to burst open—and voila—you ovulate.

Phase Three: Ovulation (Days 14 to 18)

Ovulation marks the beginning of the **luteal phase** and usually occurs midcycle. The mature follicle ruptures, releasing the ovum (egg), which travels down the fallopian tube and either meets up with sperm trying to find an egg to fertilize or begins to disintegrate, unfertilized. The egg can only be fertilized for about 24 hours once released, but since viable sperm can linger in the fallopian tube and other crannies for 3 to 5 days, your fertile window lasts 5 to 6 days, from about five days before until one or two days after ovulation.

Detecting Ovulation from Cervical Mucus

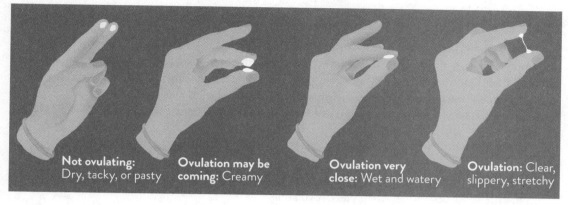

Not ovulating: Dry, tacky, or pasty

Ovulation may be coming: Creamy

Ovulation very close: Wet and watery

Ovulation: Clear, slippery, stretchy

You know you're ovulating (and fertile) when your vaginal discharge becomes plentiful, clear, and stretchy, with a texture that is usually described as being like egg whites. This is due to increased production of cervical mucus called *spinnbarkeit*. It's different in quality than the vaginal secretions you might produce when you get sexually aroused. It's notably more stretchy if you pull it between your fingers (see image above), and it's produced specifically in the few days before and until just after you ovulate.

But hey, not everyone feels comfortable touching that stuff. That's cool. You can feel the difference even when you wipe yourself after you pee—the toilet tissue practically glides over your vulva when you wipe, and you can sense that there's slippery mucus and more of it, compared to when you're closer to your period, at which time things feel drier and less slick down there. This copious, odorless cervical mucus is "engineered" to have the perfect pH to keep sperm alive for about 5 days, help healthy sperm find their way to your cervix, while "weeding out" damaged ones as a way to protect your egg from a sperm with possible bad DNA, and transform the sperm as they pass through your cervix so they have more of a chance of fertilizing that waiting

egg. It also makes for great vaginal lubrication. If you're not producing fertile cervical mucus, you might not be ovulating, or factors I share on page 62 might be interfering with its production.

Knowing if and when you're ovulating is important—it can help you prevent an unwanted pregnancy or time conception if you want to get pregnant, and if you're not ovulating, this can be a sign of stress, hormonal problems, including PCOS, or hypothalamic amenorrhea (all covered in the next chapter and Advanced Protocols).

Some women experience *mittelschmerz*—a sharp pain in either your right or left side, depending on which ovary is releasing the egg that month. If you were to look at your cervical mucus on a fertility microscope, you'd see what's called a *fern pattern*—because that's what it looks like at this time of the month. Though you may hardly feel it, your temperature elevates slightly, caused by the warming progesterone released from the corpus luteum after ovulation.

Phase Four: The Luteal Phase (Days 14 to 28)

The luteal phase typically lasts for 14 days, though from 9 to 13 days is normal. The term

Discharge: What's What, What's Normal, What's Not

Many women come to me thinking that they have a vaginal infection because they notice increased vaginal discharge. But not all discharge is infection. Often, it's natural, cyclic cervical mucus, normal vaginal cell "sloughing," or arousal fluid. Knowing the difference can spare you unnecessary worry, trips to the pharmacy for over-the-counter remedies, and trips to the doctor, while also informing you when you do need treatment.

Cervical Mucus

Produced in what are called cervical *crypts*, changes in mucus color, texture, and amount are predictable throughout the menstrual cycle, and can be used to determine where you are in your menstrual cycle and when you're ovulating.

- Just after your period, when you're not likely to be fertile, you'll notice little or no discharge.

- During the midfollicular phase, as your body starts to ramp up estrogen production, you'll begin to notice that your mucus is thicker, creamy, whitish, yellowish, and not stretchy or elastic.

- Toward the end of this phase, it becomes thinner, may be a little cloudy, and you might feel "damp."

- One or two days before ovulation, when estrogen is at its peak, and during and right after ovulation, your cervix produces abundant, clear, slippery, wet, stretchy, elastic cervical secretions that may or may not have a slight reddish tinge. This is peak fertile mucus and signals the best time for conception. The amount is different for every woman; not every woman produces a significant amount (still normal), but it is generally more plentiful than at other times in your cycle. In some women, it can be up to twenty times more than the usual amount of discharge. Because it is dependent on estrogen levels, your mucus is certainly part of your vital sign: its presence indicates you have healthy levels of estrogen, and because it increases naturally when we ovulate, it's a good sign that you're ovulating.

- After you ovulate, progesterone causes cervical mucus to get much thicker and drier and creates a mucus plug in the cervix, acting as a physical barrier preventing sperm from making their way in.

- A couple of days after you ovulate, mucus becomes scanter and stickier again, signaling a lower fertility phase.

- As your period approaches, your discharge may become more paste-like and become drier (and less hospitable for conception). If you got pregnant, it may continue to increase rather than subside.

- In our fifties and beyond, cervical mucus production naturally declines for most women, reducing vaginal lubrication—but the more you use it, the less you lose it—as we'll discuss in Part Three.

Vaginal Discharge

We also all produce vaginal discharge, mucus that keeps everything moist down there, so your vaginal tissue stays healthy. It's the difference between a lush oasis or dry desert: when your tissue is healthy and moist, infection can't take hold as easily; when it's dry and irritated, not only do you feel uncomfortable and sex gets painful, but you're more susceptible to vaginally—and sexually transmitted—infections. Each day, vaginal lining cells also slough off and get replaced, part of our vag's being a "self-cleaning oven." We notice this combo of cells and mucus as the white or slightly yellowish discharge we may see in our panties. This discharge also helps to maintain proper vaginal pH. If you have any irritation down there, the discharge will increase as your body tries to protect and soothe your tissue.

Arousal Fluid

When we're sexually aroused, we produce more abundant, typically clear or creamy mucus that keeps us lubricated. This arousal fluid can add to the mix of what's going on in terms of your secretions, but it's circumstantial, not cyclic. What's a normal amount? It's different for every woman and it varies according to where we are in our cycles, but most of us produce anywhere from a scant amount to up to 2 tablespoons per day.

Signs of a Problem

Signs that there could be a problem include a persistent and increased watery vaginal discharge that's present throughout the month. This may occur with cervical dysplasia or abnormal cervical cell changes. Other signs that there could be a problem are vaginal discharge accompanied by unpleasant odor, itching, burning, irritation, pain with sex, or frequent peeing. Here's a quick simple overview:

    Yeast infection—whitish or yellowish "curd-like" discharge, yeasty odor, lots of itching

    Bacterial vaginosis (BV)—possibly increased discharge, odor like spoiled fish, itching, redness, irritation

    Trichomoniasis—often accompanied by a foamy greenish discharge, described as a putrid odor

"luteal" refers to the corpus luteum, or "yellow body," the hollow on your ovary left after the egg was released from its follicle. Progesterone, produced by the corpus luteum, now takes over the luteal phase hormonal landscape, while estrogen starts to increase again toward its second peak, and testosterone rises as well.

What happens during this phase depends on whether you conceived. If so, the fertilized ovum will travel through your fallopian tube to a cushy uterine lining to implant and grow. This lush lining is essential for conception and requires ample estrogen and progesterone during each cycle. The corpus luteum continues to produce progesterone while the uterine lining continues to thicken with fluids and nutrients to nourish the embryo. Progesterone also causes the cervix to thicken to protect against bacteria and additional sperm.

If fertilization didn't occur, then about 10 days after ovulation, progesterone and estrogen will drop, your uterine lining will shed, and you'll have a period. This major decline in estrogen and progesterone leads to the signs and symptoms we experience leading up to our periods and is a common trigger for women who suffer from menstrual migraines and PMS.

The luteal phase has two very distinct hormonal landscapes. In the first half of the luteal phase, energy is usually high and your sex drive ramped up, and cervical mucus is slippery and abundant, making you feel wet down there. During this time, if your hormones are in a healthy flow, you might be getting wonderful sleep, getting projects done with ease, and feeling on top of the world. Around midway in the luteal phase, the week before your period, as progesterone and estrogen start to decline your cervical mucus will become more sparse,

Your Hormones, Your Gut

You may have noticed that your pooping patterns change right before your period. That's because estrogen and progesterone play a role in peristalsis, the rhythmic stretching and contracting of the smooth muscles lining that gastrointestinal tract. Estrogen *increases* muscular contractions, keeping motility humming along and your bowels nice and regular. But just before ovulation and again before your period, rapid drops in estrogen can take your intestines on a fast ride, causing cramping and speeding motility up enough to cause loose stools. Prostaglandins can also increase preperiod loose stools.

Progesterone, on the other hand, *relaxes* smooth muscle, slowing gut motility. At its highest in the week before your period, your bowels may slow down, making you feel bloated or causing a heavy feeling in your abdomen. For some women, constipation is more of the issue. Estrogen and progesterone levels can influence whether you have IBS (irritable bowel syndrome), and there's a relationship between IBS and endometriosis, which I talk more about on page 191.

Creating hormone balance can help your gut health and vice versa, as you'll learn in Chapter 9, and reducing inflammation can keep bowel-cramp-causing prostaglandins in check, as you'll learn how to do, too. As always, it's all connected!

thicker, whiter, and more "tacky" or pasty. In this form, it's more hostile to sperm, preventing them from making their way toward your uterus, which is now past its peak for optimal implantation of an embryo.

Premenstrual Ramp-Up: While uncomfortable premenstrual symptoms are not inevitable, mild and easily manageable sensations before your period aren't necessarily the sign of a problem. Called *moliminal symptoms*, these predictable changes are your body's way of saying, *Hey, in case you've forgotten, your period's about to start.*

These include:

- Increased sensitivity to pain and overall greater inflammation (due to increased inflammatory prostaglandin production)

- Loose stools or mild bloating (due to increases in prostaglandins)

- Mild constipation (due to lower estrogen)

- Mild pelvic heaviness (due to the increased weight and volume of your uterus from the increase in endometrial lining)

- Mild cramping (due to the increase in prostaglandins that contract the uterus, so the lining is shed and bleeding is controlled)

- Mild fluid retention, belly bloating or fullness, or mild breast fullness and sensitivity (due to changes in progesterone and estrogen levels causing the body to retain more water and salt)

- Cravings for sugar, carbs (likely due to a drop in serotonin), chocolate (which some hypothesize is due to a drop in magnesium), and red meat (to antidote iron lost with our periods)

The graph below shows how your hormone levels rise and fall throughout your cycle.

Cycle Sense: Meet Your Inner Guidance System

Hormonal. In so many ways, this word needs no explanation. We know what we mean when

The Menstrual Cycle

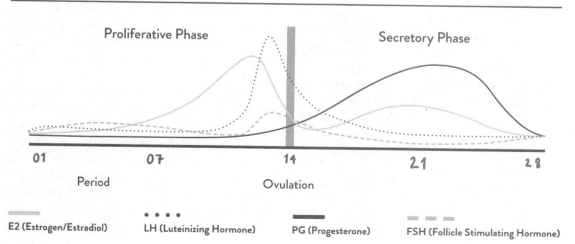

Proliferative Phase   Secretory Phase

01   07   14   21   28

Period   Ovulation

E2 (Estrogen/Estradiol)   LH (Luteinizing Hormone)   PG (Progesterone)   FSH (Follicle Stimulating Hormone)

our best friend, sister, or coworker says she's feeling it. It's woman code for "I feel hijacked by a force out of my control." But what does being hormonal actually mean? And is it a bad thing? Why do we have so many emotional, mind, and mood shifts throughout our cycles? It's time to talk about those "under-the-radar" cues I hinted at in the beginning of Chapter 2. This sixth sense is another fascinating and useful facet of your Hormone Intelligence.

Research proves that the natural fluctuations of our hormones throughout the menstrual (and life!) cycles influence our moods and energy levels, focus and creativity, sleep patterns, the types of foods we need and crave, our exercise preferences, endurance and pain tolerance, and even the clothes—and mates—we select. You can use these signs and preferences as a guidance system, and also as diagnostic and predictive tools, to better understand why you're reacting the way you are to a partner or colleague, why you want to relax into a yoga mat rather than hit the Soul Cycle studio for a week of the month, why you'd rather eat caramel popcorn than a kale-quinoa salad, or why you dropped your paycheck on that sexy new dress rather than into your savings account!

The origins of our hormonal emotions and drives are part of an ancient, intelligent guidance system that predates even cavewoman times, back to when these impulses drove us to vie for limited resources, particularly mates and food. So, that sexy dress purchased just before ovulation? It's your hormones driving you to vie for a mate who could protect and provide. The external conditions have changed—we no longer have to compete for food or mates—but inside, the biological signals still fire. They let us know that our hormones are flowing and well. I see them as a powerful inner GPS that we can use for self-awareness and to become intentional in how we use our energy and the choices we make. You'll learn what being "hormonal" means for you, and how to leverage your Hormone Intelligence to make choices that give you the greatest sense of power, confidence, and ease. You'll access a wealth of information that's as good as any hormone testing, especially when you learn, as you will in Chapter 4, exactly what imbalances mean when they do show up. Ultimately, your Hormone Intelligence becomes a sixth sense.

To learn to do this, I'm going to take you on an intimate journey into your hormonal inner life so you can learn to harness your *cycle sense*. While we can't fully change the demands of the man-made world we all live in, we can make shifts in our daily practices that keep us more in harmony with our cyclic rhythms. As you get more in tune with your body signs, this becomes even easier to do. Build your Hor-

Sending Up a Flare

Ever noticed that you more commonly get a cold or a flare of inflammation or an autoimmune condition right before your period? This is because, in the second half of the menstrual cycle, immune function becomes slightly suppressed so we don't react against sperm or an embryo should we try to conceive during our fertility window. This explains common premenstrual flares of asthma, allergies, IBS, chronic fatigue syndrome, autoimmune disease, or herpes. Addressing inflammation and bringing your hormones into healthy ranges should help decrease flare-up frequency and severity, or eliminate them.

mone Intelligence routine over time, layering in more nuanced practices in harmony with your cycle, as you identify your own rhythms, preferences, drives, and needs. I show you how to by paying attention to changes in four key areas over the four phases of our cycles:

- Mood and Mind-Set
- Sleep, Focus, and Creativity
- Food and Exercise
- Relationships and Sex

To hear these messages, we have to practice listening. That involves making time throughout the day and over the arc of your life to de-liberately get quiet, feel (rather than just think), and notice how you feel. What are the sensations going on in your body right now? Are you breathing deeply? Clenching your jaw? Your pelvic muscles? Is your posture upright? Are you knitting your brow? Use the cycle sense blueprint that follows to understand the cyclic changes you experience in your energy levels, your emotional ups and downs, creative ebbs and flows, sleep patterns, and if you want to get creative with it, you can use this information to optimize your life journey by adapting your social calendar, your diet, and when you make plans and new commitments.

One practice I find powerful and indispens-

Red Flag Symptoms

If you suddenly or regularly experience any of the following, medical care is important to rule out a potentially serious problem:

- Heavy uterine bleeding (soaking through a pad or tampon more than every two hours)
- Bleeding for more than seven days
- Period pain out of the ordinary
- New onset of severe pelvic or abdominal pain *not* during your period
- Pain gets progressively worse or lasts longer than the first couple of days of your period
- Pain, fever, and chills during any time in your cycle, including after wearing a tampon
- Dizziness, fainting, shortness of breath (can be due to anemia from a heavy period)
- Bad-smelling discharge (can be a sign of infection)
- Bleeding between normal period time
- Your period stops for three months or more and you're not pregnant, breastfeeding, or on long-acting birth control pills
- Chronic depression, suicidal thoughts

Note: Crampy pelvic pain and uterine bleeding can be due to miscarriage or ectopic pregnancy. If you've missed a period or have irregular periods, don't typically have painful periods, or are experiencing one that is worse than usual and you are sexually active, make sure to evaluate for possible pregnancy.

able in my work with women is called the Body Scan (see below). When done as a quick practice, which you can do in just a few minutes, it's a great way to do a quick check-in and ask yourself, *What does my body need right now? Am I in flow? Or are there "stuck" areas?*

Winter: Period Inner Guidance

Much like we go more inward in the winter, the start of your period is a natural time to slow down, get quiet, and take time for reflection.

Mood and Mind-Set

While we're often portrayed as irrational and out of control in movies, a study published in the journal *Biology of Sex Differences* found that hormonal changes during this phase may actually activate our willpower and enhance our ability to stick to resolutions. One study also demonstrated that, contrary to stereotypes that suggest women are "dumber" during our periods, there is no link between periods and reduced cognitive function. Brigitte Leeners, the study's lead author, said, "Our brain's ability to function isn't hindered by blood coming out of our . . . wherever." Exactly. Your period, however, is a great time to check in with yourself; as you shed layers—literally physically, but also symbolically—you can use this time to let go of anything you need to emotionally, spiritually, physically, to give yourself a metaphorical new start.

Many women are embracing their periods as a time of heightened emotional sensitivity, creativity, intuitiveness, and personal power. The term *moon time* is sometimes used by women

Body Scan Practice

Here's how to listen to your body on purpose. I recommend intentionally practicing even if just for a 1- to 5-minute self "check-in" daily. You can also take up to an hour to go deep with it and explore the sensory landscape of your body, noticing where you hold tension. I recommend this practice in which you deliberately let your mind roam over your body, looking for tense spots so you can begin to notice where you hold tension.

- Sit upright in a chair or lie on the ground and close your eyes, breathing naturally at first, then gradually more slowly and deeply.

- Feel either your feet on the ground or the parts of your body touching the ground. Just feel that contact, that grounding with the earth.

- Then deepen the breath.

- Now let your breath wander and simply notice how you feel. To take this to a deeper level, notice areas that feel tense, blocked, or stuck. Use your breath to imagine massaging out that tension or releasing the blockage. Is there anything in your life that you associate with this tension you're holding?

- Hold this awareness so that when you return to regular awareness, you can draw on that skill to use anytime without even having to go into a meditative state.

in place of the word *period* as a more poetic affirmation of this. Indeed, the words *menarche*, *menses*, and *menstruation* have their origin in the word *moon*, reflecting the cyclical nature of a woman's body in harmony with the monthly cycles of the moon. And as a result of reclaiming our power, a new wave of young women is sharing knowledge about the physical *and* sacred power of menstrual cycles. There's even a "Red Tent" movement where women gather to share stories, ceremony, helpful ideas, and comfort. A new kind of conversation has started among women, about our bodies. At last.

Sleep, Focus, and Creativity

For the first day or so, it's natural to want to slow down rather than come at the world full throttle. Low progesterone and estrogen levels can make it harder to sleep at the start of your period, and you may find yourself having vivid dreams. Giving yourself time to hit pause for a day or two, tempering your activities to the best your calendar will allow, taking some extra time for self-care, and using the sleep-enhancing practices in Chapter 8 can help you get through those early couple of period days. By day 3, many women start to feel a renewed energy as estrogen starts to climb back up. It's a great time to start to plan new projects!

Food and Exercise

As estrogen declines, so does the feel-good neurotransmitter serotonin, potentially making you feel more down and making you crave "comfort foods." Low blood sugar may accentuate this. About 75% of us skip workouts during our periods because we just don't feel like it. This makes sense when you learn that hormone shifts and increased prostaglandins make us more sensitive to pain in the week before and at the onset of our periods. Despite your compelling desire to get horizontal and pull a cover over your head, regular, moderate exercise improves your sense of well-being and reduces period symptoms from bloating and cramps. So instead of bailing on your workouts, during this week, consider a gentler approach to your routine: try a nature walk, yoga, or gentle Pilates.

Relationships and Sex

Lower estrogen and testosterone—and cramps, bloating, or just wanting to be alone—may mean you prefer to pass on sex right now, or you may feel awkward about the messiness. If you want to, pass. But period sex is safe, many women find orgasms during this time to be extra-heightened, and orgasms can relieve pelvic tension. (Note: While you're unlikely to conceive if you have sex during your period, it's not impossible, so don't pass on contraception unless you want to get pregnant!)

Spring: Follicular Phase Inner Guidance

The follicular phase feels like springtime. It's the easiest phase of most women's cycles emotionally and physically, though stress about fertility may weigh on you if you're trying to conceive.

Mood and Mind-Set

Peaking estrogen ushers in a welcome calm and optimistic headspace, while testosterone enhances energy, confidence, and motivation as well as muscle strength and sex drive. You might be eager to socialize, connect with girlfriends (your ancient hormonal blueprint is driving you to have a social safety net in case you conceive a child), or go out on the town. You might not only feel great but also enjoy estrogen-driven clearer skin and more symmetrical features that make you look prettier and sexier to yourself! Studies show a keener ability for recognizing facial expressions and more empathy as a result.

Sleep, Focus, and Creativity

Higher estrogen levels may help sleep come easier now (though great sleep evades some women until progesterone comes on deck in the second half of the cycle). The estrogen boost can lead to sharpened focus, decision-making, and memory. It may be a great time to apply for that job you've been wanting, take that interview, apply to that graduate program, or dig into creating that business plan you've been putting off.

Food and Exercise

As you head toward ovulation, you're more likely to feel at home in your body. You're likely to have fewer cravings and less of an appetite, and may even naturally weigh a couple of pounds less. An energy boost and an urge to be more active might inspire you to enjoy higher-intensity workouts, so it's a great time to use that gym membership card that's been gathering dust, spend some time with your personal trainer, ride your bike, jump rope, lift weights, or dance it out until you're sweaty!

Relationships and Sex

For several days before you ovulate, rising testosterone and estrogen most likely increase your sexual drive—in a big way. This can also make you suspend your better judgment—at a time when you're also more likely to get pregnant, so be wise.

High Summer: Ovulation

When ovulation is happening according to plan, it's often felt as a time of ripeness. Not only is your egg mature and ready to burst forth, but the hormones that accompany this phase are reflected in mood, mind, energy, and drive.

Mood and Mind-Set

Ovulation usually puts us at the peak of energy, desire, mood, and optimism. Our mental alertness and focus are high, our ability to learn new information is super sharp, and one study showed that we're especially adept at innovative problem solving. We're more inclined to get together with our girlfriends, go out and mingle, and take a bigger chance on life!

Sleep, Focus, and Creativity

The peak in estrogen we experience midcycle can be a great boon to sleep, though some women need progesterone on board to get their z's on—but good news, progesterone starts to rise soon after you ovulate, and that's when delicious sleep happens.

Food and Exercise

Leading up to and during ovulation we tend to eat less and exercise more, our evolutionary biology pushing us toward mate hunting over food hunting! Consequently, we find ourselves with fewer cravings, along with hormonally powered higher willpower and energy. Ovulation can be a good time for that three-day mini cleanse you've had on your to-do list, and it's a great time to engage in more social forms of exercise—hitting the gym or taking that yoga class—even if online.

Relationships and Sex

This is where stuff gets interesting! High estrogen and testosterone levels boost sexual desire and pleasure way up—it's the time of month that it's easiest to experience orgasm, including that toe-curling kind. It's nature's sneaky way of trying to get us to reproduce. We unconsciously turn the flame way up, and potential mates are like moths. We're much more likely to dress in sexier clothing (whatever that means for you) and accessorize—which can also lead us to binge shop, so beware! This is also a time when we're naturally drawn to socialize, particularly in places where potential mates might be found. You might be thinking, *Well, I'm already coupled up, so I definitely wouldn't do this.* Guess again. Married women are even more likely to go for sex appeal as a

What If I'm on Hormonal Birth Control?

I can't overstate the liberation the Pill has brought women. Freedom to choose when to get pregnant gave us a whole new level of access to a workplace that has historically discriminated against mothers (and continues to). I'm neither against use of the Pill for medical reasons, nor do I in any way judge women who choose to use it. In fact, there are some symptoms that are improved—at least temporarily—with the Pill. But this freedom does come with a price that is almost universally downplayed by the medical establishment.

There are the obvious, common side effects that many women experience—bloating, breast tenderness, weight gain, mood swings—symptoms you might choose to just put up with if you really want to be on the Pill or other hormonal contraception (i.e., the patch, hormonal IUD, injections, and the "ring"). But there's more.

Hormonal contraception interferes with the conversation your brain is having with your ovaries and uterus. It alters your hormonal physiology so that you don't experience the cyclic shifts in estrogen and progesterone that create most of the physical, emotional, and behavior shifts that indicate where you are in your cycle. It also may change the signals we communicate to and receive from others. While all this research is still new, a whole body of research led by Martie Haselton, PhD, at UCLA is exploring how the Pill / hormonal contraception may alter our normal cycle sense, including our social judgment, ability to read facial expressions and recognize stranger danger (think random dude in a bar), our sexual desire and possibly even mate selection, though whether this is the case, and if so, its significance remains uncertain.

Because some hormonal birth control sort of flatlines your cycle and prevents ovulation, you won't get much of a midcycle surge of creative, juicy energy, or the "highs" that come with ovulation. In other words, it reduces our ability to use our cycles and hormonal signs as a vital sign—it short-circuits your hormone intelligence.

On the other hand, you won't experience the lows of progesterone and estrogen that cause so many of the symptoms women experience as hormone imbalances and problems, which is suppressed by contraception and thus prevents you from getting pregnant. I talk more about the pros and cons of hormonal birth control, and how to come off it, in Chapter 10.

biological way to make sure your mate stays loyal in a crowded sea of fertile women vying for a mate!

That boost in physical appearance and clearer skin continues, and our ovulatory scents (sweat, vaginal odors) become more appealing to other humans. Additionally, during ovulation, we are innately driven to be attracted to partners with what are called "high fitness genes." This can manifest in a strong jawline or high intelligence, or simply how someone smells to you. The problem is that if your mate doesn't quite fit this description, your eye is more likely to wander to a person who does—and we're more likely to have an affair at this time of the month. Wild, right? Another reason to be aware of what's driving us biologically!

Men are also more receptive to our ovulatory signs. Interestingly, we're also endowed with more physical strength and heightened physical awareness. Martie Haselton, a professor of psychology at UCLA who studies the biology of ovulation, believes this is nature's way of giving us extra superpowers to protect ourselves from overly aggressive potential mates or outright aggressors who are picking up on the fertile signals and sex-scent hormones (pheromones).

Late Summer into Autumn: Luteal Phase Inner Guidance

You've ovulated, and now, unless you've conceived, you're on the journey toward your next period. This phase typically causes the most dramatic downshifts in our mood and energy.

Mood and Mind-Set

Early in the luteal phase we're still "high" on estrogen and testosterone and by midluteal phase, progesterone, too. However, about a week before your period, declining estrogen levels can lead to lower moods, lower energy, and a feeling of being "depleted." That sunny ovulation energy may give way to a more inter-

We Can't Heal If We Can't Feel

The very nature of the word *hormonal* is linked to women's emotions, with the suggestion of them being out of control. But we live in a culture where we're taught to keep our emotions suppressed, which we do with hormonal birth control, antianxiety medications, and antidepressants. The cultural caricature of women as "hysterical" or in a perpetual state of PMS makes us judge and suppress our own emotions, or blame them on our hormones.

What if, instead, we were able to express our emotions, be heard, and get what we need? While I'm not suggesting we spill our rage all over our spouse, mom, coworker, or the too-slow grocery checkout person (please don't), we do have to stop silencing and "tone policing" ourselves. Anger can be a powerful force and, like a storm, can leave the air feeling clearer, more energized. It's been a major force for political change since time immemorial, and one important study discovered that it's not being unhappy in a relationship that makes us sick, it's being unhappy and silencing yourself!

nalized feeling, the desire to spend more time quietly and introspectively, and if you do have PMS symptoms, this is when you may start to dread—or feel—them. You may feel more emotionally heightened, reactive and easily irritated, weepy, or sensitive to critical comments. During this time, your emotional filter is likely to lower, too, and with it, your emotions. If you've been squashing them down as we so often do, especially anger, they may come tumbling out now.

The end of the luteal phase (and the first day or two of your period) is the energy low point of the month for most women, so give yourself a pass—this is normal. Shifts in your brain waves during this time may make you crave quiet, alone time and some R&R, so learn to weave some downtime and space for introspection into your calendar, even if it's just an evening to turn it all off and chill. So if you feel a natural inclination to quiet down, heed your body's signal—it'll help you preempt irritability, resentment, and burnout, as well as getting sick due to lowered immunity. Knowing you can look forward to even a little space can do wonders for your energy and mood. It's a great time to give yourself permission to pause, slow down, and rest if you feel you need it.

Sleep, Focus, and Creativity

During the first half of the luteal phase, progesterone starts to rise, so you may notice that you feel more peaceful and easygoing and get deeply restful sleep. In the few days leading up to the start of your period, however, as estrogen and progesterone levels take a dive, sleep can get disturbed and dreams vivid, even weird—some women report violent or bloody dreams. I call it dreaming in red. My own dreams have included vampire attacks with me invariably waking up to the start of my period. Many women find this to be a highly intuitive time, a time when their inner life is closer to the surface, revealing unmet needs and frustrations. You may find that you're in a creative "zone," ripe for turning inward, journaling, or artistic expression. Paint, write poetry, journal; however it nourishes you to, express yourself.

Food and Exercise

The final days of the luteal phase can throw a curveball into healthy eating and exercise. Studies show that our food intake increases by as much as 10% in the second half of the luteal phase, with a higher preference for sweet and fatty foods, possibly due to higher energy demands from our body. Also, since the feel-good neurotransmitter serotonin requires estrogen as a building block, and estrogen is in lower supply right now, your genius brain gets you craving pasta, pastries, and sugar, because serotonin can also be produced from carbohydrates. This is also the classic time for chocolate cravings, which may (or may not) be due to a desire for more magnesium during this time. If you know that your need for carbs goes up before your period, you might be more inclined to see that craving as a sign of where you are in your cycle rather than a green light to sugar binge; you might then choose that healthy sweet potato over the bag of Oreos (or Newman-O's). And if you do need a little "something-something," I've got you covered with healthy indulgences, including chocolate-containing ones, that are hormone healthy.

Higher progesterone levels also cause you to desire fatty foods—not necessarily a bad thing if they're the right kind—and in the late luteal phase, you may crave red meat and other iron-rich foods to avoid anemia during your period. (One study published in the *American Journal of Epidemiology* found that women with the worst PMS symptoms have the lowest iron levels.) So use this awareness the right way: rather than crushing that bag of Justin's Peanut Butter Cups or pulling into the Burger King with a squeal of tires, feed your body what you're craving: healthy, whole-food carbs; quality, unprocessed fats; and iron-rich foods.

While keeping up your usual exercise is great if you're motivated, you may find yourself wanting something gentler. As women recover from muscle damage more slowly during this time, make sure you balance high-intensity exercise with a good warm-up and wind-down, and trust your instincts if a more relaxed, gentler exercise routine appeals to you more during this phase. But beware that slowing down too much may make you feel more tired, and lower levels of activity are associated with longer periods. Women with PMS who exercise regularly and frequently have fewer symptoms than women who do not exercise. High exercisers experience fewer behavioral and mood changes, better concentration, and less pain. So don't let your exercise routine go altogether; instead, trade a hard run for Pilates, bench-pressing for downward dog, that long run for a long walk.

Many of us have experienced having bloating, heaviness, and low self-image in the days leading up to our periods. The bigger your hormone swings, the more acutely you might feel this. If you have a history of an eating disorder or challenges with your body image, this can be an especially difficult time of the month. Research published in the *International Journal of Eating Disorders* shows that premenstrual hormonal and serotonin shifts, along with the physical sensations of bloating, constipation, and fluid retention, can activate weight obsession and sink self-image, while hormone shifts also increase depression. Know that this will pass, make sure to connect rather than isolate—and, of course, seek help if needed.

Relationships and Sex

As estrogen drops, you might find your libido does, too; increased vaginal dryness might also make intercourse less comfortable, tanking your sex drive further. That said, some women find that the increased pelvic pressure and fuller sensations in their genitalia just before and at the start of their periods increase their desire, with increased pelvic blood flow leading to hell-yeah orgasms for some women. During the luteal phase, we're biologically driven to nourish relationships we depend on for security, and one of the ways studies find that we do this is by giving those people gifts. This may lead us to spend more money on friends and loved ones (and even charitable giving) during this time. It's thought that this behavior harkens to times when our survival as mothers depended on fostering social alliances that historically would have been beneficial in the event of a pregnancy.

How to Be Your Own Cycle Interpreter

One of the most powerful ways to tune in to your Hormone Intelligence is to map (track) your menstrual cycle. I began tracking mine nearly forty years ago, in my teens, and it's been some of the best "me-search" I've ever done because I learned to read my own cycle signs—and cycle sense—early on. I know when my body is on track hormonally, and if I do get off track, I can quickly course-correct.

Tracking your cycle involves charting the data from your choice of two of the following 3 parameters:

- the calendar days of the month you menstruate

- changes in your cervical mucus throughout the month

- your daily basal body temperature

Every woman's cycle is a little different, so mapping your cycle can help you learn what your hormones are trying to tell *you*. It's the epitome of Hormone Intelligence! Recording what's going on day to day allows you to get a 30,000-foot view of your cycles over time and will give you important information not only about whether your cycle and related hormones are working optimally but if other signs and symptoms are cycle related. It's one of the most effective ways to determine whether you're ovulating, and intentionally tracking your cycle can help you sort out whether pelvic pain, low sex drive, acne, sleep problems, migraines, bloating, and other symptoms are cyclic—and therefore hormonally driven. Your cycle and symptom map can become a powerful hormone-tracking tool—better than any app! Even if you already know you have a hormone imbalance or gynecologic condition, it's useful to learn what's normal for you and what isn't, and tracking your cycle can give you clues to your hormone imbalance based on the length of your cycle, the length of your periods, whether you're ovulating, and more.

The Essentials of Cycle Charting

Three methods are involved in cycle charting, all of which fall under the umbrella of the fertility awareness (FA) method. How many you practice is up to you, but for the clearest picture of hormonal health, I recommend women track at least the first two methods for a minimum of three months to get a good sense of their typical cycle—that is, how it is functioning currently. As they follow the program to address any imbalances, my patients keep charting until their cycle is regulated, any symptoms have resolved, or they're pregnant, if that is their goal!

Most women find that after some time, they no longer need to record changes in mucus, or even chart anything at all: their Hormone Intelligence just kicks in as a sixth sense. Just a few years into charting my cycle, I ditched the pen and moon calendar (there was no such thing as an app in 1983), because I reliably knew that when I had an energy boost and found myself choosing a slinkier top to wear, getting jazzed about a new idea, or wanting to jump my boyfriend, I was ovulating. Flash forward to the few days before my period, and sure enough, I always managed to find myself wearing my favorite red sweater.

If, however, you plan to use cycle charting as your method of birth control, you'll want to be on your A game, getting the method down with the diligence of a scholar for several months, while using condoms as an additional barrier method.

Method 1: Menstrual Cycle Charting (+ Optional Inner Guidance Journal)

This is the simplest of the three methods and it's totally free. You simply record the first day of your period and last day of your period on a

A Gift for You

At avivaromm.com/hormone-intelligence-resources you'll find a chart you can download and print, to help you track your cycle and many more wonderful resources.

calendar for at least three consecutive months. You can take this one step further by jotting down your daily moods, cravings, energy level, and other Hormone Intelligence signs, watching for patterns. You might start to notice patterns in how you dress, ebbs and flows in your personal drives, creativity, ambitions, and your sexual attractions! You're data mining your inner guidance system!

Method 2: Cervical Mucus Tracking

As I showed you on page 47, the changes in cervical mucus color, texture, and amount are predictable and can help you to identify when you're ovulating. A quick reminder:

- After your period, you'll notice little or no discharge.

- During the midfollicular phase, as your body starts to ramp up estrogen production, you'll begin to notice that your mucus is thicker, creamy, whitish, yellowish, and not stretchy or elastic.

- Toward the end of this phase, it typically becomes thinner, maybe a little cloudy, and you might feel "damp."

- In the 1 to 2 days before ovulation, when your estrogen is at its highest level, and during and right after ovulation, your cervix produces abundant, clear, slippery, wet, stretchy, elastic cervical secretions that may or may not have a slight reddish tinge. This is peak fertile mucus and signals the best time for conception. The amount is different for every woman, and not every woman produces a significant amount (still normal), but it is generally more plentiful than at other times in your cycle. In some women, it can be up to twenty times more than the usual amount of discharge.

- After you ovulate, you produce progesterone, which causes cervical mucus to get much thicker and drier and creates a mucus plug in the cervix, acting as a physical barrier preventing sperm from making their way in.

- A couple of days after you ovulate, you'll likely notice that your mucus becomes scanter and stickier again, signaling a lower fertility phase. As your period approaches, your discharge may become more paste-like and drier (and less hospitable for conception). Or, if you got

Dry Spell?

If your estrogen is low or you're not ovulating, your cervix also won't get the message that it's time to produce fertile cervical mucus, so you'll mostly have drier days. Additional factors that can alter cervical mucus include antidepressants, antihistamines, oral contraceptives, the chemotherapeutic drug tamoxifen, breastfeeding, cervical inflammation, cervical surgery including procedures like biopsies and LEEPs (loop electrosurgical excision procedures) to evaluate for cervical dysplasia, douching, or vaginal and sexually transmitted infections. Low folate, zinc, and vitamin A may also play a role in low cervical fluid production. A decline and eventual cessation of discharge with menopause is normal. If it happens before you're about forty years old, this could be a sign of primary ovarian insufficiency (POI).

pregnant, it may continue to increase rather than subside.

The idea of checking your cervical mucus may gross you out, but it's something you're probably already doing without being aware of it. And no, it doesn't require sticking your fingers up your vagina (though that is one way to check).

Here are three ways to do it:

Option 1: Check out the color and texture of the discharge on your underwear each day.

Option 2: Wipe your vaginal opening with white toilet paper or tissue before you go pee. Look at the color and feel the mucus with your fingers.

Option 3: Insert a clean index finger just inside your vaginal opening then look at the color and notice the texture of mucus between your index finger and thumb.

Check your cervical mucus each morning for the next six weeks. Record what you notice on your cycle chart: your bleeding days, dry days, wet days, sticky days, cloudy days, and slippery days. If you don't have a 28-day cycle, or any regular cycle, that's okay; track the pattern according to *your* cycle. If your cycle is irregular, or you're not ovulating, seeing mucus production come online indicates that you're moving toward a more natural cycle. Note that after sex, semen in the vagina makes it harder to assess the volume and quality of your cervical mucus, so consider that when you're tracking. If you're in a hetero relationship, you can do "other things" or use a condom for the first month that you're learning this method.

Method 3: Basal Body Temperature (BBT) Monitoring

BBT monitoring takes a bit more work than the previous methods, but I recommend it if you're unsure whether you're ovulating. This method uses a basal body thermometer, which has a range from 96°F to 100°F, so you can see each tenth of a degree, to measure the subtle but trackable progesterone-driven postovulation body temperature increase I mentioned on page 47. Digital options and apps make this method easy. You take your temperature each morning before you get out

Can't I Just Use a Cycle Tracking App?

You can use a smartphone app to track your menstrual cycle; just know that most apps are designed on the premise that all women have a 28-day menstrual cycle with regular mid-cycle ovulation—which isn't the case! Therefore, using these for pregnancy protection can be risky. A 2016 study found that at least 20% of these apps contained inaccurate or erroneous information. So if you use an app to help keep track of your personal cycle deets rather than tracking them on paper or on a spreadsheet, awesome, just please always heed your own Hormone Intelligence alongside it, using the methods and insights described above.

of bed, and before you move around, eat, or sip anything. Make sure to record your results on your cycle tracker (download yours at aviva romm.com/hormone-intelligence-resources).

Here's what you're looking for: One to two days after the LH surge and ovulation, you'll see a rise in body temperature by about 0.5°F that lasts for about 10 days. Temperature drops back down just before your next period comes. Recording your BBT for at least three months will give you a sense of whether and when you're ovulating. Your BBT is very sensitive to even subtle changes in your biology, as might happen with fever, stress, lack of sleep, moving around early in the morning, or even getting up to pee before you check your temp. It can also be influenced by travel, time zone changes, sipping anything hot or cold—any of these things could skew your readings, making it less than 100% reliable as a primary method of birth control!

At Your Cervix

Not only does your cervical mucus change throughout your cycle, so does the position and firmness of your cervix. When you ovulate, thanks to estrogen's effects, your cervix is higher in your vaginal canal, noticeably softer and mushier to the touch (like your lips), the os (opening) is slightly wider, and your cervix points more to the back of your vaginal canal rather than hanging out more midline. Progesterone does the opposite, causing your cervix to sit lower in your vagina and feel firmer. To get a sense of these changes, you have to check every single day, and not a whole lot is noticeable until you're ovulating. This is *not* a necessary part of developing your Hormone Intelligence, but it's another way to be intimate with the marvelous changes your body goes through each month.

The Adventure Continues

As predictable as our cycles generally are when our hormones are in balance, when things go awry, they also do so in predictable ways. So now that you know vital signs of healthy, optimal cycles, and how to leverage your Hormone Intelligence, let's talk about how to use your symptoms as a sixth vital sign to get to the bottom of what's going on with your hormones, cycles, and gynecologic health. You don't have to be a medical doctor to be your own best medical detective.

what your symptoms are saying

(AND WHY IT'S IMPORTANT TO LISTEN)

and i said to my body. softly. "i want to be your friend."
—**Nayyirah Waheed, poet**

We all know that normal body temperature is 98.6°F (37°C), give or take a little. We also know aches, a headache, and chills tell us we might have a fever. When the reading on a thermometer confirms our suspicion, we feel some relief—*that's why I feel so crappy*. If it's just a cold we get extra rest, have hot tea, vitamin C, and perhaps a warm bath. If it's a raging fever with worrisome symptoms, we seek a diagnosis. Your temperature is a vital sign that provides a wealth of information that allows you to make decisions about your health.

Your menstrual cycle and gynecologic symptoms are no less important. They give us important clues about our hormones and our health, telling us when everything is normal, as I showed you in Chapter 3, and when it's not, as you'll learn in this chapter. As you read, keep in mind that whatever your cycle is doing, your body is not broken. Your hormones are responding to something going on in your ecosystem that needs attention, and this is exactly what we'll be focusing on in Part Two.

When Your Menstrual Cycle Is "Off the Blueprint"

Menstrual cycles vary from normal in a few predictable ways: irregularity, excessively heavy or excessively light periods, or cycles accompanied by pain or PMS symptoms. On page 67 you'll find a chart showing you how common symptoms correspond to the gynecologic conditions we'll be exploring further together in this chapter, and the plan. It's very common to have more than one condition, and to have many symptoms. For example, many women have both PMS and PCOS or endometriosis, and then may also experience a fertility problem and later go on to experience challenges as they enter perimenopause. I know that sounds bleak—preventing or reversing this is exactly why you're here!

Menstrual Cycle Problems: What They Are, What They Tell You

Our endocrine systems are sensitive to travel, weight loss, stress, major life changes (having a baby, a breakup, starting a new job, moving, divorce, or an illness)—all of which can throw off your hormones and cycles. So it's normal on rare occasion, and with an explainable cause, to have an irregular, longer, shorter, or missed period. Breastfeeding, hormonal contraceptives like the Pill or an IUD, and perimenopause also alter estrogen and progesterone and cause irregular cycles. Remember, too, there's no perfect cycle.

But if you go less than 26 days or more than 34 days between one period and the next, if your month-to-month variation in cycle length is greater than 4 days, if your cycle length is more than 7 or less than 3 days, or if you have excessively heavy or excessively light periods, you technically have irregular cycles. New shifts that can't be explained by specific circumstances and that persist for more than 3 consecutive months suggest the need for extra attention. If you've had irregular cycles for as long as you can remember, then there's a good chance you have an underlying hormone imbalance, or it's quite possible that you have PCOS or endometriosis, so definitely complete those respective questionnaires later in the chapter.

Let's look at the most common menstrual cycle problems and why they're important to identify and repair.

Long Menstrual Cycles

The Basics: Your periods are 35 days or more apart.

Why It Matters: During a normal cycle, your period is brought on by the natural drop in progesterone that occurs after ovulation. Long menstrual cycles are a common sign that you're not ovulating regularly, or at all. PCOS is responsible for this 40% of the time, though other causes of anovulation can also be involved. Long cycles also mean that your uterine lining proliferates for a longer period of time; this can lead to much heavier, crampier periods, but also, unchecked over even just a couple of years, is associated with an increased risk of endometrial cancer. PCOS and not ovulating can be a problem if you're trying to conceive; women with periods closer to 29.5 days have the highest likelihood of conception. So it's important to try to get your cycle closer to a 26- to 34-day range.

Short Menstrual Cycles

The Basics: Periods less than 26 days apart most months.

Why It Matters: As much as we might be all kumbaya about having periods, short periods means you're having more than one a month—enough to make any woman cry! On top of the nuisance of it, frequent periods can be a sign of high estrogen, a risk factor for endometrial and breast cancer, can be a sign of a short luteal phase (controversially called *luteal phase dysfunction*), which is due to low progesterone, or can be a sign that your ovaries contain fewer

Common Symptoms, Common Conditions at a Glance

Symptom ⌄ / Condition ➤	Menstrual Cycle Problems	PMS	Endo-metriosis	PCOS	Fertility Problems	Uterine Fibroids	Ovarian Dysfunction / Premature Ovarian Insufficiency
Heavy periods	✔		✔	✔		✔	✔
Skipped periods	✔			✔	✔		✔
Painful periods	✔		✔			✔	
Chronic pelvic pain			✔			✔	
Anxiety, depression, mood swings		✔	✔	✔			✔
Digestive symptoms		✔	✔			✔	
Hair loss / hair in unwanted places				✔			
Acne		✔		✔			
Trouble getting/ staying pregnant	✔		✔	✔	✔		✔
Cyclic breast pain, swelling, cysts		✔					

eggs and perimenopause is approaching—okay if you're over forty-two years old, but prior to that might point to primary ovarian insufficiency (POI). More frequent blood loss increases your risk of becoming anemic, which can seriously negatively affect your mood, mind, energy, and exercise, and severe anemia puts you at increased risk of cardiac problems.

Skipped Periods (Amenorrhea)

The Basics: Skipping three or more consecutive periods or menstruating fewer than eight times in a year.

Why It Matters: A skipped period here or there can simply be a response to stress, travel, or big changes in your life, in which case it's simply a reminder to make sure you're not pushing too hard in your life; but generally, once the stress is passed, periods will get regular again on their own. Skipped periods are the most common first sign you'll notice if you're pregnant, and breastfeeding is another common and normal reason—the hormone prolactin, which helps you to produce breast milk, suppresses estrogen and progesterone, and your period as a result. Birth control pills and other forms of hormonal contraception, antidepressants, blood pressure medications, and certain chemotherapy drugs can prevent ovulation and suppress your period.

Skipped periods, if you're not pregnant, breastfeeding, or heading into menopause, are most commonly due to a phenomenon known as **hypothalamic amenorrhea (HA)**. Due to evolutionary hardwiring, which we'll talk more about in Chapter 7, when you're under a high amount of stress, your body puts the lid on reproductive functions to conserve energy for your well-being. You just don't have extra to spare, so you don't ovulate and you don't have a period. HA is very common in women in their teens, twenties, and thirties and is the result of significant life stress, overexercising, being underweight, or a combination of any of these. If you're a high-intensity athlete or work out a lot, eat restrictively (even if for health reasons), or are below optimal body weight for your height, there's a good chance that this is the reason you're skipping periods.

Suspect HA if you have the following:

- A BMI <18.5 (you can calculate yours with any free online BMI calculator)

- Weight loss of ten or more pounds in less than three months' time

- Restrictive eating, preoccupation with your weight, a very low-calorie diet

- An intense athletic training practice (high-intensity workouts, distance running, ballet, gymnastics, hot yoga, etc. >5 days/week)

- Tremendous personal stress

- A diagnosis of osteopenia or osteoporosis (bone loss), or history of a stress fracture

HA is a potentially serious problem; in addition to skipped periods, there are usually accompanying nutritional deficiencies, and women with this condition are at increased risk for bone loss (and fractures), even at a young age. The good news is that these are reversible with the core plan and the Advanced Protocols in this book.

Additional underlying causes of skipped periods include thyroid problems (see Chapter 7 for additional information). Surprisingly, approximately 40% of women with untreated **celiac disease** have menstrual cycle disorders; skipped periods is the most common one. Finally, primary ovarian insufficiency (POI) is another reason for skipped periods. PCOS and

Anovulation Symptom Self-Assessment

How do you know if you're not ovulating? Here's a list of symptoms:

- ☐ Menstrual cycles consistently or frequently shorter than 26 days, or longer than 34 days
- ☐ Periods that last longer than 8 days
- ☐ Skipped periods
- ☐ Heavy periods
- ☐ Low or almost no midcycle, fertile-type cervical mucus (see page 47)

- ☐ Lack of ovulatory rise in BBT (see page 63)
- ☐ Sleep problems (due to low progesterone)
- ☐ Depression
- ☐ Difficulty conceiving (if you've been trying)
- ☐ Symptoms of PCOS (see page 76)

HA share some similarities and can co-occur, but if it's solely HA, you won't have the hair loss, unwanted hair, or other symptoms of PCOS, and you're more likely to have the symptoms bulleted on the opposite page. Day 3 follicle-stimulating hormone (FSH) and estradiol levels (see page 32) can help distinguish between the causes of ovulatory dysfunction—so ask your primary care provider to run these tests and explain the results.

Rare causes include a tumor in the hypothalamus, pituitary, or in an adrenal gland, usually accompanied by other nongynecologic symptoms (ranging from headaches to weakness) or Asherman's syndrome, a scarring of the endometrial lining that is due to having had a D&C for a postpartum hemorrhage or miscarriage, which causes scant or absent periods. These require medical attention and are beyond the scope of this program.

Skipped Ovulation

The Basics: Irregular ovulation or not ovulating at all.

Why It Matters: If your periods come regularly and you experience noticeable cyclic changes including mittelschmerz (page 47), cervical mucus changes, breast fullness late in your cycle, etc., then it's likely that you're ovulating. Postovulatory basal body temperature elevation confirms that you're ovulating. Like a skipped period, skipped ovulation once in a blue moon isn't necessarily a problem. But if it's your usual pattern, it's a big deal.

In addition to HA, described in the previous section, causes include sleep problems, hypothyroidism, PCOS (74% of women with PCOS don't ovulate regularly or at all), and primary ovarian insufficiency (POI). Anovulation can also indicate low estrogen, which has long-term risks (see page 33). If you're not ovulating, you're not producing adequate progesterone. As progesterone also regulates

other hormones, including androgens, it plays a role in preventing PCOS and its symptoms. And of course, if you're not ovulating, you can't get pregnant. You also won't get the benefit of the midcycle's inner guidance cues I discussed in Chapter 3. Ovulation is an important barometer of your overall health, of healthy brain-ovary communication, and of healthy ovarian function, so even if you never plan to get pregnant, if you have ovaries (even just one), it's important to restore regular ovulation.

Heavy Menstrual Bleeding (HMB, Also Called Menorrhagia)

The Basics: Periods lasting longer than 7 days, blowing through more than 6 pads or tampons per day, soaking through more than two pads or tampons in two hours, passing large clots.

Why It Matters: Many women have gone to their doctors concerned about "terribly heavy periods" only to be told that "all women think their periods are too heavy."

Heavy periods are also almost always a sign of a hormone imbalance: either high estrogen or low progesterone. **High estrogen levels** lead to a significant buildup of the uterine lining. When that sheds, heavy bleeding occurs—and usually with it, heavy cramping, because the uterus contracts more intensely to expel that blood. Low progesterone, usually the result of ovulatory dysfunction or PCOS, prevents regular periods and, as a result, also leads to significant buildup of the uterine lining and subsequent heavy bleeding when your period does start. Other causes include **endometriosis** (page 77) and **adenomyosis** (page 80), **uterine fibroids**, and though not a common cause, thyroid problems (see page 145). **Primary ovarian insufficiency** and perimenopause are associated with changes in menstrual cycles, sometimes leading to heavier periods.

While having a period on the heavier side

may be normal for you, a chronically heavy period can result in anemia, causing fatigue, loss of concentration, and depression, and can affect your work and lifestyle. Severe anemia can also cause other symptoms such as breathing difficulties and a racing heart, particularly following strenuous physical activity. Many women would rather stay home to avoid fear of a "bleed through." Heavy periods are not something you should have to just "deal with."

Light Periods

The Basics: Scant menstrual flow or periods that last fewer than 3 days; blood flow less than 5 to 10 mL over the course of your whole period.

Why It Matters: While few women would complain about a light period, they can be a sign of hormone imbalance. Light periods can occur due to low estrogen or hypothalamic amenorrhea (HA, discussed on page 68), or can be a symptom of PCOS, hypothyroidism, or primary ovarian insufficiency (see page 311). Other less common causes of light periods include cervical stenosis—"stiffness," usually due to damage from a cervical procedure, or intrauterine adhesions (IUA), which can be the result of a past D&C.

If you're trying to get pregnant, light periods can suggest a problem for conception. Studies have shown that when the endometrial lining is less than 7 mm thick, chances of conception decline dramatically and risk of miscarriage increases. In one study, pregnancy rates increased gradually from 53% among women with a lining of <9 mm, to 77% among patients with a lining of ≥16 mm. The Pill also keeps your uterine lining from getting lush and thick in preparation for possible implantation. An ultrasound can determine uterine thickness accurately.

Don't Ignore Heavy Bleeding!

- Bleeding disorders: It's estimated that up to 20% of women with very heavy periods may in fact have an inherited bleeding disorder, von Willebrand disease. It usually shows up in a woman's teens or early twenties, and a very heavy flow can be the first sign of it, so torrential periods in young women warrant a blood test for this condition.

- Miscarriage: Because up to half of all pregnancies end in miscarriage, often before the woman even realizes she was pregnant, an unusually heavy flow could be a sign of a miscarriage or ectopic pregnancy. In this case, your period will usually return to normal in one or two cycles after the pregnancy loss; so unless it stays abnormally heavy after three cycles, just watch and wait.

- Pelvic infections including endometritis and pelvic inflammatory disease (PID), can cause abnormal bleeding, which can occur any time during your cycle, not just your period.

- A very common worry is, "Could it be cancer?" Endometrial cancer may cause irregular bleeding in the form of spotting, but it is not usually a cause of heavy periods.

Bleeding Between Periods (Metrorrhagia)

The Basics: Spotting (light brown and scant) or bleeding more like a period, between periods.

Why It Matters: Spotting shortly after becoming pregnant (implantation bleeding) is commonly misinterpreted as bleeding between periods, and bleeding between periods can also be due to a miscarriage. Other common causes include starting or stopping any hormonal birth control (the Pill, IUD, ring, patch, or an implantable device) or skipping a dose of the Pill. Because hormonal birth control overrides true periods, this is a breakthrough bleed rather than a bleed between periods. Emergency contraception (i.e., the morning-after pill) may also cause bleeding, often like a heavy period. Uterine fibroids and cervical polyps can cause bleeding between periods, and PCOS can cause such irregular periods that it can seem like you're bleeding between periods.

Short, frequent periods may be misinterpreted as bleeding between cycles—it can be hard to discern, but if the bleeding is more like a period, it's very likely that's what's going on. Both endometriosis and adenomyosis can cause bleeding between periods—it can be heavy or spotty, but it's not usually a consistent pattern like your period (i.e., a heavier first day of flow that tapers); and you won't have usual period symptoms, though you may have cramps and not feel like your happiest self (who would if they're having pain and extra bleeding!). Sexually transmitted infections (STIs) and pelvic infections can cause vaginal bleeding, and cervical and endometrial cancer can both cause vaginal bleeding, so it is important to get proper screening for persistent or heavy bleeding, and bleeding that can't be explained by one of the more common causes.

Period Pain (Dysmenorrhea)

The Basics: *Dysmenorrhea* is the medical term for painful menstruation, and there are two categories.

Primary dysmenorrhea refers to typical painful menstrual cramps, not due to an underlying diagnosable medical problem. It only occurs around the time of your period, feels achy or crampy and lasts for as long as 3 days, and in severe cases may be accompanied by nausea, vomiting, diarrhea, backache, headache, and dizziness.

Secondary dysmenorrhea is period pain that's symptomatic of a disorder in the reproductive organs. It may occur only around your period but may also be associated with abdominal or pelvic pain or pressure throughout the month, constipation or pain with bowel movements, urinary problems, or pain during sex. These symptoms suggest an underlying condition, usually endometriosis (or adenomyosis), though it could be uterine fibroids, or another cause of chronic pelvic pain. Secondary dysmenorrhea tends to get worse, not better, with age if the underlying conditions aren't addressed.

Regardless of which you have, your period shouldn't feel like a life sentence of suffering. You should not spend days of the month on ibuprofen and your period should not make you cry because of the pain. The words *feels like steak knives* should not cross your mind! If they do, something's up that definitely requires more attention.

Why It Matters: Primary dysmenorrhea is almost always due to the overproduction of inflammatory prostaglandins (PGE2). They cause your uterus to get all up in a bunch with spasms, cramping, and pain that makes you want to curl up with a heating pad and the TV remote until the pain ends. On the flip side, if you're producing low levels of anti-inflammatory

Don't Miss Early Warning Signs in Young Women

During the first five years after menstruation begins, it's normal to have irregular cycles, skipped periods, hormonal ups and downs, and mild acne. It takes a little while for hormones to settle into regular rhythms. Understanding your teenage daughter's normal menstrual cycle changes can help you to reassure her and guide her to develop her own Hormone Intelligence. In addition, learning what to expect in her many years of cycling—and how to recognize when symptoms seem to be off her normal arc—can help her turn problems around quickly.

But pain severe enough to require medication, heavy periods (more than six pads or tampon changes per day), acne, severe depression or anxiety, or more than a few pounds of weight gain are not just "normal"; these are symptoms of underlying hormone imbalances, and catching these *now*, as a teen, can not just save her years of suffering and misery but can also allow you to catch conditions like endometriosis and PCOS that are almost always missed in this age range but that can lead to problems later.

prostaglandins (PGE1 and PGE3), you'll also experience more pain. Elevated estrogen is yet another reason your periods might be painful; remember when I said a thicker endometrium means more uterine cramping? A thicker uterine lining forms, causing the body to cramp that much harder to shed it, meaning a more painful, often heavier period. In Part Two you'll learn how our inflammatory responses get so out of control, and what to do about it, and the Advanced Protocols, which you can start anytime, will give you solutions for period pain and secondary causes.

Premenstrual Syndrome (PMS)

"How many women with PMS does it take to change a light bulb?" The punch line to that old joke is, "That's not funny." And for 85% of all menstruating women—the percentage of women in the United States who experience premenstrual syndrome (PMS)—it's no laughing matter.

PMS has long been misunderstood. While it's been recognized as a "real thing" for over sixty years and as an official medical diagnosis since the 1990s, many physicians still don't believe it's anything but in women's heads—so a lot of women get dismissed and never get proper treatment. The fact that antidepressants (SSRIs) are the best conventional medical therapy reinforces this misconception. Further, because so many women experience it, some in the medical community have suggested discarding the term *PMS* and accepting the symptoms as normal! This attitude trivializes the daily significance of PMS for the millions of women who suffer from it—and might just be making you cringe inside at the idea someone would say, "Just live with it; it's normal." But PMS is not all in your head. Repeat. It's not all in your head—and it's not something you should live with.

The Basics: More than 150 physical, behavioral, emotional, and cognitive symptoms have been ascribed to PMS. Interestingly, the actual physiologic causes of PMS are still unknown. While it is generally described as a hormonal imbalance, studies looking at hormone levels in women with and without PMS show pretty much the same results; however, it's thought that in women with PMS, there is a variation in how even those normal hormone levels are interacting with their stress hormones and neurotransmitters (chemicals that control mood).

That's why it can't be fixed with the Pill—and in fact, why from a conventional medical perspective, antidepressants have been found more effective. What we do know is that many factors have been shown to increase a woman's risk of having PMS, and nutritional, lifestyle, and other approaches have been proven to reduce or stop PMS.

On average, women experience it for about 6 days each month, in the week leading up

PMS Symptom Self-Assessment

How do you know if you have PMS? Although the criteria for diagnosis of premenstrual disorders are variable, there is general agreement that if you have 5 or more symptoms during the week prior to your period, resolving within a few days after your flow starts, it's technically PMS.

One or more of the following symptoms must be present:

- ☐ Mood swings, sudden sadness, increased sensitivity to rejection
- ☐ Anger, irritability

- ☐ Sense of hopelessness, depressed mood, self-critical thoughts
- ☐ Tension, anxiety, feeling on edge

Plus one or more of any of the following symptoms to reach a total of five symptoms overall:

- ☐ Difficulty concentrating
- ☐ Change in appetite, food cravings, overeating
- ☐ Diminished interest in usual activities
- ☐ Easy fatigability, decreased energy

- ☐ Feeling overwhelmed or out of control
- ☐ Breast tenderness, bloating, weight gain, or joint/muscle aches
- ☐ Sleeping too much or not sleeping enough

If you have premenstrual symptoms that get in the way of your best life, something is definitely affecting your total ecology—you don't need a diagnosis to prove that!

If you don't have periods, for example, you have your ovaries but had a hysterectomy, or you are using a hormone IUD, then you don't have your periods to use as a gauge; but the PMS/PMDD is probably still occurring cyclically. To find out, and thus also confirm that your symptoms are due to PMS or PMDD, track them—if your symptoms occur every 24 to 38 days or so, you have your cause.

to their period, but for some women, symptoms begin shortly after ovulation and persist through the onset of their period. Symptoms that are more than mild cues that your period is coming are outlined in the following paragraphs. When symptoms start to get in the way of your mood or physical comfort, or interfere with your ability to function, this isn't normal anymore and it could be PMS.

The most common emotional symptom of PMS is "mood swings" but these come in as a close second:

- increased tension
- irritability
- anger (or rage)
- impatience
- low mood or depression
- anxiety
- sleep problems
- insecurity

PMS: Women's Cycles + Culture Clash

I want to propose a radical idea: perhaps part of what is happening in PMS, at least for some women, is the fact that we *do* have different needs going on in the days leading up to and on the first couple of days of our moon times. Perhaps the conflict between external, worldly demands (work, family, social obligations) and a more inherent desire to hibernate, nest, retreat, and go within, creates conflict—and when we don't hit pause when we need to, we get irritable and out of sorts. The authors of a leading endocrinology textbook, *Clinical Gynecologic Endocrinology and Infertility*, pose the compelling question:

"Is PMS due to an individual pathologic problem or is it due to cultural beliefs, beliefs that lead to the menstrual cycle being associated with a variety of negative reactions, or a combination of both? What if our societies and cultures had celebrated menstruation as a time of pleasure (and even public joy) rather than something private (to be hidden) and negative? Would we have PMS today? The answer may lie in the unraveling of the role of our shared beliefs about menstruation in society, rather than the functioning of those beliefs in individuals" (page 92).

Of course there are many reasons we can feel sad, angry, irritated, frustrated, anxious, or depressed that do not have a hormonal or biological origin; however, cyclic changes in your mood that are disruptive to your life, as well as chronic depression or anxiety, can most certainly be an indication of hormone imbalances. They are often overlooked symptoms of PMS, PCOS, and endometriosis. Like all hormonal imbalances, depression and anxiety can also alert you to root cause imbalances including inflammation, a thyroid problem, high stress levels, blood sugar imbalance, not getting enough of the nutrients you need, microbiome problems, and even environmental toxin exposures, which have been linked to problems with mood.

- fatigue
- low self-esteem
- low motivation
- poor memory or concentration
- not feeling social

The most common physical symptoms are abdominal bloating and an extreme feeling of fatigue. However, breast tenderness, cravings (for sugar, carbs, chocolate, salty foods, or other foods), headaches, acne, premenstrual hot flashes, and dizziness are common. Less common but also possible are general aches or pains, nausea, or increased inflammatory or allergic symptoms, including allergic reactions, upper respiratory tract infections, or flares in an autoimmune condition. You might not know this: If you've had a hysterectomy but still have your ovaries, underwent an endometrial ablation and now have amenorrhea, or have a levonorgestrel IUD, which usually causes women to stop having periods after about six months, you can still be experiencing PMS; you just don't have periods to gauge this by (see the PMS Symptom Self-Assessment on page 73 for how to know).

Why It Matters: PMS is associated with a number of nutritional factors and it can reflect environmental exposures and inflammation. It can also have a really tough impact on your life, compromising work and relationships (as one of my patients said to me, "Oh no, I don't have PMS—but I do have three days every month where I tell my husband we're definitely getting divorced!"). At least 5% of menstruating women are incapacitated by severe PMS—every month. Missed days can mean missed paychecks; skipping the office party can mean a missed promotion; skipping your kid's soccer practice or the parents' meetings

can lead to guilt—and other parents' judgments. If PMS is running—or ruining—your life, I've got your back in the Hormone Intelligence Plan and the Period and PMS Advanced Protocol in Chapter 12.

Menstrual Migraines

The Basics: Up to 70% of women with migraines also experience menstrual ones; however, it is possible to *only* have menstrual migraines, and not have them otherwise, called "pure menstrual migraines."

Why It Matters: Menstrual migraines are the result of the dramatic drop in estrogen after levels have been high for days, which occurs twice in your cycle—just after ovulation and again just before your period. This drop drags your serotonin levels down, too, and this is what is thought to cause migraine pain. Most women who experience hormonal migraines get them premenstrually, but others get them after ovulation, and some both. Having migraines generally predisposes you to experience hormonal migraines. Compared with nonmenstrual migraines, the menstrual type tends to be more severe, lasts longer, and is less responsive to usual acute medication therapies. Menstrual migraines can be severely incapacitating, and overall reflect possible hormone imbalance, or the mitochondrial imbalances we'll discuss in Chapter 11.

PCOS

The Basics: PCOS is a complex, multifactorial metabolic and endocrine system condition, which also happens to affect our menstrual cycles and fertility.

Why It Matters: PCOS affects as many as 10% of women of childbearing age—or more than five million women in the US alone—making it the most common endocrine problem in this age range. It's a glaring example of a gynecologic condition with significant ramifications if untreated, yet 50% of women with PCOS may be undiagnosed.

In PCOS, insulin triggers the ovaries to secrete, while inhibiting SHBG (page 106) production, leading to the increased circulating testosterone that causes frustrating weight gain, distressing hair loss, hair growing in unwanted places (your chin, breasts, or lower belly), and cystic acne. These symptoms can have a major impact on self-esteem and a woman's social life—many are too embarrassed to date or go out with friends. Other symptoms you might not realize can be associated with it include depression or sleep apnea (50% of women with PCOS have some degree of sleep apnea), which can leave you feeling exhausted and miserable and can interfere with your daily functioning. Not to be too scary, but it's important that you know that sleep apnea is also associated with an increased

PCOS Self-Assessment

How do you know if you have PCOS? Because it manifests with different symptoms and even different biochemical imbalances, it can be hard to diagnose and there's no laboratory test that proves you have it. Ultrasound findings, helpful if the classic "string of pearls" (numerous ovarian follicles in various stages of development) is seen, don't alone prove that you have PCOS, nor does an absence of findings prove you don't. However, a diagnosis can be made on an approved set of findings and symptoms called the Rotterdam Criteria.

If you have two of the following three symptoms, by definition you have a diagnosis of PCOS:

- ☐ Infrequent periods more than 35 days apart
- ☐ Polycystic ovaries seen on ultrasound
- ☐ Symptoms of excess androgens (acne, hair loss, hair in unwanted places—upper lip, chin, chest or belly, nipples, etc.)

Additional common symptoms strongly suggesting PCOS include:

- ☐ Irregular cycles
- ☐ Anxiety, depression
- ☐ Binge eating
- ☐ Skipped periods, sometimes for months at a time
- ☐ Darkened, velvety-textured skin around the neck, in your armpits, or in your groin
- ☐ Weight gain or trouble losing weight
- ☐ Skin tags
- ☐ Trouble getting pregnant
- ☐ Reliance on the Pill to treat symptoms like irregular cycles or acne

risk of accidents, high blood pressure, obesity, and cardiovascular disease. Additionally, sleep apnea causes insulin resistance, which, in a vicious cycle, can perpetuate PCOS. Even if you don't have sleep apnea, PCOS doubles the likelihood that you'll have sleep problems—especially difficulty falling asleep. As many as 70% of women with PCOS have insulin resistance beyond that which would be expected by their body weight.

With PCOS, your brain continues telling your ovaries to mature follicles, but high androgen levels interfere with ovulation. As many as 85% of women with PCOS experience some menstrual cycle disruption, including irregular periods and anovulation. Menstrual cycles are typically very long; some women skip periods for months at a time, and periods are often then heavy and painful. Chronic buildup of the uterine lining due to having eight or fewer periods a year is a risk factor for developing endometrial cancer, while heavy periods increase the risk of anemia. A 2015 study showed that infertility is ten times more common, and subfertility is very common, while miscarriage is 20 to 40% more likely in women with PCOS.

Insulin also causes your body to store body fat, which is why it's difficult to lose weight. Because PCOS also leads to weight challenges, this condition can have a terrible impact on self-image. On top of this, the inflammatory and hormonal changes associated with PCOS increase anxiety and depression, making these body image issues, not to mention those due to hair loss and acne, that much harder to cope with. Speaking of weight, PCOS affects women of all sizes; however, the fat shaming that has now been well documented to be present in conventional medical practice may lead overweight women with PCOS to be subjected to advice from their doctor that they should diet and exercise more if they want to lose weight and feel better, whereas thinner women may have their PCOS diagnosis entirely missed or dismissed—so pervasive is the belief that this is a "fat woman's" disease. PCOS is also a recently identified cause of binge eating disorder, a problem affecting millions of women, leading to a traumatically difficult relationship with food; unable to control food intake, women blame themselves for "weakness" and poor willpower, when it is the condition causing this symptom in many.

PCOS is also associated with a higher risk of developing subclinical hypothyroidism and elevated thyroid antibodies, and much higher risk of developing other autoimmune conditions, with over half of all women with PCOS developing metabolic syndrome or diabetes by age forty. A host of cholesterol abnormalities are also increased, affecting almost 70% of women with untreated PCOS, rates of fatty liver disease are increased, and as a result of all these metabolic problems, heart attack risk is four to seven times greater. According to a 2015 study published in the *Journal of Clinical Endocrinology & Metabolism*, women diagnosed with PCOS are twice as likely to be hospitalized for heart disease, diabetes, mental-health conditions, reproductive disorders, and cancer of the uterine lining.

It's a big deal not to be glossed over or treated simply with a pharmaceutical; getting to the root causes while treating the associated symptoms is critical to long-term health. The great news is that it's a reversible condition—and Hormone Intelligence is designed to help you do exactly that!

Endometriosis

Endometriosis ("endo") is one of the most common hormone-related conditions. It affects 1 in 10 women—about 176 million human beings on the planet—and can start in our teens and twenties, but may show up later. Despite its prevalence, it takes an average of nearly ten

Endometriosis Self-Assessment

If you experience the symptoms I list below regularly, it's possible that you have endometriosis. Period pain and chronic pelvic pain can be found in as many as 20 to 90% of women who are eventually diagnosed with this condition. A definitive diagnosis requires a biopsy sample obtained by laparoscopic surgery. If you have presumptive symptoms, it's not essential to get a formal diagnosis unless you plan to pursue surgical treatment. Endometriosis can also, though less commonly, be asymptomatic and first be evident in women only when a woman is diagnosed with a fertility problem.

Symptoms include:

- ☐ Heavy periods
- ☐ Significant lower back pain with periods
- ☐ Cramping between periods
- ☐ Clots with your period
- ☐ Nausea, vomiting, or abdominal pain, especially around your period
- ☐ Abdominal cramping accompanied by diarrhea and/or constipation
- ☐ Pain with bowel movements or urination
- ☐ Painful sex, particularly with penetration
- ☐ Pelvic pain that gets worse after sex or a pelvic exam
- ☐ Lower back pain or pain in the back of your legs, which is typically worse around your period
- ☐ Depression

- ☐ Difficulty getting pregnant
- ☐ Ovulation pain
- ☐ Pelvic burning, aching not limited to menstruation
- ☐ Bleeding after bowel movements or intercourse, especially on your period
- ☐ "Referred pain" especially in your shoulder blades or top of collarbone
- ☐ Bloated or swollen abdomen
- ☐ Irritable bowel syndrome (IBS)
- ☐ Urinary symptoms, i.e., increased frequency, urgency, or pain when you pee
- ☐ Allergies, asthma, migraines, or an autoimmune condition (i.e., thyroid disease, rheumatoid arthritis, lupus, celiac, psoriasis, multiple sclerosis)
- ☐ Fibromyalgia
- ☐ Feeling tired or unwell, especially around your menstrual cycle

As there is a genetic predisposition associated with endometriosis, if your mother or sister has it, it's more likely that you do, as well. The Endometriosis Advanced Protocol begins on page 279. If you have moderate to severe symptoms, I highly suggest incorporating those recommendations along with the core plan, from the beginning.

years before most women receive a diagnosis. In the meantime, many miss school and work and temper career aspirations, and because it can interfere with fertility or cause such extreme pain that women might choose a hysterectomy before having had a child, it can preempt motherhood. The pain also leads women to take a wide range of medications, including narcotics, and often undergo multiple surgeries.

The Basics: In endometriosis, tissue that normally lines the inside of the uterus—the endometrium—grows outside the uterus, commonly on the ovaries, bowel, or the tissue lining the pelvis. Just like the lining inside your uterus, it's triggered by your monthly hormone cycle to thicken, break down, and shed with each menstrual cycle. This shedding is similar to menstruation, but blood in the abdominal cavity gets trapped, irritating surrounding tissue. Eventually this causes the formation of scar tissue and adhesions between the abdominal organs. This can cause chronic abdominal and pelvic discomfort or pain, constipation, and urinary and fertility problems. Endometriosis is classified into four stages corresponding to the extent and spread of lesions throughout the body. Aside from greater interference with fertility at more aggressive stages, stages and symptom severity don't necessarily correspond; the stages are a classification used for surgical purposes.

Why It Matters: The human impact can be severe. Endometriosis commonly sends women to emergency rooms in agony. Even less severe endo can disrupt sex, work, school—and life! It leads many women down a road of surgery after surgery but, if not done properly, lesions can grow back and surgery can add to scarring and adhesions. Women with endometriosis are more than three times as likely to fill an opioid prescription as women who don't have it, to use higher doses, and to use opioids concomitantly with benzodiazepines. Most

are not told that the combination of narcotics and "benzos" dangerously increases the risk of overdose tenfold!

Endometriosis involves much more than the endocrine system. It's a chronic inflammatory condition with complex alterations in immune function leading it to misfiring, producing excess inflammatory chemicals and triggers (i.e., natural killer cells, a type of a white blood cell and a component of innate immunity) that cause tissue damage. At the same time, cells that usually mediate the damage are skipping out on their jobs; instead of scavenging damaged cells, they're promoting inflammation and damage. The good cells have gone rogue, acting like the cells they're supposed to be protecting us from!

This altered immune function and chronic inflammation also puts women with endometriosis at greater risk for other conditions including eczema, allergies, asthma, autoimmune conditions, and chronic fatigue syndrome. Chronic inflammation and altered immune function are implicated in a variety of cancers, and women with endo, as a result, also have a higher risk of developing both ovarian and breast cancers. Endometriosis can damage the fallopian tubes or ovaries, causing fertility problems, though most women with mild to moderate endometriosis will eventually be able to get pregnant without treatment. Women with endo are more likely to get headaches, aches, and pains. I know this is some scary stuff to hear, so keep in mind I'm sharing this so you know how important it is to get in the driver's seat if you think—or know—you have endo. And why it's such a tragedy that doctors are missing the diagnosis so often, and in many women for so many years, when catching it early can help prevent and reverse damage.

Where do our hormones come into this picture? As estrogen increases cyclically, so does endometrial tissue proliferation inside—and outside—of the uterus. That tissue is fed by estrogen; just like when your period comes and the endometrial lining sloughs off, so does this tissue wherever it is in the body—but when it's in your abdomen or other locations (it can find its way almost anywhere in the body—even the lungs and sinuses), that blood acts as a major irritant, which over time can lead to damage of surrounding tissue, scarring, and adhesions, which lead to many of the related symptoms, including pain. The estrogen connection explains why women don't develop active endometriosis until we start our menstrual cycles, and why it improves after menopause when we have much less estradiol, the most potent form of estrogen.

Progesterone plays an interesting role: as an immune system regulator, it suppresses immune system overactivity and possibly even autoimmunity. But in women with endometriosis, the endometrial tissue is *resistant* to progesterone (thought to be the result of chronic underlying inflammation in the endometrial tissue). Consequently, normal immune suppression isn't happening.

But what causes all this to happen? Endometriosis is a "perfect storm" condition with multifactorial roots including altered immunity, imbalanced growth, abnormal endocrine signaling, and genetic factors. The latest evidence shows us that for some women, the tracks of abnormal immune and endocrine signaling may even be laid down in their bodies before birth, due to environmental exposures their mothers had even before they were pregnant with them, or during pregnancy itself. It is also associated with a wide range of triggers that could have occurred at any time during life, altering immune and hormonal functioning, including changes to your microbiome, hidden toxin exposures, and more. There are also many known factors, including specific nutritional and dietary factors, exposure to specific environmental toxins, and some very interesting gut-related conditions, as you'll learn all about in Part Two.

Fertility Challenges

If it's taking longer than you thought it would for you to get pregnant, there's a good chance you're freaking out a little bit or a lot. Fertility challenges affect at least 75 million women in the US—about 12% of women.

The Basics: Defined as the inability of a couple to conceive after twelve months of regular intercourse without contraception in women less than 35 years of age; or after six months of regular intercourse without contraception in women 35 years and older. I use the terms **subfertility** and **fertility challenges** to describe difficulty in conceiving unless a woman has been proven to be medically unable to have a child. True infertility is rare, occurring in at most 2% of couples.

Why It Matters: Fertility is a major window into your overall health. Exposome medicine

Adenomyosis: A Sister to Endometriosis

Adenomyosis is not well understood, but can be considered a sister disorder to endometriosis. The main difference is that in adenomyosis, instead of abnormal endometrial tissue growing outside of the uterus, it's growing into the uterine muscle layer, which can make medical treatment, particularly surgical options, more challenging—all the more reason for trying a natural approach first whenever possible.

Fertility Self-Assessment

Symptoms that put you at risk for a fertility challenge include:

- ☐ Short luteal phase (<12 days long)
- ☐ Short or long menstrual cycles
- ☐ You're not ovulating
- ☐ You're not having ovulatory-type cervical mucus
- ☐ Hypothalamic amenorrhea

- ☐ PCOS
- ☐ Endometriosis
- ☐ Hypothyroidism
- ☐ Premature ovarian insufficiency (POI)
- ☐ Perimenopause

When Is "Still Not Pregnant" a Problem?

Statistically, 70–85% of women trying to become pregnant, at all ages within their reproductive years, will become pregnant within twelve months. If intercourse is happening twice a week, an estimated 89 to 95% of couples aged 30 to 39 trying will become pregnant within 24 months. Among couples trying to conceive after 12 months, even with an infertility diagnosis, pregnancy rates are as high as 63%. So if you've been on the baby-making train and are still within these windows, your fertility may be totally fine and I don't suggest putting a label on yourself just yet. Follow the Hormone Intelligence Plan and use the tips in Chapter 15 to support natural fertility and conception for 6 months—because the healthier and more nutritionally optimized you are when you get pregnant, the better it is for baby. If you've been trying for longer and really do merit a fertility diagnosis, please keep the faith; I've helped many women get pregnant over the years, and the protocols I share in this book have been refined over decades of practice.

In women, the most common known causes are: anovulation (which can be due to PCOS, hypothalamic amenorrhea, or other causes), low progesterone (which prevents the endometrium from being optimally prepared for implantation), but about a third of the time, the causes remain medically completely unknown. This can leave you with the devastating feeling that there are no answers or nothing you can do, but there is so much hope. Statistically, most women will ultimately conceive.

Keep in mind, male partner factors account for 30 to 50% of all fertility problems. Male fertility problems have been increasing due to environmental endocrine disruptors, which you'll learn all about in Part Two. If you're trying to conceive, your partner can come along on the Hormone Intelligence journey with you, optimizing his nutrition and reducing environmental toxin body burden, for a start.

fills in the gaps of what can't be explained by conventional medicine. For example, we know that "hidden" factors account for fertility challenges at least 10% of the time and also contribute to the known causes. These "unidentified" issues include: diet and nutritional deficiencies, chronic inflammation, stress, occupational and environmental exposures, smoking, and medications, including ibuprofen, as well as just coming off the Pill, to name a few. In my medical practice, where fertility care is one of my favorite parts of my work, I rarely treat fertility challenges per se; rather, I help women to nourish all their ecosystems to optimal health—that's where the magic usually happens.

Uterine Fibroids

The Basics: *Uterine leiomyomas*, or fibroids, are noncancerous growths of muscle tissue in the uterus. They vary in size from practically microscopic to the size of jumbo grapefruit, or bigger. They grow singly or in clusters and can grow in a variety of locations in the uterus or cervix.

Why It Matters: If fibroids sound like an "old lady" uterus problem, guess again. Fibroids start growing in our twenties, thirties, and forties when we have lots of growth-stimulating estrogen hanging around to feed fibroids like Miracle-Gro, and a lot of women already have small ones growing by this time. By the time we get into our perimenopausal years, they've gotten big enough to start causing symptoms, if they haven't before, so we think of them as problems in women our mom's or grandmom's age. One in three women experience symptoms including abnormal uterine bleeding, pelvic pain or pressure, and increased need to urinate, and they may affect fertility and pregnancy. They are the most common cause of hysterectomies other than cancer.

While I'm not going to deep dive into all the nuances of fibroid types and locations, I want to emphasize that while a genetic component is common, they're another vital sign that some-

---

Uterine Fibroid Self-Assessment

If you regularly experience the following symptoms, you could have fibroids. However, these are also similar symptoms of endometriosis, so complete that self-assessment as well. It is also possible to have both conditions at once.

Symptoms include:

- ☐ Heavy periods
- ☐ Severe menstrual cramps
- ☐ Bleeding between periods
- ☐ A feeling of fullness in the lower abdomen
- ☐ Pain during sex
- ☐ Low back pain
- ☐ Constipation
- ☐ Abdominal pain
- ☐ Urinary frequency, urgency, or difficulty peeing

The Uterine Fibroids Advanced Protocol starts on page 293.

thing is up with your hormonal ecosystems, usually imbalances in blood sugar / insulin and elevated estrogen. I also don't want you to end up with a hysterectomy in your fifties or beyond, when this can often be prevented with steps you can take now.

Hot Flashes, Vaginal Dryness, Low Libido—At Any Age

The Basics: Menopause is the complete cessation of our menstrual cycles, a natural eventuality we all face, usually in our early fifties. Perimenopause is the time leading up to menopause, and *primary ovarian insufficiency* (POI) is a medical condition in which a woman 42 years of age or younger experiences diminished ovarian function leading to cessation of ovulation and fertility.

Why It Matters: As we age, our ovarian function naturally declines; we produce less estrogen and progesterone and we stop ovulating. This decline begins in our late thirties, with mild symptoms becoming apparent sometime in our early to late forties, depending on our level of ovarian health and reserve, at which time we're in perimenopause. Skipped periods, especially when accompanied by hot flashes, night sweats, insomnia, low sex drive, vaginal dryness, depression, anxiety, and memory problems, can be signs of perimenopause and are due to ovarian dysfunction. This may also be detected if a fertility workup reveals low ovarian reserve. Why does this happen? In Part Two, there's a whole chapter dedicated to exactly this!

POI carries significant risk factors including premature aging and increased risk of osteoporosis, heart disease, and dementia later in life. But even severe symptoms in women in their natural perimenopause years—particularly severe hot flashes—suggest an elevated risk for heart attacks, cognitive decline, and breast cancer. In Chapter 11 I'll share strategies for nourishing your ovaries with the goal of restoring function and even reversing primary ovarian insufficiency (POI). Whatever your

Perimenopause and Primary Ovarian Insufficiency (POI) Self-Assessment

How do you know if you're in perimenopause—or experiencing primary ovarian insufficiency? The symptoms are the same—it's the timing that's different.

Symptoms include:

- ☐ Hot flashes, night sweats
- ☐ Irregular or skipped periods
- ☐ Vaginal dryness, pain during sex
- ☐ Recurrent bladder infections
- ☐ Sleep disturbance
- ☐ Decreased libido
- ☐ Mood swings, depression, anxiety
- ☐ Weight gain around your middle
- ☐ Change in breast shape or size (can increase or decrease)
- ☐ Bone loss (fractures, loss of height)—your medical provider can confirm with bone density testing

age, the healthier your ovaries, the later this decline is likely to occur, and the better your health span is predicted to be.

How Do Cycles and Symptoms Tell Us So Much?

Do you remember in the beginning of the book I told you "it's all connected"? It is, which is why our hormones tell us so much about our health and environment. Like that orchestra I talked about in Chapter 2, when the conductor isn't properly leading the symphony, when one instrument is out of tune, or one musician is off tempo, beautiful music can quickly become discordant noise.

While it may seem impossible that multiple different hormone imbalances and conditions can be addressed with one approach, in fact, all the hormone imbalances we are currently facing are the result of a common set of factors. These interact with your personal genetic predispositions to create the hormone imbalances you're experiencing.

That's why ignoring them, hoping they'll go away, or suppressing them with pharmaceuticals, surgeries, and procedures that still don't address the roots of the problem is not the answer. Your hormonal health is a direct reflection of your total health—physical, emotional, mental, and spiritual health, all of which are shaped by our environment. When you look at all of them, you take in the total ecology of your health. Rather than trying to "fix this dang hormone problem!" what we actually want to ask is, *How can I shift my inner and outer environments so that they support my overall health?*

The bottom line is that your hormonal life should never have you in chronic or even regular discomfort, you should never be in pain (okay, admittedly, contractions in labor are the exception—they're a pretty strong sensation!), and you should never have severe *anything*—mood changes, cravings, bloating, headaches, sleep problems, you name it. Being a woman should not, in any way, interfere with your quality of life.

It's Not as Simple as Sprinkling on Some Hormones

It would be nice if hormone imbalances could be fixed with some hormone fairy dust, or at least pills and supplements that easily get you to "standard" hormone levels. Unfortunately, even though medications can temporarily help with severe symptoms, hormones alone as treatment have largely failed to prove effective for most gynecologic conditions—and nearly always comes with a price: risky side effects. But there's another reason that simply sprinkling on the hormones doesn't work: many of the conditions we assume are caused by hormone imbalances are way more complex than hormone levels being too high or low. Here's a crazy fact: conventional science and medicine aren't sure what causes nearly every gynecologic condition in this book! That's why it's so important to expand your thinking about healing hormone imbalances beyond the confines of conventional medicine to a broader scientific view that takes a more global ecological approach. That's where we can find the answers we're looking for.

Take **PMS**. We all know what it is and what causes it. It's a hormone imbalance, right? If only it were that simple. Most studies find that hormone levels are usually normal in women with PMS. For reasons not yet known, women with PMS seem to have an irregular *response* to progesterone and the "feel good" neurotransmitter, serotonin. That's why giving progesterone doesn't "cure" PMS, or even relieve symptoms. You can have all the hormones, but if you can't respond to them, it won't do any good. We do know, however, that stress hormones, environmental chemical exposures, and dietary factors can cause or worsen PMS, while certain antidepressants that boost serotonin, vitamin B6, and exercise do improve PMS symptoms, often substantially. This may be because these changes increase our hormone response, rather than increasing our hormone production.

PCOS is another example of a hormone condition that's not strictly hormonal. While high testosterone is a major player causing the suppressed ovulation resulting in low progesterone, as well as the physical symptoms we see, PCOS is the result of a complex constellation of factors, including insulin resistance, which can be a result of diet, obesity, stress, microbiome imbalances, environmental exposures, and chronic inflammation.

Even **low libido**, which most medical doctors, including holistic ones, assume is caused by a hormone imbalance and is typically attributed to low estrogen or low testosterone, can also be due to a host of intersecting factors that have nothing to do with hormone imbalances. For example, libido dips when we're exhausted or under stress. It can be affected by a history of sexual trauma, body image issues, or relationship issues. It can be a simple matter of a lack of self-confidence. Dr. Lorraine Dennerstein's research has shown that a woman's feelings for her partner, and her relationship satisfaction, contribute more to her sexual desire than hormonal changes in menopause. In fact, research shows that hormones are the least likely culprit in cases of low desire in women at any age, and that relationship quality, happiness, and beliefs about sex and desire play more of a role in low libido than do hormone levels.

Each of these conditions shares common, intersecting pathways within the landscape of your body, with continuous cross talk between all its systems. Your immune, nervous, metabolic, and digestive systems are all also influenced by external factors—stress, environmental toxins, your nutritional status, the health of your microbiome, and more. That's why most conventional, and even "alternative," approaches to hormone health that rely simply on testing and treating with hormone medications—even so-called natural bioidentical forms, aren't enough to fix what is likely to be so much more than a "hormone problem."

Hormone Intelligence is a new way of relating to your cycles and symptoms, and your environment. I believe that every woman has the power to restore balance and ease in her body. Learning to use your body's innate Hormone Intelligence, you can more quickly move the needle on your hormone health. But before you begin the plan that will change your life, I want you to know how incredible and special your body already is, and how important—and powerful—it is to embrace being your own healer.

you are your own best healer

It takes years as a woman to unlearn what you have been taught to be sorry for.
—Amy Poehler

Ten years of medical training may mean that your doctor knows anatomy and physiology better than you do, but nobody knows *you* better than *you*. After all, you've had how many years of training in yourself? By now, at least a few decades! One of the most vital steps you can take toward reclaiming your hormone health is to know your body and trust your intuition. But this is hard against the backdrop of centuries of medical and scientific dismissal of our emotions, intuition, and body wisdom.

Looking back even a couple of centuries in the history of women's health, we find that healing was once in the hands of women. But by the late eighteenth century, things changed; medicine became a profession that not only systemically eliminated women healers from its ranks, barring women from entering medical training, but also made it difficult for women healers to practice at all. Health care became the provenance of men, and women's natural body processes became a prime target for medicalization. We can't, nor would we want to, go back in time, but we can put all this knowledge (old and new—wisdom and science) together in a new medicine for women that bridges the best of all worlds. And we need to in order to avoid overtreatment, but also to claim more sovereignty over our health, and peace with our bodies.

I want to take you one level deeper, to help you access your own inner knowing and reclaim the belief that your body can heal, that nature's medicines have a place in healing, and that within you lies the ability to transform your health, no matter how far from that you feel today. Clarissa Pinkola Estés, author of the bestseller *Women Who Run with the Wolves*, called this "digging into the psychic archeology of the female underworld," a recovery of our natural instinctive psyche. I also consider it a recovery of women's wisdom about healing. I've seen so many times how cultivating this mind-set can unleash a powerful internal force that activates the body's healing potential. As we repair our hormones, we have an opportunity to repair aspects of our inner landscape as women. It may at times require being a warrior for your own health—a bit defiant and non-conformist, being willing to break taboos and question the gospel that conventional medicine is the only reliable, effective, or even the safest first option, and having a fierce belief in the power of your own body. I welcome you to break the spell of seeing doctors as gods, as having greater power over or wisdom about our bodies than we do. It's an illusion based on centuries of dominance, not truth.

Rewilding Ourselves

Our culture makes it hard for us to come home to, love, and feel truly comfortable in our bodies. We're taught to accept a disconnect from our wild, sacred selves as normal. We are taught to deny or suppress our natural power and instincts, taught to judge our hormonally driven mood shifts as a problem to be solved, rather than messages to be listened to. Separated from nature's rhythms, we also become disconnected from our inherent rhythms. Reclaiming hormone inner balance requires realigning these rhythms—our chronobiology, which you'll learn about soon—and reconnecting to our own wild, unfettered nature, which I talk more about in this chapter.

We all have a shadow side, suppressed by stereotypical roles that have held women down for centuries, keeping us from the true freedom and expression of our unique selves. Your feelings are there for a reason—and it's not enough to dismiss yourself, or let yourself be dismissed as "just hormonal." Whether they're a call from your body for better hormone balance, a call from your life for greater balance, or a call from your soul for more freedom, passion, and creativity, this book invites you to reconnect to your body, your fire, your passion, your SELF. It invites you to embrace what has been considered *taboo*.

5 Ways to Reclaim Your Wild

- Stand barefoot outside for five minutes, close your eyes, breathe deeply, and just feel your feet in the grass, on the soil, on this glorious Mother Earth.
- Sit on the ground and feel the energy of the earth moving up through you all the way to the top of your head.
- Put on drumbeat music (Afro beats, Caribbean, world music) and let your body move.
- Grow and garden, a house plant, herbs in your windowsill, and pay attention to their life cycles.
- Sit outside under the moon, preferably with women-friends, create a moon-ritual, or—dare I say it—go outside on the next full moon night and loudly and full throated let it all loose and howl!

Become Woman Wise

Hormone Intelligence also reconnects us to women's "old ways," or "women's wisdom," stripping away the distraction and clutter of modern living, the shame around our bodies, the taboos around self-healing (and self-loving!), and embraces the healing roots that have always been in women's hands, even when we've forgotten them: women's mysteries, birth, herbs, and more. You have the wisdom and the power already inside of you. I invite you to awaken to your own inner guidance system—your *wisewoman*, as I call her. Call her what you like, she is the voice of your Hormone Intelligence, the guardian of your personal ecosystems. I believe we each have our own, alive and waiting for us to hear her call, to rekindle that flame of connection if it's grown faint. As we walk through this program together, I am going to show you how to connect with this knowing, and the healing power of nature's rhythms, so you can take back your hormonal health once and for all.

How to Get the Health Care You Deserve

Does tapping into women's ways mean you'll never need medical help? Unlikely. Complex problems like PCOS, endometriosis, or a fertility challenge may get you to seek medical help. But with the knowledge and tools you gain in this book, you never have to feel helpless, dismissed, disrespected, or diminished. Health care should be kind. Respectful. Open-minded. Your experience of your symptoms

Honor Your Womb

Whether you still have yours or your uterus has been removed for medical reasons, I invite you to consider that you still have a *womb*, a divine seat of power centered in your abdomen. Light a candle if you'd like, and even some incense if that's your jam (it's definitely mine!), though it's not required. Now, sitting or lying down comfortably, eyes closed, lay one hand on top of the other, just above your pubic bone, and let some warmth get generated. Take a moment to honor the transformative power that is inherent in your body—wherever you are in your life cycles, whatever is going on in your body, hormones, health. Feel that warmth flowing into your belly and back to your hands, in a continuous, pulsating wave, back and forth. Now let yourself go deeper into the sensation, just feeling that natural ebb and flow of energy.

As you allow yourself to relax even more deeply, notice any emotions that arise. Do you feel gratitude? Sadness? Pain? Joy? Power? Grief? A mixture of feelings? If you've had a cesarean, a hysterectomy, or trauma, are you able to send healing warmth into your belly, or womb if it's there? Allow the feelings to rise up while you send love in. Honor your womb and yourself for what you/she have been through. Take a few minutes in this space. Now rub your hands together vigorously, shake them a few times, and put them on your heart. Hold this space for a minute. Then open your eyes. Optionally journal what came up for you.

should be validated. And you should be offered a wide range of helpful, reliable, and safe solutions—not simply the medication du jour.

As has probably become clear by now, the medical establishment doesn't always operate in your favor. But you can work with this reality; healing options exist on a spectrum, and different choices will be appropriate for you based on the severity of your symptoms, how much they're impacting your quality of life and needs at the time, and the known effectiveness and safety of the treatment options for whatever you're experiencing. There are very few women who leave a medical appointment feeling better about their bodies, more knowledgeable about what is going on, or, for that matter, respected.

In this next section I share guidelines to help you get in charge of your health care, find the best provider for you, and get the care you deserve and need.

Here are my top six tips for getting the medical care you need and deserve.

1. Work with a Woman

The data is clear: women doctors listen more, interrupt less, make fewer mistakes, and their patients are overall happier and live longer. Need I say more?

2. Remember, You're the Boss

You do not have to accept any test or treatment you don't want and should not be pressured into a decision. You have the right to say, *I'd like to think about that for a few days and I'll get back to you.* You're allowed to ask for evidence and data and to disagree. You also have the right to get another opinion—you're not "cheating" on your health care provider; you're doing due diligence for your health and safety. A provider should understand that, particularly when it comes to big decisions. When it

comes to any recommendations, you should be able to ask:

- Do I *really* need this?

- How likely is it that taking this treatment is going to help me, and how much?

- What are the risks or side effects? How likely are they? Are they dangerous?

- What are the alternatives I might consider, including watching and waiting, or more natural therapies?

3. Trust Yourself

It can be hard to trust yourself, especially if your medical provider is telling you that you're just fine. From the time we're kids we're raised on the doctor-as-god, expert-knows-best model. You might even start to question your own judgment. If you're having symptoms that are affecting your well-being, something has changed from your usual baseline, or you just feel that something is off, trust your instincts and seek help until you get the right answer.

4. Be Your Own Advocate

This is where that warrior woman might have to "rise up." Studies show that as women, we're especially likely to try to "please" our care providers. We're unlikely to say, "Please don't do that," we try not to complain and may therefore minimize our symptoms, and we don't correct doctors when they repeat our own health information incorrectly. If you think something is up, speak up. You have to. Nobody is going to do it for you and you've got to get comfortable making yourself heard. Whether you're in your primary care provider's office or the emergency department, tell them something is up, that you don't usually have these symptoms, and you need proper medical attention. Don't get sent home without a diagnosis. You have to, by all means, make sure that you are being taken seriously. This means being a strong self-advocate.

5. Bring an Advocate

Bring an advocate with you, preferably a woman, preferably a friend, someone who isn't a pushover when it comes to authority and who's going to have your back. People do weird things around authority. I've seen situations where a woman brings her boyfriend and the doctor is male, and the boyfriend and the doctor side with each other. It gets weird, so have somebody you can trust, and if you have somebody who you trust of your own gender, that can be even more effective.

6. Know When It's Time to Break Up

Sometimes you might have to do the hard work of breaking up with your doctor. If your provider can't offer what you need, expand your team or find another provider. You deserve to be respected. If your doctor or any practitioner is insensitive or condescending, won't listen, makes you feel small, invisible, unheard, insecure, or if you have to fight to get what you need, that's not good medicine. It's when mistakes get made. There are statistics showing that when doctors are hurried, they're not paying attention. When they're not making the effort to make good relationships, big important diagnoses get missed.

There are also many types of practitioners who can complement conventional care if you are working with a medical provider who is not knowledgeable about the therapies you're interested in including as part of your care, or if you don't need medical care and just need the natural therapies. This includes acupuncturists, nutritionists, herbalists, health coaches, fertility awareness teachers, pelvic floor therapists, and body workers. If trauma is part of

your history, a therapist can be an invaluable member of your health team.

Create a Healing Mind-Set

Success in any new endeavor, or when changing any habit, requires a success mind-set. Top athletes know this. Sometimes making changes is hard; sometime we make changes, start to see success, and are tempted to slip back into old patterns. I want to give you a few tips to help get—and keep—your head in the game. Here are some things to remember as you go through this six-week plan.

Put Yourself on the Front Burner

Even if you're hardwired to put everyone else first (a learned behavior for most women and practically all moms!), it's time to focus on *you*. It's time to make a conscious decision to devote the time you need to make this plan happen for yourself. Fortunately, all the things you'll be doing are wonderful so it's not toooo hard! So get ready to indulge yourself, all in the name of health. You deserve to do this, and the people you love should also want you to feel your best.

Give Yourself Some Love

I've worked with so many women who came to me feeling "less than" a woman or than her ideal of herself because she was diagnosed with PCOS, endometriosis, a fertility problem, or breast cancer, or had lost a breast, ovary, or uterus. None of this makes us less whole, less than women, less than ideal. But 30-plus years as a healer has taught me something so important that this book is not complete without me telling you: Yes, it's normal to feel frustrated, overwhelmed, disappointed, sad when your body isn't com-

Woman Wise: What Do You Believe About Your Body?

Einstein said, "There are only two ways to live your life. One is as though nothing is a miracle. The other is as though everything is a miracle." Anthropological studies show us that our attitudes and beliefs about menstruation, birth, and menopause are not only culturally shaped, but can influence how we experience them. Until now, the messages you've gotten about having a period, pregnancy and birth, or aging were likely less than positive.

We all develop stories about our body based on our histories, experiences, and what we've been told by our culture. Our brains and our hormones are profoundly connected, and as such, our beliefs about our bodies and being a woman shape our biology, and how we experience our cycles, our blood, our discharges, our odors, our body shapes. Few of us were taught that our bodies are powerful organisms capable of healing and transformation. Instead, we were taught to see being women as a disadvantage, our hormonal ebbs and flows as a burden, our lady parts as gross at best, disaster zones at worst. All this makes it hard to be a body-positive girl in a body-negative world aimed at making us feel we are permanently broken, and permanently dependent on people in white coats to rescue us.

We're changing that story here and now.

Use this journaling practice to uncover hidden beliefs that could get in the way of tapping into your healing capacities. Write out your responses to the following questions, answering them based on what you believe:

- My mother's attitudes about her body are/were:

- My mother's attitudes about periods are/were:

- My mother's attitudes about sex are/were:

- My mother's attitudes about being a woman are/were:

- My family gynecologic history (mother, aunts, grandmothers on both sides) as I've heard it:

- My beliefs and attitudes about my body's ability to heal are:

- My belief and trust in the therapies I'm trying are:

- What (or who) triggers my doubts or my beliefs about healing or the treatments I'm using:

- My beliefs about my symptoms and the meaning I give them are:

fortable to be in right now, even to grieve when you receive a diagnosis that doesn't fit your view of who you are. But being at war with your body, hating on yourself, wishing you were someone different, smack-talking your body—none of this activates your healing capacities; it just makes you more miserable. Healing starts when you realize you're actually a whole, amazing human being (even if you have symptoms or a diagnosis).

Get Curious

It's really easy to get stuck on a label or diagnosis we have. To heal our hormones, to love our hormones and the very unique part of being women that they create, we have to step out of self-judgment and into a place of curiosity about the wonder and possibility of what can happen when we try something new. How do you feel when you eat a breakfast that has more protein and good-quality fat compared to that muffin and cuppa coffee? How's your energy at 10 a.m.? 4 p.m.? What advice works for you and what isn't working?

Take It Slow

Healing from the inside out, remapping your hormones is not an all-or-nothing overnight event; it takes time, happens in baby steps, slowly and steadily in response to simple acts, done over time, that gently, cumulatively, shift your physiology. This means that while I'm asking you to make changes over six weeks, you should go at the pace that feels right and doable to you. Honestly, most programs are based on the fact that books sell better when they are based on a short time frame; that is, my publisher would have been in heaven if this book was "two weeks to total hormone repair." In the real world, taking it slow, making all the changes over a realistic timeline, a few at a time, is more sustainable than trying to do it all at once, or frankly, in just six weeks. So give

yourself space to breathe into it, enjoy the process, and trust me, you'll get there. And when you do, you'll be able to stay there.

Reframe Success

There's no report card that comes with this book. No grades. It's just you, anyone you invite to join you, me, the book, the journey. You don't have to do this plan perfectly to succeed. Jump right in, get started, and do your best. It's not a race, it's not a contest, and there are no prizes for perfect attendance (well, other than feeling *spectacular*!). My point is, don't beat yourself up if you aren't perfect. Instead, keep reminding yourself why you are doing this and just *keep going*. Have to stop and restart? This is a lifestyle, not a sprint.

Celebrate Your Wins and the Small Gains

Instead of looking all the way down to the finish line, celebrate those mile markers along the way. Your brain loves celebrations, but it especially loves rewards, which can keep you in a positive mind-set and inspire you to keep going. Rewards validate the hard work you do to achieve even small goals, so remember: No perfectionism! I recommend counting a win at the end of every day and building some rewards for yourself into your plan (not involving junk food!) for motivation and fun. The reward can be as simple as a little extra "you time," or something more fancy, like that dress you've been eyeing or those boots, or a pedicure or a massage or just a day to yourself reading a book and sipping tea in peace. With every step forward, you win, and you deserve to celebrate that!

Ride the Waves

A question I get all the time is "How long does it take to see improvement?" It's the adult version of, "Are we there yet?" You will likely start to see changes in the first couple of weeks, particularly improvements in energy, digestion, sleep, and mood; and you will likely see significant changes after six weeks.

Rewrite Your Hormone Story

Feeling out of control of your body for a long time can make you feel like you don't have much control over your life, future, or happiness. So many of the women who contact me via the internet about their health concerns (some become my patients) have been struggling with symptoms for so long, they've forgotten to focus on what it feels like to be healthy. When I ask, "What does being healthy look like to you?" I am sometimes met with a long list of symptoms, as if the question itself didn't even register. Most women have never considered what health "looks like" to them. Many of us have even wrapped our identities in the blanket of our symptoms, illness, and diagnosis.

How the Hormone Intelligence Plan Works

Although hormone imbalances show up uniquely for each woman, there is a consistent, identifiable set of underlying factors, or root causes, that predictably alter not just our hormone balance, but all the interrelated networks, including our immune system and nervous system, for example, that affect hormone signaling. Confused signaling eventually shows up as hormone symptoms, sometimes small ones that we might write off as normal discomforts and inconveniences, like menstrual cramps or premenstrual headaches, and sometimes big, loud, disruptive ones that de-

mand our attention like chronic pelvic pain, irregular cycles, fertility problems, PCOS, endometriosis, heavy monthly bleeding, and more. I'm going to uncover exactly what these roots are, including the science behind them, and give you a step-by-step plan to put out the fires that are sounding your hormone smoke alarm.

In Part Two, you'll find the six-week plan to rebalance your hormones, heal your gut, cool inflammation, and deeply nourish your body, mind, and spirit to reverse and resolve the symptoms and conditions that got you to pick up this book, and to create optimum hormone and gynecologic health for a lifetime—even if that's all you were looking for. You'll learn all the ways you can restore health and balance in each ecosystem to reclaim hormone balance and heal gynecologic problems. In addition, if you want to start with a more advanced plan from the beginning, whether to jump-start treating more problematic symptoms or to personalize your plan, look ahead into Part Three, "The Hormone Intelligence Advanced Natural Protocols," to find your symptoms or diagnosis, and feel free to supplement the core plan you'll be following over the next six weeks.

In the next six chapters, which I recommend you take a week at a time, you'll journey through the six root causes along the way to health transformation:

1. **Eating for Hormone Health.** First we'll make sure your food is nourishing hormone health. You'll soon understand why.

2. **The Stress-Hormone Connection.** Next we'll address one of the most potent hormone disruptors: stress. You'll learn some simple but amazing ways to work with this inevitable aspect of life.

3. **Reset Your Body Clock to Sync Your Hormones.** After that, we'll reset your circadian rhythm. You'll get to know yours—and how to sync it up to what is most natural for you.

4. **The Gut-Hormone Connection.** What about the gut? Most people have some level of digestive distress some of the time, but digestive problems are especially common in women with hormone imbalances. I'll explain why, and show you what you can do to get your digestion running smoothly.

5. **The Detoxification-Hormone Connection.** Sadly, we're living in a sea of toxic exposures, but there are powerful things you can do to reduce your toxic load and tune up your detoxification system for maximum toxin-eliminating power.

6. **Rejuvenate Your Ovaries.** I'll explain how to rev up your own cellular repair system—and reverse at least one type of aging!

At the beginning of each chapter, you'll find your to-dos for the week pertaining to that chapter. While the plan is meant to be done in total, you may find that one or more root causes is more affected than others, and so you may choose to focus on that one with more emphasis. Peppered throughout the book you'll find additional helpful guidance on specific symptoms such as bloating and other digestive problems, ovarian cysts, hormonal hair loss, sleep problems, and more.

Then, in Part Three, "The Hormone Intelligence Advanced Natural Protocols," I give you targeted, specific tools to reduce and reverse the "Big 7" gynecologic conditions this book focuses on: period problems (including PMS), PCOS, endometriosis, fertility challenges, uterine fibroids, and sexual and vaginal health, as well as discussing how to naturally support symptoms of perimenopause (and primary ovarian insufficiency, or POI).

While the plan in Part Two may be all you need to resolve symptoms and start to reverse bigger conditions, I highly recommend adding in some of the solutions from the Part Three Advanced Protocols right from the beginning of your Hormone Intelligence six-week journey if you have particularly troublesome symptoms, need specific symptom relief now (i.e., period pain), or feel more urgent in your timeline (you're on the verge of fertility treatment, endometriosis surgery, or other interventions) and want to accelerate the natural plan from day one. You can also layer more solutions into the plan at any time.

Get Ready to Treat Yourself

The Hormone Intelligence Plan provides you with a clear blueprint that will help you to understand how your symptoms are a rallying cry from your body to get to the root causes of what's actually going on. And I hope you have a sense that I'm with you—and cheering for you—every step of the way. Are you ready to start a fascinating conversation with your hormones? Are you ready to tap into your Hormone Intelligence? Then let's do this thing! You're going to love what happens.

find balance

THE HORMONE INTELLIGENCE PLAN

Love yourself first, and everything else
falls in line. You really have to love yourself
to get anything done in this world.

—Lucille Ball

nourish

EATING FOR HORMONE HEALTH

We are indeed much more than what we eat, but what we eat can nevertheless help us be much more than what we are.
—**Adelle Davis**

Every cell in your body involved in hormone balance is guided by a genetic code that relies on the information provided by the right foods. Specific vitamins, minerals, proteins, fats, carbohydrates, and fiber are required to manufacture, transport, utilize, break down, and eliminate hormones, as well as do all this for their important counterparts in your hormone health, for example, the neurotransmitters that support mind and mood. What you do—or don't—eat, and what makes its way into your food from our modern food system, influences everything: your menstrual cycle regularity and whether you experience PMS, menstrual pain, endometriosis, PCOS, fertility, uterine fibroids, breast health, and stressful moods. It shapes your long-term health, too—when you go into menopause, your bone strength, heart and brain health, and how you age.

The relationship between the foods we eat and our hormones is so powerful that I want to shout it from the rooftops so every woman knows she can restore and support hormone balance with simple dietary changes—the very ones you'll find in this chapter and going forward in the Hormone Intelligence Plan. It's why food is the first root of Hormone Intelligence. Based on reclaiming a plant-based, slow-food tradition, preparing more of your own foods, and connecting how you eat and how you feel, the Hormone Intelligence Diet is what I think of as the LBD (little black dress) of diets—it's classic and timeless, and it works for almost everyone and every occasion.

Food Addresses All the Roots

While we each have unique nutritional needs, the Hormone Intelligence Diet has all you need to reset food-related imbalances in each root cause of hormone imbalance. How is it that one plan can do this for so many women and so many conditions? Simple: it's based on *the most studied and proven healthiest diet on the planet*, the Mediterranean diet, but modified for women's hormone health. It contains the nutrients, plant-based chemicals, and ingredients you need to nourish all the axes, glands, and organs that shape hormone health: your brain, ovaries, uterus, adrenals, thyroid, while also supporting your gut, detoxification system, sleep, mind, and mood—supporting the *inner ecosystems* that create hormone balance. It also has all the components that health experts agree on, regardless of the diet camp they're in. And it eliminates hormone-hindering foods.

The plan in this book is going to fire up your metabolism, cool the flames of inflammation, and nourish your cells, glands, and tissues so they can support your hormone balance. It's also going to expand how you feel about food, removing the food battles, confusion, and overwhelm about what to eat. You're going to learn that food can be a healthy pleasure, while finally getting in the driver's seat of eating for optimal hormone health.

There are thousands of studies demonstrating the connection between women's hormonal and gynecologic health, diet, specific foods, and nutrients. I'm not going to linger over why sugar and processed foods are unhealthy. If you're like most of my brilliant patients, you've read a book or two. I know that you know that. But I *will* provide you with the research that shows *how* they muddy your hormone signaling, because knowing why helps us stick to our goals. If you don't want to read the why, you're welcome to skip to the second part of this chapter (starting on page 113) and dive right into the guidelines. Or keep reading, and begin the plan at the same time by getting ready to start with the Week 1 meal plan today!

The "D" Word

Before we begin, I want to talk about the word *diet*. It's more loaded than a hot dog with "the works." Food is part of our personal, primal nourishment story, of having enough, of being fed, of feeling safe and cared for. For many women, food is part of a history of trauma,

---

Hormone Intelligence: Eating for Hormone Health

- Learn what to eat for hormone balance—and why.
- Clear out foods that sabotage hormone health, bridge your phytonutrient gap, and eat for energy balance.
- Use the weekly meal plans and (delicious!) recipes in Part Four to support you through the next six weeks—and beyond. Try new things in the kitchen, have fun, and enjoy a new way of eating and relating to food.
- Go easy on yourself, using the Six Hormone Intelligence Food Principles (starting on page 113).

suffering, and body battles. Dieting is also part of the culture of body loathing, body shame, and fat shaming we all live in. I get it.

Many health-conscious women now also suffer from a condition called *orthorexia*, an obsession with clean eating accompanied by food restriction and control. Perhaps control is something we crave when our health and hormones feel like they're spinning out of control. The problem is that restrictive eating and constantly stressing aren't good for your hormone health, as you'll learn in this and upcoming chapters. So when I use the word *diet* in this text, *I am absolutely not talking about restrictive eating.* I'm not talking about weight loss, either, though this plan will help your body naturally find its hormone-healthiest weight. I use the word *diet* as a shortcut for "a way of eating."

My hope is that this plan will help you to relax about food and create not just a healthier hormone conversation, but a healthier relationship with eating and conversation with your body. I hope you'll embrace the joy of healthy eating in a new way that's expansive, while still learning what foods optimally support your hormone balance and which interfere, which is exactly what we'll explore in this chapter. No more fad diets, cravings, or crashes—just simple, delicious foods, with a plan that's backed by science and powered by nature.

The SAD Situation that Disrupts Hormone Signaling

Let's start with what's getting in the way of hormone health—which usually starts with the Standard American Diet (ironically, the SAD). It's the primary diet in the Western world, and it's responsible for most preventable chronic diseases. Tucked in among the problems it causes are women's hormone conditions. Let's take a closer look at how the SAD—both the foods (and *nonfoods!*) that it serves up and what it depletes us of—is undermining women's hormone and gynecologic health.

Ultra-processed Foods

Ultra-processed foods are the items we find in grocery stores and fast-food restaurants that contain ingredients either not found in nature, or that have been so altered from their original state that they don't resemble anything that could have ever come from a garden. They're engineered by the food industry to have tastes, textures, and ingredients that trigger the reward centers in your brain, leaving you wanting more and more. In other words, they're designed to be addictive and have been recognized by many of the world's leading nutritionists as "drugs." A hallmark of these "foods" is that they're high in calories and low in nutrition—a combo known as "empty calories." Some of us call them *Frankenfoods*. I call them *nonfoods*.

The hazards of ultra-processed foods could fill up a book of their own: up to 90% of chronic diseases may have their roots in the SAD. According to a 2019 study published in the *British Medical Journal*, 60% of the average American's daily diet is composed of them, including, to name a few: chips, ice cream, candy, mass-produced breads and pastries, breakfast cereals, pizza, chicken and fish nuggets, sausages, and basically all fast foods. And the more ultra-processed foods in one's diet, the lower one's average intake is of the good stuff, which may explain the phytonutrient gap I'll soon explain. While ultra-processed foods may seem convenient, there are steep costs and one is your hormone health.

Is All Meat a Problem?

Meat has been part of the human diet since our first ancestor way back when sprouted canine teeth. In every culture in the world, hunting and fishing have been a part of how we survived. The problem with meat is severalfold: overconsumption, reduced quality, and environmental contamination with chemicals and pharmaceuticals that are hazardous to our hormones. Excessive meat intake, particularly red meat, even the high-quality grass-fed, antibiotic-free stuff, can negatively impact your hormone balance. Even moderate red meat intake (more than once per week) can increase estrogen levels to harmful amounts, explaining in part why greater meat consumption is a risk factor for endometriosis, uterine fibroids, obesity, heavy menstruation, abnormal uterine bleeding, cyclic breast lumps and pain, and numerous reproductive organ cancers.

The Harvard Nurses' Health Study found that, among women in their thirties with no prior fertility problems, those in the highest meat consumption group were 40% more likely to experience ovulatory dysfunction; in fact, eating just one serving of red meat on a daily basis was associated with a 32% increased risk of ovulatory problems. Endometriosis rates are higher in women who eat more red meat and less fish and vegetables. Increased inflammatory markers, including one called *homocysteine*, have been associated with a 33% increased risk of ovulating

Inflammation: The Deepest Root

Inflammation is a process in which the immune system gets mobilized to protect you against foreign bodies (a splinter, viruses and bacteria, injuries, chemicals, toxins). It's meant to be a short-lived response—the injury or invader is neutralized, and the body heals the damage. When inflammation becomes chronic or systemic (versus local), it causes damage and with it symptoms and disrupted physiologic functioning. Inflammation plays a role in most if not all of the symptoms and conditions we're talking about together.

It can impact ovarian health, ovulation, fertility, and implantation; it's part of the underlying immune disruption causing tissue damage and pain in endometriosis; it's a cause of the insulin resistance and high androgens causing PCOS; it causes PMS and menstrual cramps; it plays a role in uterine fibroids and chronic pelvic pain; and it's linked to depression, anxiety, and difficulty losing weight.

There's a long list of reasons that inflammation goes awry. On that list are: Processed foods, added sugars, poor-quality oils, artificial ingredients, and artificial sweeteners are culprits; in addition to more that you'll learn about in upcoming chapters. What you eat day in and day out profoundly influences your epigenetics, the areas around your genes that affect your susceptibility to a wide range of conditions, including PCOS, endometriosis, and fertility. But your family health history doesn't have to be your destiny. Food is information for your cells: the right foods provide you with the right information; the wrong foods can disrupt your hormones at every turn.

only sporadically. Another study found that red meat consumption correlated to poorer outcomes with IVF.

Further, to be profitable, the meat industry wants to raise the biggest, fattest animals as quickly as possible. They do this with antibiotics, more of which are used for this purpose in cattle than are used for infections in humans, and growth hormones. As a result, measurable amounts of each end up in your meat and impact your body weight. Diets that are higher in meat are usually lower in overall nutrient and fiber consumption, driving the growth of a less hormone-friendly microbiome and more inflammation. Processed meats, red meat, and ham, even in small amounts, have been linked to measurable increases in inflammatory markers in the blood, and insulin resistance. And get this: some processed meats are categorized as carcinogens by the FDA!

The Skinny on Fats

Good fat, bad fat? High fat, low fat? Sounds like a Dr. Seuss rhyme, doesn't it?

Fat phobia is a real thing, caused by decades of fat fearmongering by the FDA. But fat is an essential building block of your sex hormones as well as cortisol, produced through reactions that use cholesterol, made from fat. You have to eat fat to produce your hormones. Women on very low-fat diets, as well as those who exercise excessively or are underweight, are more likely to experience ovulatory problems and infertility. Women with PCOS who are low in healthy fats and protein are more likely to struggle with insulin resistance and elevated androgens.

Fats provide a sense of satiety, are energy dense, support blood sugar balance, and provide an essential building block needed for hormone production—cholesterol. But the fats that most Americans are getting as part of the daily diet aren't the healthy kinds. They're pro-

inflammatory; getting the right ones you need for hormone health, and avoiding the harmful ones, is key.

Trans fats. In league with *Frankenfoods*, trans fats are industrially manufactured by pumping hydrogen into vegetable oils, called *hydrogenation*, to create a solid fat that is rancidity resistant, giving foods that contain them an unnaturally long shelf life. They're so harmful that some states have banned their use! They're terribly pro-inflammatory and contribute to virtually every problem I talk about in this book.

The Nurses' Health Study found a strong association between trans fats and endometriosis, versus a lower risk of endometriosis in women who consumed fats from fish and avocados instead. More inflammation also means more pain, so not only is endometriosis more prevalent, it may be more severe, as may be menstrual cramps, depression with PMS, and all the other symptoms and conditions linked to inflammation.

Another study found that for every 2% increase in calories consumed in the form of trans fats (a matter of a couple of tablespoons) in the daily diet, ovulatory infertility increased by more than 70%, the greatest risk occurring when trans fats took the place of hormone-healthy fats in the diet.

Stay away from anything with the term "partially hydrogenated" on the package, all ultra-processed foods, and items such as: commercial pie crusts, boxed pancake mixes, cake mixes, packaged cakes, frozen dairy desserts, half-and-half, cake icing, and microwavable popcorn. Also, avoid all ultra-processed foods and you'll likely be avoiding trans fats.

Vegetable Oils and the Problem of High Omega-6s, Low Omega-3s

Our ancestors ate an abundance of essential fatty acids (EFAs), essential because we don't synthesize them in our bodies—we have to get them from dietary sources. EFAs are needed for hormone production and cell membrane function—and thus healthy hormone signaling. They protect us from inflammation, support immune health, and regulate pain.

Throughout human history, until about the last seventy years, our diets provided an estimated 1:1 ratio of two important types: omega-6 to omega-3. Both omega-6s and omega-3s are important *polyunsaturated fatty acids* (PUFAs), but when omega-6s outweigh omega-3s, it's a setup for inflammation. Our modern diet tipped the balance: now we're getting as much as a 20:1 ratio of 6s to 3s.

Where are the 6s coming from? Vegetable oils including canola, grapeseed, corn, soybean, cottonseed, sesame, peanut, and generic vegetable oil and margarine, most fast foods, and packaged snacks, even some sometimes seemingly healthy ones like most energy and granola bars. Commercially raised beef, poultry, and eggs are also a source (because they're fed a diet high in PUFA containing corn and soy) leading to high tissue levels.

Low omega-3 and high omega-6 levels are associated with dysregulation in the endocannabinoid system, which is linked to insulin resistance and pain. Conditions associated with low omega-6 levels include:

Need Milk? Dairy and Your Hormones

I'm not fanatical about going dairy free; in fact, in some of the Blue Zones—places around the globe with the highest rates of healthy centenarians—yogurt, milk, and some cheeses are part of the daily diet. But dairy products may be one of the most significant routes of human exposure to excess estrogen. Unlike pasture-fed animals a hundred years ago, modern dairy cows are usually kept pregnant or lactating year-round to raise their milk yield, and they continue to lactate during the latter half of each subsequent pregnancy, when the concentration of estrogens in milk is higher. Studies have shown that about 60–80% of estrogens come from milk and dairy products in Western diets. Recently it was found that these compounds even at very low doses may have significant biological effects. For example, a five-year study conducted by the Centers for Disease Control and Prevention (CDC) between 1999 and 2004 found that regular intake of cow's milk in girls five to twelve years of age led to early onset of menstruation in much higher rates than experienced by non-milk-drinkers.

Cow's milk (and related dairy products) contains *insulin-like growth factor 1* (IGF-1), a hormone similar to insulin that stimulates the growth of cells while preventing unhealthy cells from doing what they're supposed to do naturally—die. The dairy industry also allows the use of the growth factor *rbGH*, which amps up IGF-1. IGF-1 is associated with breast and other cancers, and may play a role in uterine fibroid growth.

Low-fat dairy products: According to research from the Harvard School of Public Health, women consuming low-fat dairy products had less success getting pregnant, and there was an association between cream and yogurt intake and increased risk of anovulation and anovulatory infertility. What causes this? It's unclear but likely candidates are the fact that dairy products cause inflammation in about 50% of people who consume them (a

- Anovulation, ovarian dysfunction
- Cyclic breast pain and lumps
- Endometriosis
- Fertility challenges and decreased IVF success
- Heavier menstrual bleeding
- Menstrual pain
- Osteoporosis
- PCOS
- PMS, especially with depression
- Prenatal problems including preterm labor
- Primary ovarian insufficiency

Increasing omega-3s in the diet can reverse problems. How do you ensure a healthy 3:6 ratio and ample 3s in the diet? I'm going to show you in this chapter!

Sorry, Sugar, You've Gotta Go

We're hardwired to love sweets. The sweet taste has been an important stimulus for humans to go in search of nutrient- and energy-rich foods since time immemorial. However, our ancestors' "sweet tooth" was satisfied with the limited sources they had access to, in small amounts, seasonally: berries, roots, tubers, and honey.

The average American now has 24/7 access to not just sugar, but refined sugar, and consumes

protein specifically in cow's-milk dairy products, not in sheep or goat milk,—A1 casein—has been shown to be an inflammatory trigger for endometriosis) and because of the tendency of environmental chemicals, including herbicides, pesticides, persistent organic pollutants (POPs), phthalates (like BPA), PBDEs (more on these in Chapter 10), and others, to bioaccumulate in animal fat, dairy products are often a veritable repository of hormone-disrupting toxins. The link between dairy products and estrogen-related cancer, including endometrial cancer, is well established, as is an association with ovarian cancer.

But don't you need dairy for bone health? While calcium is needed, dairy is not. In one of the most rigorous studies to date, researchers tracked nearly 78,000 women for twelve years and found that those who drank two or more glasses of milk daily broke more bones than women who rarely consumed milk. Those consuming the most vitamin D–rich fish (e.g., salmon and sardines) had a 33% lower risk of hip fracture.

Several studies have shown some benefits to eating dairy: One found a reduced risk in fibroids, a couple of studies showed improved fertility with consumption of three servings of full-fat dairy daily, and another found reduced menstrual pain, also at this daily amount. However, these have been contradictory, with the strongest evidence finding no benefit and most studies concluding that any benefits seen are not from the dairy, but the fact that eating dairy is associated with a higher intake of vitamin D, calcium, and fat—important for hormone health.

Over the next 6 weeks we are going to "86" the dairy, with the exception of ghee. If you love milk in your chai, don't worry, I've got your back. On page 361 I teach you how to make delicious, creamy, nondairy milks—so good that you won't believe they're not the real thing. Concerned about your calcium? Hormone Intelligence eating will meet your needs, and a daily multivitamin will fill in any gaps.

about 160 pounds of sugar and 200 pounds of white flour each year. That's a combined pound a day—far above even what our great-grandparents ate—in their lifetimes! Eighty-one percent of Americans consume more than the highest daily acceptable level of sugar every single day. Breads, sugary drinks, pizza, pasta dishes, and "dairy desserts" like ice cream are the main sources. The problem for your hormones? Something called insulin resistance.

Bear with me as I deep dive into insulin resistance for a minute; it's important to know about, as it affects over 80 million Americans, about a quarter of us, and it has a profound effect on inflammation and hormone health. And lest you think so, you don't have to be overweight to be affected. "Normal weight" women are 40% more likely to suffer from chronic diseases as a result of metabolic problems and chronic inflammation that can be traced to insulin resistance.

Insulin resistance is a state in which your cells have become insensitive to the hormone insulin. When this happens, they can't take sugar up into your cells like they're supposed to and you end up with high blood sugar, which is inflammatory and damaging to your cells and blood vessels, and is a major player in many gynecologic conditions.

There's a special role for insulin resistance in PCOS. When your cells no longer respond to insulin, it has nowhere to go, so it remains in circulation. This triggers the ovaries to produce androgens and inhibits the liver from producing sex-hormone-binding globulin (SHBG), whose job it is to bind extra hormones. The result is increased free testosterone—and PCOS. Through a process called *aromatization*, extra androgens are also converted to estrogen. High estrogen and testosterone levels confuse signaling between the pituitary and the ovaries so that your ovaries get stimulated to produce follicles but not to ovulate—one of

the core problems of PCOS. Between 50 and 70% of women with PCOS demonstrate measurable insulin resistance beyond that which would be expected by their body weight or degree of obesity. I describe additional symptoms and problems associated with anovulation on page 68. Of note though, low progesterone and high estrogen are a setup for fertility problems and can contribute to endometriosis.

Insulin resistance goes hand in glove with disruptions in metabolic hormones we don't dive into in this book: leptin, ghrelin, and adiponectin. But it's important to note this can lead to sugar cravings, binge eating, and weight gain, while preventing you noticing when you feel full. Elevated leptin also disrupts ovulation. It's high leptin levels that partly explain why women with PCOS can spend years battling their weight and binge eating disorder.

There's just no other way to say it: Sugar is addictive and we have all been strategically targeted by Big Food to be sugar addicts. You do not have to be its victim anymore! To balance your energy and your hormones, refined sugar and refined carbs have to go. But you have to be careful with less obvious choices that might seem healthy, for example, some smoothies and fresh-pressed fruit and even veggie juices can pack a shocking wallop of hidden and even natural sugar. My patient Kiki was skipping breakfast and lunch, instead going to a juice bar on her way to work, thinking she was making a healthy choice. When we looked online at the ingredients together, we discovered that each "healthy shake" contained over 30 grams of sugar—six teaspoons per smoothie! Nut milks and nut-milk beverages, specialty bottle teas, and other health-food beverages can be similarly sugar loaded—and they're expensive! Check labels before drinking!

Artificial sweeteners are not a hormone-healthy alternative. Even just one week of using them led to an increased risk for developing Hashimoto's, in one study. Studies have also found a harmful impact of artificial sweeteners on the gut microbiome, which as you'll learn in Chapter 9 is central to hormone balance.

Avoid the "-ols," sweet-tasting alcohol sugars hidden in many foods, including popular functional food nutrition bars. They're used to sweeten foods without the calories. Xylitol is an example you're probably familiar with. They're an IBS trigger, and may be particularly problematic for women with premenstrual bloating or endometriosis. One study found that eating 50 grams of xylitol or 75 grams of erythritol led to bloating and diarrhea in 70% and 65% of people respectively.

Are natural sweeteners okay? Natural sweeteners, including honey, maple syrup, date sugar, coconut sugar, and stevia (if made from 100% stevia leaf, no solvents used to extract it) all have their place in a healthy diet when you're feeling great. You won't find much of these in the meal plans, though you will find some treats that I feel are fine to enjoy once a week, or if you need something sweet during your premenstrual phase, because as you now know, mentally and emotionally, restricting isn't good for you—or for sticking with a plan. There's also the occasional recipe that includes a teaspoon of maple syrup or honey to round out the taste. However, this is always an optional ingredient; omit it if any sugar just leads you to crave more.

The Weight of the Matter

For most of us, that number on the scale (or our clothing size) is a major self-esteem buzzkill—unless it's where we want it to be. But those goals are often based on unrealistic, false standards that have nothing to do with health. So I'm loath to even bring up the topic of weight.

The fact is we can enjoy glorious, sumptuous health at many different sizes and shapes.

But, much like there's evidence that being underweight or having low body fat can lead to hormone problems, there's also evidence of problems that can arise when a woman is substantially overweight, particularly problems that result from excess estrogen and insulin resistance. For example:

- High body fat is a major trigger of premature puberty, triggering breast development and menstruation, as well as elevated leptin levels, setting young girls up for problems with inflammation and confused hormonal messaging around hunger and fullness.

- As BMI climbs over 25, studies show that women experience reduced egg and uterine lining quality, take a longer time to get pregnant, and once pregnant, are more likely to experience pregnancy complications including a greater risk of early and recurrent miscarriages, gestational diabetes, preeclampsia, and a slightly higher risk of preterm birth.

- As weight goes up, chances of IVF working go down in women pursuing fertility treatment. These effects are exclusive of whether a woman has PCOS, though they are more pronounced when there is PCOS.

- A high BMI is also associated with increased risk for fibroid development, more severe perimenopausal symptoms, and breast cancer.

The upside is that these are all reversible. In one study, by losing an average of 22.5 pounds, 90% of women with anovulatory cycles resumed ovulation, and their menstrual cycles normalized. In another study, women struggling with PCOS and obesity had dramatic improvement in fertility when lifestyle changes and weight loss were undertaken before starting fertility treatment with Clomid.

There are tremendously complicated factors that lead to women being both under- and overweight, and I want to make something very clear: none of them are your "fault." We live in a society that, on the one hand, creates horrible pressure on women to be thin and perfect, while creating an environment that has itself been described as "obesogenic," meaning that our food, environmental toxin exposures, stress, lack of sleep, trauma history, microbiome disruption, sedentary lifestyles, and hormonal problems themselves all contribute to struggles we have with our weight. The total ecology in which women live is giving our brains and bodies mixed messages. And it plays out in our hormones—and weight. We're going to shift all that together.

Soda, Wine, and Coffee, Oh My!

Staying hydrated is one of the six pillars of the Hormone Intelligence Diet. But sometimes we don't hydrate optimally. I don't mean to be a party pooper here, but have a read so you know why sodas, alcohol, and coffee aren't part of the six-week plan.

Soft Drinks

Sugar-sweetened beverages are a risk factor for a number of hormonal problems; fertility problems rise to the top. A 2018 study published in *Epidemiology*, which surveyed 3,828 women aged 21 to 45 living in the United States or Canada and 1,045 of their male partners, found that drinking one or more sugar-sweetened beverage daily—by either partner—is associated with a decreased chance of conception by 25 and 33%, respectively, per month for women and men. According to the Harvard Nurses' Health Study, women who consumed two or more sodas a day were up to 50% more likely to experience ovulatory infertility than women who drank less than one soda a week, while another study found that drinking one sugar-sweetened beverage daily—by either partner—was associated with a 20% reduction in fertility. Of note, energy drinks have been related to even larger reductions in fertility. Remember, ovulatory infertility doesn't just affect women trying to get pregnant; if you're not ovulating, that affects your total hormone picture, including your cycle length, regularity, how much you bleed with each period, and how much it hurts!

Studies link soft drink consumption with premature puberty, and there's more. Women who drink more than one cup of soda daily have been found to have a 15% higher estradiol concentration than those who don't drink soda. Perhaps this in part explains why a study of over 23,000 women found that those who consumed the most sugar-sweetened beverages, compared with women who consumed the least, had a 78% higher risk for endometrial cancer. Given that women with anovulation, and particularly those with PCOS, are also at increased risk, it's just one more reason for women to avoid sugar-sweetened beverages.

Red Wine: It's Good for Me, Right?

Enjoying a drink once in a while, even up to once a week, may be no problem if your hormones aren't giving you too much trouble, but, sorry to say, even that perfect organic cabernet from Northern California or Southern France, even when consumed in moderation, can impact your hormones. If you're trying to get your hormones in balance, alcohol might not be your best pal for now. Here's what we know:

- Elevated estradiol levels have been found after alcohol consumption, with persistently high levels in the luteal phase, which can lead to increased breast symptoms, heavier periods, and more menstrual cramping.

- Even mild to moderate alcohol intake on a regular basis has been associated with hormonal changes including more period pain, and decreasing intake can reverse it.

- Regular alcohol intake has been associated with hormone imbalances and weight problems that are associated with increased risk of developing PCOS, fertility problems, uterine fibroids, and more severe menopausal symptoms.

- There's increased risk of nonalcoholic fatty liver disease (NAFLD) in women with PCOS even from small amounts of alcohol intake.

- Regular drinking has also been associated with endometriosis.

- Alcohol, especially beer, also appears to be associated with an increased risk of developing fibroids.

- Drinking alcohol depletes nutrients necessary for ovarian function including B vitamins, selenium, and zinc.

Although studies on alcohol and fertility are contradictory (a few studies have found increased fertility after light wine drinking, while another found that wine, but not beer or spirits, slightly reduces fertility), a convincing number of studies suggest that even low to moderate alcohol intake may negatively affect fertility. Pooled data from nineteen studies involving 98,657 reproductive-age women found that, in relation to nondrinkers, any amount of regular drinking was significantly associated with a 13% reduction in time it took to get pregnant, whereas moderate to heavy drinking led to a 23% reduction.

The International Agency for Research on Cancer estimates that for every alcohol-containing drink consumed by a woman daily, her risk of breast cancer goes up 7%; a woman who consumes two to three drinks a day has a lifetime risk of about 15 to 25% increase over those who don't drink. Alcohol is also inflammatory for the gut, disrupts your microbiome, and impairs liver function—affecting all your root cause pathways that you're trying to repair and restore.

Note that your cycles may influence when and how much you drink; studies now suggest that women are more inclined to drink in the luteal phase (duh—researchers could just ask women instead of doing these studies!), that luteal phase brain changes make us *enjoy* the alcohol more, and that they may also affect your mood more than drinking in the follicular phase (no, drinking in the follicular phase instead is not the solution!). When you lean in for a drink to make you feel more relaxed and sexier, remember that alcohol itself is a depressant, and drinking in the second half of your cycle might worsen anxiety and depression during this phase. If you're already someone who struggles with PMS, this can make it worse.

Do you have to become a complete teetotaler forever? That will be up to you. If you do have a drink, pay close attention to how you feel after—and the next day. Puffy face? Fingers? Irritable or blue mood? A sure sign that alcohol is not a bestie for your hormones right now.

Coffee Break? Or Coffee Breakup?

There's a reason I've saved coffee for last. It's the one recommendation (aside from 86-ing the alcohol) I give that I sometimes hear my patients groan over, or say, *I'll give up anything, Dr. Romm, but not the coffee!* We do love our coffee. So much so that 90% of women drink *at least* one cup a day. Often, it's not even for the taste. In fact, most women, to make coffee tasty, add coffee's playmates: sugar and cream or milk, upsetting blood sugar balance, creating insulin resistance, and possibly getting a slow steady drip of unhealthy fats in your diet.

So why are we drinking it? Because so many of us are so freakin' exhausted trying to keep up with it all—and it's a pleasure boost that helps us to get through. We love the energy caffeine gives us, especially when we're not sleeping as well as we'd like, and we love the focus it gives us that keeps us on target and on time with the projects we're all juggling.

I'm not opposed to coffee; in fact, it has strong cognitive health benefits, especially as we get older. The problem is that there are downsides for your energy, mood, and hormones—the anxiety, jitteriness, and blood sugar crashes that come an hour or two after we drink it, and the overstimulation we feel when we're trying to get to sleep at night. And the hidden effects. A study published in the *American Journal of Clinical Nutrition* tells us that caffeine levels from just a few cups of coffee can increase our risk of hormonal conditions. For some reason, in some white women, coffee leads to lowered estrogen levels, which can predispose them to decreased fertility, menstrual cycle irregularities, sleep disruptions, and over time possibly even bone health. In Black and Asian women, the same amount of caffeine may cause elevated estrogen levels, which can lead to symptoms of estrogen excess in some women—breast pain, heavier periods, migraines as estrogen levels plummet premenstrually—reminding us that we also can't take a one-size-fits-all approach to our dietary choices.

Caffeine also affects your sleep. Caffeine, even as much as six hours before bed, can have significant disruptive effects on nighttime rest.

As you'll learn in Chapter 8, you can't reset your hormones without high-quality sleep, and enough of it.

Coffee intake can rob your body of calcium and other nutrients you need for ovulation, fertility, and hormone health. Numerous studies have been done on coffee and fertility, and there's a lot of conflicting information. The overarching data suggests that a cup of coffee per day probably doesn't affect fertility, including IVF. However, we do know that caffeine can increase our stress hormones, jack our blood sugar, and lead to insulin resistance, all of which can aggravate PCOS, which in turn affects fertility. Some studies have also linked over 100 mg of caffeine in coffee daily in early pregnancy with increased miscarriage risk.

Many women find that coffee causes PMS and monthly painful breasts, and it worsens their hot flashes. One study found that caffeinated beverage intake increased the incidence and severity of PMS in a study of college-age women. That's because it causes the release of stress hormones. And one common question I get about coffee is "Does coffee cause cramps?" Very few studies have looked at the impact of coffee on menstrual pain symptoms, but one study found a very significant correlation. I can tell you from my clinical practice that I see a very strong association, and interestingly, the only time in my life that I personally experienced menstrual cramps was in medical residency—when I was drinking coffee to keep up with all-nighters. While I might attribute the pain to the stress of residency and lack of sleep, the cramps immediately went away in the following month after I gave up the liquid fuel! Kicking the coffee habit means you're not starting your day with these potential hormone-disrupting ingredients or getting a slow drip of them with additional cups of coffee throughout the day.

Freaking out a little at the thought of giving

up coffee? I feel you—and I promise you that while there may be three or four initial days in which you go through some coffee withdrawal, if you stay hydrated, practice some simple bedtime and morning self-care, and stick with the meal plans, within five days you'll start to feel better, and within a week you'll have more energy than you've had in years, with better sleep, clearer thinking, and happier blood sugar.

Wait, what about Bulletproof and similar coffee products? Nope. While adding saturated fat to your coffee may slow your caffeine jag a little, that extra daily dose of saturated fat can be enough to cause unhealthy cholesterol levels (I've seen that happen more than once!)—and you're still getting the same amount of caffeine. Want a delicious coffee alternative? Try one of my favorite recipes on page 369.

What We're Missing: The Phytonutrient Gap

The problem isn't just the hormone-harming food exposures we're getting; it's what we're not getting that our body requires for creating hormone health and for buffering the impact of environmental and dietary exposures on our hormone health. As a result of this, and massive changes that have taken place in the SAD over the past 60 years, at least 80% of Americans are not getting the daily nutrients they need for even basic health from their diet.

Phytonutrients and phytochemicals (*phyto* comes from the Greek word meaning "plant") are plant-based elements we require not only for nutrients, but for detoxification, protection against inflammation, and DNA repair. Over 25,000 phytochemicals have been identified to date and include compounds like polyphenols, proanthocyanidins, and carotenoids, and they're only in fruits, vegetables, grains, legumes, nuts, and seeds. The *phytonutrient gap* describes the difference between what you need to get for optimal health and what you're getting—and most of us aren't getting enough of what we need for optimal hormone signaling.

A large study done by the US Centers for Disease Control and Prevention (CDC) found that in every state in the US, less than 16% of people are getting the amount of fruits and vegetables they need for basic health, 75% of women do not meet current adequate intakes for calcium, and 90% of women have inadequate intakes of folate and vitamin E from food sources alone. Keep in mind the CDC standards are based on bare-bones minimums for preventing disease—not nearly the amounts needed for *optimal* health. We deserve to go for the gold—optimum health!

Here's just a short list of the nutrients most American women are typically low in according to 2009 statistics from the US Department of Agriculture:

- Vitamin E
- Folate
- Calcium
- Magnesium
- Zinc
- Vitamin B6
- Iron
- Vitamin B1

Everything from when we start our first menstrual cycles to how quickly and easily we get pregnant once we start trying, to our age at menopause, can be positively—or adversely—affected by our level of fruit and vegetable consumption. Here's just a bit of the study data on this:

- Women eating a primarily plant-based diet with high-quality fats, plenty of fresh vegetables, some fruit, high-quality fiber, and some eggs (if tolerated) were less likely to experience menstrual pain.

- Following a vegetarian diet for just two cycles reduced menstrual cramp duration and severity, regulated hormone levels, and improved weight loss to the tune of almost four pounds on average.

- Higher blood levels of folate from eating more green veggies were associated with higher luteal phase progesterone levels; this translates into more regular periods, higher levels of fertility, and better moods and sleep.

- Healthy protein intake improves ovulation in women with anovulatory cycles and improves AMH (anti-Müllerian hormone), important for women who are trying to conceive, and also a sign that ovarian function is healthier, meaning it can prevent primary ovarian insufficiency and improve fertility.

- A diet rich in fruits, vegetables, and omega-3 fatty acids from fish, and containing ample calcium and vitamin D is connected with lower risk of developing endometriosis; higher intake of red meat, coffee, and trans fats appears to increase risk.

- A 2004 study published in the journal *Human Reproduction* found that women who consumed three or more servings of fruit per day recorded a 14% lower likelihood of developing endometriosis than women who consumed one portion or less daily.

- Women who consumed one or more servings of citrus fruits daily dropped their risk of endometriosis by over 20% compared with those who consumed citrus fruits only once a week.

- Higher rates of anovulatory infertility have been seen in women with heavier meat-based diets than in those who consumed plant proteins, while decreasing animal protein in the diet led to a 50% decrease in the risk of ovulatory infertility.

- Consumption of green vegetables and fruits (especially citrus fruits) is associated with a decreased risk of developing uterine fibroids.

- Women with the highest intake of yellow and green vegetables, and especially fruits like tangerines, persimmons, and oranges, as well as bell peppers and butternut squash, which contain a special chemical called β-cryptoxanthin that increases our vitamin A—found to extend women's reproductive life span and health span—are the least likely to experience early menopause, according to several large studies conducted around the world, including one with over 30,000 women. This is significant; for each year of earlier onset of menopause, women experience a 2% increased likelihood of death due to cardiovascular disease.

- Lower intake of fruits and leafy green vegetables is associated with premature loss of ovarian reserve, found in 10% of women experiencing difficulty conceiving by their mid-thirties.

The Hormone Intelligence Diet is designed to bridge the phytonutrient gap, giving you the rainbow of veggies and fruits you need each day to take back your hormone health.

How to Eat for Hormone Health: Six Hormone Intelligence Food Principles

Eating for hormone health involves six simple steps that will become second nature for you. You'll start to make your food choices in the context of asking yourself two simple questions: What kind of information is this food going to give me? Is this going to give me the information that's going to make me feel as fabulous as I deserve to feel? You'll start saying yes to only the ones that do. And you'll never want to go back to anything else, because you'll notice how fantastic you feel (and look!).

Step 1: Eat Real Foods Only

The one unequivocal commitment I ask you to make over the next six weeks is to **nourish your body** with a commitment to eating only healthful, real foods, in a wide variety—as you'll learn more about in a minute. In a nutshell: the closer a food is to how it looks in nature, the healthier and the fewer ingredients, the better. If you think about it, real food doesn't have "ingredients"—it's just the food. Eating only real food also means going mostly

How to Quit the Sugar Habit

- Toss all the sugar-laden items that are hanging around—in your pantry, fridge and freezer, and the back of that drawer! Avoid sugar traps, like your colleague's M&M bowl that you pass on the way to the ladies' room. Take another route, or just step away from the candy (remember your WHY!).

- Make it a habit to keep your blood sugar steady at all times with the meal plans, and a snack if you need it.

- Get enough sleep and manage your stress (we're all over this in the next two chapters).

- Always have healthy snack alternatives on hand and if you just "have to have" something sweet, have some dark chocolate (yes, you can keep that in the back of your desk drawer!), berries, or believe it or not, some nuts or a hard-boiled egg, because protein can kick the sugar craving.

- Hydrate—we often confuse thirst hunger for a craving.

- Sublimate: Have a list of activities other than eating that you can do, like take a walk, dance, step away from a task that's boring or stressing you, and so on.

After just a week, you're going to have more energy and better moods. You'll think more clearly and feel more steady all day long. You'll sleep better. Your sugar and junk food cravings will disappear. You'll lose unwanted pounds. You won't be bloated. You're going to get rid of those awful cramps. Your blood sugar will be so steady and sleep so much better that you won't need to turn to it for quick energy, either.

organic (as much as possible), so that you're eating a low body burden diet, free of pesticides, residues, and food additives. You'll learn why this is important in Chapter 10, but we're not going to wait until then to get started.

Step 2: Rock-Steady Energy (and Blood Sugar)

Protein, fats, and slow-burning carbohydrates ("slow carbs") are your steady energy rock stars. In the right amounts, at the right times, they keep your blood sugar steady and your energy humming, while preventing sugar cravings and 3 p.m. energy crashes and stopping you from ever getting "hangry" again.

When your blood sugar is balanced, so is everything else—your energy, gut health, nervous system (and mood), immune system, and your hormones. Steady blood sugar is important for healthy cortisol levels, which you'll learn about in the next chapter. It also prevents and reverses *insulin resistance*, a major problem for your hormone health.

Step 3: Eat More Plants

"Eating your vegetables" is a big deal when it comes to hormone health, and you're going to be seriously bumping up your intake of leafy greens, berries, and a variety of brightly colored, fresh, vibrant fruits and veggies. They're pure nutrient warehouses, filled with the vitamins, minerals, and fiber your body needs for thousands of hormone-related functions, 24/7.

While this is not a vegetarian or vegan diet plan, plants are the heart and soul of it— because they're what create glowing wellness. If you are vegan or vegetarian, there are modified plans for you that make this plan easy to follow, and if you're open to adding fish or eggs, you can modify the meal plans by mixing and matching with the many vegan and vegetarian options in Part Four.

Step 4: Hydrate Enough and Wisely

Many of us are chronically underhydrated, sipping coffee and tea throughout the day, but forgetting our most important beverage for cellular health: water. Not drinking enough water leads us to feel more fatigued and increases our inflammation, and even mild dehydration has been found to negatively impact problem solving, mood, and attention and to increase sensitivity to pain, cause headaches and muscle cramps, and possibly to affect cervical mucus viscosity, leading to problems with fertility, in particular, the ability of sperm to navigate thicker cervical mucus and reach their destination. We may also confuse thirst for hunger, leading us to nosh when what we need is to hydrate. Just in it for vanity? Studies compared the impact of taking collagen versus drinking on skin health and wrinkling: water not only surpassed collagen's effects hands down, but the benefits of water drinking were ongoing whereas collagen benefits didn't continue with continued use.

Step 5: Indulge Now and Then (The 95/5 Rule)

It's a scientific fact: our brains rebel against overrestriction. Overrestriction sets you up for failure. It raises your cortisol and makes you more likely, not less likely, to "binge out." Therefore, please, indulge now and then. Just use the 95/5 Rule. Eat the "YES" foods for Hormone Intelligence 95% of the time. Then 5% of the time, eat whatever-the-hell-you-want-to with these caveats: it's real food and preferably doesn't include alcohol. Mathematically speaking, if there are approximately twenty-one meals each week, twenty of those should be from the plan. That gives you one meal each week to play with more freely.

Above all, the 95/5 Rule includes a *no shame, no guilt clause.*

When you do indulge, enjoy it! Ideally, stick within the basic rules of the Hormone Intelligence Diet—to which end I've given you a whole set of **Healthy Indulgences** (sounds so naughty, and they're so good) recipes right in this book. They do include some honey, maple syrup, or coconut sugar, and of course, chocolate (after all, I wouldn't have survived as a women's hormone expert if I didn't consider dark chocolate a food group of its own)!

Eating for Hormone Intelligence 101

The Hormone Intelligence Diet is remarkably simple; it's the way of eating I personally live by and have taught to over 10,000 women, many of whom say it changed their lives. Here's the overview, which you don't even need to plan for, because it's all in the Hormone Intelligence meal plans that are done for you:

Every MEAL should include:

- 1 serving of protein (i.e., essential fatty acid–rich, low-mercury fish, poultry, eggs, legumes, or beans)
- 1 serving of healthy fats (avocado, olive oil, coconut oil, ghee)
- 1 to 2 servings of veggies, fruits, or a combination

Plus every DAY you'll enjoy:

- 6 to 8 servings of vegetables, and up to 2 servings of fruit
- 1 to 2 servings of slow carbs, which could include a grain or an "energy veggie" (see page 122)
- Nuts and seeds (or nut or seed butters)
- Water

Several times WEEKLY you'll enjoy:

- A portion of lacto-fermented veggies (see page 125)

Every WEEK make sure you're getting a wide variety for foods:

- Ask yourself, am I changing it up?
- Eat a variety of different colors and textures and flavors
- If you want one, enjoy 1 Healthy Indulgence (starting on page 364)

Using these guidelines, meal planning becomes easy, and eventually, very intuitive. You'll instinctually reach for a protein and a fat when you're hungry, you'll keep a rotating bounty of vegetables and fruits and grains at the ready. Your body will reward you by feeling amazing and symptom free. Starting on page 116, we'll unpack each of the categories of the Hormone Intelligence Diet, and I'll walk you through your tips to success. Then you'll be on your way!

Step 6: Be Kind to Yourself

I want to acknowledge something that I think a lot of books and practitioners minimize: making dietary changes is not simple for everyone. We all have deeply powerful personal, social, emotional, and physical relationships with and drives to food that are practically hardwired in. You may have a history of anorexia or other personal associations with food that are painful or challenging. I get that. Go gently and listen to your inner wisdom about what's best for you. Take it slowly, and consider creating a group of women to go through the plan with—that can often make it easier.

Most of us were also not raised to understand the connection between our food and how we feel day to day. Eating well shouldn't be so hard, but our preferences and tastes are often based on what we were fed at home growing up. So yeah, sometimes it might feel hard in the moment not to eat something. But you're worth it!

Real life also somehow manages to "happen" just when we set out on a new self-care plan. You get stuck at work unexpectedly and have to eat what's brought in. It's your kid's birthday and you have a piece of cake. There's the fight with your sweetie and two glasses of wine, the holiday dinner and Grandma's cookies, the bachelorette party or night out with the girls—and who-know-what happens—and of course, there are the five days before your period that derail your best-laid plans. One of the most important aspects of the Hormone Intelligence Plan is working with the rhythms of your life, another is self-compassion. That's the best way to "hack" all this. To keep the upper hand, you've got to anticipate life's moves. At the end of this chapter I'm going to give you some troubleshooting tips for when "life happens," but before you jump into those, grab your journal or calendar and write down how life might show up for you in the next six weeks, and plan ahead—trips, work meetings over lunch, that cocktail party, birthday party, and so on.

What to Eat for Hormone Health

Now that you understand the overarching principles of the Hormone Intelligence Diet, let's get granular about the foods you'll be enjoying on your journey to hormone balance.

Hormone-Healthy Protein Sources

Protein provides a major source of energy, giving you hours of fuel per serving and keeping you feeling satisfied. Feeling sated prevents sugar cravings and binges, and studies show that swapping out empty carbs in the diet for healthy protein can dramatically improve blood sugar and hormone balance, helping to reverse PCOS symptoms, improve ovulation in women with anovulatory cycles, and improve AMH (anti-Müllerian hormone), important for women who are trying to conceive and also a sign that ovarian function is healthier, meaning it can prevent primary ovarian insufficiency. Protein-rich foods also provide amino acids and sulfur-rich compounds, the building blocks we need to make compounds used in detoxification, and for producing the neurotransmitters that support our mood and prevent and reverse PMS and depression.

The type of proteins you eat matters. Here are the best choices.

Fish

Omega-3 fats, which are found abundantly in fatty fish like salmon, have numerous benefits for hormonal and gynecologic health, including improved ovulation and progesterone levels, decreased premenstrual symptoms and pain, reduction in the risk of developing endometriosis, and less need to take ibuprofen for endometriosis pain. Your hormones take a hit when you don't get enough and the right balance of essential fatty acids in your diet, particularly the omega-3s, and this may especially impact fertility, period pain, and endometriosis.

Among women trying to conceive naturally, a diet higher in seafood leads to greater fertility. In a study of 500 couples tracking their time to conception based on fish intake, women who ate more than eight servings of fish per menstrual cycle were 40 to 60% more likely to conceive compared to women who rarely ate seafood. The greatest benefits occurred when both partners in a couple ate eight or more servings per fertility cycle. It may also prevent complications of pregnancy including preterm birth and preeclampsia. Higher intake of omega-3-rich foods, or supplementation, may also prevent or reduce menopausal symptoms and postmenopausal osteoporosis.

The mechanism by which EPA and DHA decrease menstrual and endometriosis pain is by decreasing prostaglandin E2 and prostaglandin F2α production, therefore reducing inflammation within the uterine lining. This is also why numerous small studies have shown that eating fish two to three times per week—especially loading up on salmon or sardines, which are the richest in omega-3s (and the lowest in heavy metal contamination)—or taking about 1 to 2 grams of omega-3 fish oil per day can prevent and reduce menstrual pain in just three months. While fresh fish is ideal if you can get (and afford!) it, frozen salmon and water- or olive-oil-packed canned salmon or anchovies are also healthy choices. Just make sure they have no salt added.

The Hormone Intelligence Diet includes low-mercury, omega-3-rich fish three times a week. If you don't eat fish, make sure to include a fish- or algae-based EFA product in your supplement "daily dose." Though this doesn't provide protein, it can bridge the EFA gap and keep your hormones in well-oiled health.

Eggs

Eggs are one of the most nutritious foods on the planet. And no, they don't cause high cholesterol. With a side of veggies, they're a quick,

Hold the Mercury!

Mercury is harmful to your hormones, and a lot of fish are high in this common contaminant in rivers, lakes, and the ocean. A study on fish consumption and fertility illustrates this: in a study comparing time to conception in women eating fish in Sweden (which is considered to have some of the lowest-mercury waters) to those eating fish from Lake Ontario, notoriously contaminated with heavy metals, the women in the Lake Ontario group had a longer time to conception. All seafood now has some mercury so it's important for all women, especially those trying to conceive (or pregnant), to eat ONLY fish with the lowest mercury levels. Omega-3 supplements from reliable companies are rigorously tested to also provide the lowest possible heavy-metal contamination. Some of the fish that contain the least mercury and the most omega-3 are: salmon (fresh and canned), anchovies, and sardines.

complete, and easy meal unto themselves, versatile enough to have at breakfast, lunch, or dinner. If you eat both the white and the yolk, they're also a rich source of brain-, cell-, and hormone-healthy fats and nutrients. They've been shown to improve insulin sensitivity—no surprise as they create a great feeling of energy balance. They're a frequent flyer in the Hormone Intelligence Diet, but I do provide alternatives if you can't eat them. If you're trying to conceive, eggs are an important source of choline, needed for baby's brain growth—learn more on page 288.

Beans, Beans, They're Good for Your . . . Hormones

Legumes and beans are plant-based sources of protein that also provide powerful protective phytoestrogens (see page 123) that block and reduce the effects of hormone-disrupting environmental chemicals and also eliminate breakdown products of estrogen, keeping hormone levels healthier. They're rich in zinc, folate, and amino acids needed to support detoxification. Eating legumes two to three times/week, which is built into the meal plans, improves blood sugar and weight without even dieting or increasing exercise. How's that for simple! Canned or precooked bottled beans can be used; make sure to purchase organic products with no salted added. If you're preparing dried beans, soak them prior to cooking to prevent gas, and season all beans with cumin, oregano, or other aromatic spices, as you'll see in Part Four recipes.

Nuts and Seeds

Nuts and seeds are incredibly hormone healthy. Almonds, pecans, and walnuts can prevent and reverse high cholesterol and promote heart health and are an important part of any plan to reduce insulin resistance. Seeds have many powerful benefits for hormone health, including providing some hormone-regulating effects, and they include ovary-nourishing nutrients like selenium and zinc. Nuts and seeds provide a delicious, quick source of healthful protein and fat. You'll find recipes and quick snacks that include nuts and seeds in Part Four.

Poultry and Red Meat

Meat is more of a complement than a main attraction in the Hormone Intelligence Diet, but it does have an important role in supporting women's health and is thus included sparingly. PMS is more common in women with low iron, and low iron may also be a problem for women with heavy periods, heavy bleeding from fibroids, or a history of iron-deficiency anemia. Poultry and red meat are a quick, easy source of iron. Meats are also rich in vitamins B6 and B12, zinc, selenium, and the metabolism-boosting nutrient coenzyme Q10, all important for healthy ovulation, fertility, and thyroid function. You won't be eating a lot of meat on the diet, but when you do, take care to treat yourself to the highest-quality options if you can. Do your best to use only ethically and ecologically raised antibiotic-free, grass-fed, meats. They're better for you, the animals, and the planet.

Hormone-Healthy Fats

It's time to let go of fat phobia. Fat's bad rep comes from decades of misleading information from the nutrition and diet industry. High-quality fats are a mainstay of hormone production and balance. Without fat, you can't produce estrogen, progesterone, testosterone, and cortisol. Fats are also essential components of cellular membranes, including those in your nervous system, so they're essential for a healthy mind and healthy moods. One study found a marked reduction in pain after just three months of treatment with omega-3 fatty acids, so much so that the women in the study were able to decrease use of pain medication after just three months of supplementing this nutrient that most of us are low in. Women with a high omega-3 PUFA (polyunsaturated fatty acids) intake also have a lower risk for endometriosis. Researchers from the Harvard School of Public Health monitored the fat consumption of 147 women undergoing IVF treatment and discovered that those who ate the highest amounts of monounsaturated fat were 3.4 times more likely to have a child after IVF. They concluded that avocados contain the best kind of monounsaturated fat while saturated fat was found to decrease the number of "good eggs." And high-quality fats do not make you fat—it takes healthy fats to burn fat.

Healthy fats also help you:

- Feel satisfied and full after meals

- Maintain steady energy and blood sugar

- Absorb vitamins A, D, E, and K

The best choices include a variety of mono-unsaturated, polyunsaturated, and saturated fats, as well as essential fatty acids.

Olive Oil: My go-to daily oil is olive oil. I use it in salad dressings, stir-fries, on my greens, and for most of my cooking needs.

Avocados: Rich in monounsaturated fats and magnesium, they can be eaten in an almost endless number of ways, from guacamole to salads, right out of the shell, or, for a pleasant surprise, try the Chocolate Avocado Mousse on page 365.

Nuts and Seeds: A great source of healthful protein, nuts and seeds are also a premium source of hormone-healthy fats. They provide not only an abundance of omega-3s, but a rich, satisfying taste.

Fish: Three 4 oz. servings of high-quality salmon each week can meet all your omega-3 needs. Sardines are another great, high-omega-3 option that are easy to eat and don't require any preparation.

Saturated Fat: In small amounts, organic butter, ghee, or coconut oil are hormone healthy, and ghee is great for gut health (see page 196).

Oils should be cold-pressed, organic, non-GMO, and ideally sold in dark containers to protect them from oxidation (rancidity) due to light exposure; butter and ghee should be organic.

"Slow Carbs"

Carbohydrates (a.k.a. "carbs") are sugars, starches, and fibers found in fruits, grains, vegetables, and dairy products. They're classified as simple or complex based on the type and length of sugars they're made up of.

Energy balance requires a healthy steady rise, not too high, the right amount of insulin, and cells that are sensitive to insulin, allowing it to trigger the cascade of events that shuttle energy into those cells. Complex carbohydrates are found primarily in whole grains, which contain nutrients like B-vitamins, and are rich in fiber. Their complex structure gives them a slow, steady burn that doesn't jack up your blood sugar. Legumes and brown rice also contain resistant starches, indigestible fibers that increase and support healthy gut flora, maintain better blood sugar balance, improve insulin sensitivity, and contribute to easier weight loss.

Refined simple carbs turn into sugar quickly after we eat them and provide only short-lasting energy. They're generally devoid of nutrition, can actually rob nutrients, and can wreak havoc on your blood sugar, leading to insulin resistance.

Let's take a look at the slow carbs that are the mainstays of the Hormone Intelligence Diet.

Whole Grains

Going "against the grain" is trendy, with many "carbophobic" women now eating zero-carb diets. But history shows us that our ancestors got most of their energy not from meat, as the Paleo contingency tells us, but from plant sources rich in natural forms of complex carbohydrates, including roots, berries, and grains, and much of the anti-grain information is fake news from the wellness world.

Slow carbohydrates:

- Provide steady energy

- Are loaded with vitamins and minerals

- Provide healthy fiber

- Feed a healthy microbiome

- Keep cortisol in balance and promote calm moods

Studies also demonstrate that eating complex carbs benefits hormone health.

Eating complex carbs premenstrually **reduces PMS cravings and lifts mood and memory**. A moderate amount of complex carbohydrate intake **improves insulin sensitivity, reduces excess androgens, and restores ovulatory function**. Further, a lot of women with hormone imbalances, especially PMS and PCOS, develop worse symptoms and struggle with a no-carb diet.

A modest reduction in unhealthy carbohydrate intake plus increased protein and healthy fats, without even losing weight, decreased testosterone and inflammatory markers and improved insulin sensitivity. These shifts reverse PCOS symptoms and decrease the long-term medical risks of this condition (page 76). In one study, just eight weeks of improving the carbohydrate balance in the diet led to a 23% **reduction in testosterone** levels, and incidentally improved cholesterol levels, lowering the "bad" kinds and increasing the protective type.

Fertility may be affected by the choice of carbs in your diet; in one study, women who consumed simple carbs like white rice and potatoes were far more likely to suffer from **anovulatory infertility** than women who consumed slow carbs like whole grains, vegetables, and beans. For women undergoing IVF, the data shows those who have higher whole grain consumption enjoy higher live birth rates after correcting for discrepancies in age, race, duration of infertility, and more. A reduction in unhealthy carbs may improve AMH levels and ovulation in women with anovulatory cycles; **improved ovarian function** is associated with fertility and reduced risk of primary ovarian insufficiency (POI).

A low-carb diet triggers the brain's warning signals (see Chapter 7) and may also decrease thyroid function.

According to a 2009 *JAMA Internal Medicine* article, people on a low-carb diet for a year had more anxiety, depression, and anger, believed to be due to the important role of carbohydrates in serotonin production. Further, women placed on a very low-carb diet, in a 2009 study, had decreases in **focus, attention, and memory** after just one week. The good news is that when carbs were reintroduced, cognitive function quickly improved.

Restrictive dieting that limits all carbs tends to backfire for women with hormone imbalances, especially prior to the perimenopausal years. (Many women in perimenopause find that they feel better when they drastically reduce carbs, likely because the decline in estradiol changes metabolism and increases fat storage, which carbs can contribute to.)

Eating whole grains and legumes, even just twice a week, has been shown to **improve weight loss** and—unlike so many diets—keep it off, including **dropping belly fat**.

Eating healthy carbs from grains or energy vegetables about four hours before bed increases your natural production of melatonin, which helps you to fall asleep more easily, increases the amount of time you get deep sleep, and as a result, improves your cortisol curve and hormonal balance (including fertility and excess estrogen clearance), and helps with fat burning.

Fiber keeps your bowels moving, meaning less bloating and constipation, and helps you maintain healthier estrogen levels. Results of a recent meta-analysis suggest that high intake of whole grains might even be inversely associated with a reduced risk of breast cancer.

When we look at the studies on no-carb

Gluten and Your Hormones

While we're talking about carbs, it's the perfect time to talk about one of the most commonly consumed in the Western diet: wheat. It wasn't until about 10 years ago, after switching several of my patients to a gluten-free diet and seeing dramatic results, sometimes in as short as a few weeks, that I dug into the research on gluten and hormonal health.

It turns out that celiac disease, a commonly missed diagnosis, is associated with more than 55 medical conditions, including gynecologic problems. Celiac disease has been associated with delayed onset of the first period, habitually skipped periods, infertility, recurrent miscarriages, endometriosis, Hashimoto's, and early menopause. A substantial number of women have "subclinical" or "silent" celiac disease—meaning no digestive symptoms—have fertility problems. It's also associated with numerous nutritional deficiencies, including protein, fats, zinc, vitamin D, iron, and selenium, that have a direct impact on hormonal and gynecologic conditions, including those I've just mentioned.

A more common condition, nonceliac gluten intolerance (NCGI), though not an autoimmune disease, can also cause gynecologic symptoms. For example, in one study of 207 women with severe endometriosis pain, 75% experienced significant decreases in pain after twelve months on a gluten-free diet. Another study compared 300 women who either went gluten free or took medication; at the end of the study, the group following the gluten-free diet experienced significant reductions in pelvic pain, even without having celiac disease.

While I do not put every patient on a gluten-free diet, it's a simple, worthwhile first-line approach to try and thus is part of Hormone Intelligence. By following the plan, you'll discover whether gluten-free is best for you personally, while you get your hormones back on track.

versus low-carb versus slow-carb diets, it's low and slow carbs that win the race in the long run for most women with hormone imbalances. So when it comes to hormone health, a diet with a modest amount of slow carbs is the healthiest choice for most women. One or two servings per day of grains, and one or two of energy veggies—combined in a meal with healthy protein and fat, prevents blood sugar spikes and keeps insulin levels healthy, while providing you with steady energy.

Vegetables and Fruits

Every single one of my patients gets an identical piece of advice from me: EAT MORE PLANTS. As I shared, going plant-based is the heart of getting hormone-healthy. So let's get you started with the A-list.

Leafy Greens: A Girl's Best Friend

Leafy greens, particularly those in the *Brassicaceae* family—broccoli, cabbages, kale, Brussels sprouts, cauliflower, and collards—are especially important Hormone Intelligence allies. Leafy greens are rich in powerful nutrients and phytochemicals, like sulfur and indoles needed for detoxication of environmental toxins, and are the best fiber for a healthy microbiome needed for toxin elimination, which you'll learn more about in Chapter 10.

Energy Veggies

Starchy vegetables, particularly sweet potatoes and winter squashes, provide important sources of energy, nutrients, and fiber, so I refer to them as energy veggies. The starch they contain is good for keeping your bowels regular and your microbiome happy—which means healthier estrogen levels. They're relatively high in sugar compared to leafy greens, so you'll find them often, but in moderation, in the meal plans, eaten with protein and fat for energy balance.

More Plants, More Fiber

Not only are most of us living with a phytonutrient gap, but as part of it, we've been living with a fiber gap. Our paleo ancestors got about 100 grams per day of fiber from plants in their diet; most Americans are getting about 15 grams per day! Not only is this a major risk for colon cancer, it's bad news for your hormones.

But what is fiber? And where does fiber come from? There are two different types of fiber—soluble and insoluble. Both are important: *Soluble fiber* attracts water and turns to gel during digestion, slowing digestion and thus keeping you satiated for longer. Soluble fiber is found in whole grains, legumes, nuts, seeds, and some fruits and vegetables, as well as in psyllium seeds. *Insoluble fiber* is found in foods such as whole grains (in the hulls) and numerous vegetables. It adds bulk to your stool, helps with elimination, and supports microbiome health.

Fiber is critical for excreting estrogen metabolites, breakdown products made when the liver breaks down estrogen, and is meant to be dumped into and then excreted via your bowels. Compared with meat eaters, vegetarians, because of their greater consumption of fruits, veggies, whole grains, and legumes, are more effective at stool excretion of what are called *conjugated estrogens*—the estrogen byproducts that have been detoxified and packaged by the liver for excretion, and thus they have overall lower rates of excess estrogens and related hormone conditions. They also have lower rates of insulin resistance, important for preventing PCOS and reversing it in up to 70% of women with this condition.

Hormone-healthy fiber is found in all our plant foods. Especially beneficial forms are

The Wonder of Phytoestrogens

Plants are wondrous. Like us, they make hormones—in plants they're called *phytoestrogens* and are found abundantly in leafy green vegetables and legumes (i.e., lentils, chickpeas, tofu, tempeh, and soymilk) and flaxseed. Their structure is very similar to estradiol, but it's a much weaker form. This allows phytoestrogens to either bind to our estrogen receptors, gently blocking them, protecting us from more potent and potentially toxic forms of estrogen (called *xenoestrogen*) we get exposed to from our environment. They may also have beneficial mildly estrogen-stimulating actions, a plus for women with low estrogen in menopause.

Numerous beneficial effects have been attributed to diets rich in natural sources of phytoestrogens, including long-term lowered risks of menopausal symptoms like hot flashes and osteoporosis, lowered risks of cardiovascular disease, obesity, metabolic syndrome and type 2 diabetes, cognitive function decline, and breast and colon cancers. Contrary to popularly publicized studies suggesting that soy is harmful to fertility (incidentally, those studies were done on cows and cheetahs), the data clearly demonstrates that soy intake in women does not cause harm when trying to conceive naturally and is helpful when a woman is undergoing ovulation induction for fertility treatment—including with Clomid for IUI and IVF.

Soy is not without controversy; care should be taken in using soy products if you have a history of estrogen receptor positive cancer. To avoid excess phytoestrogen consumption, limit soy consumption to twice weekly and make sure all soy products are organic and non-GMO.

found in dark leafy greens in the Brassicaceae family including kale, collard greens, broccoli, and many more options that are broken down into indoles, which help with hormone detoxification. Fiber found in flaxseeds, in the form of lignins, is especially important for hormone health. It increases sex-hormone-binding globulin (SHBG) and keeps hormone levels healthy by helping you excrete excess circulating estrogen and testosterone. And fiber found in legumes also helps to support healthy gut flora while promoting healthy sex hormone and insulin levels.

Fiber is essential for digestion. Studies demonstrate a strong connection between inadequate fiber intake and insulin resistance, and strong evidence shows us that high dietary fiber intake can improve insulin sensitivity. Fiber is also an important factor in improving satiety when we eat, thus preventing us from overeating. A 2009 study of 252 women showed that increasing dietary fiber significantly reduced the risk of gaining weight and fat, regardless of the amount of physical activity and dietary fat intake. For every 1 gram of increased fiber in the diet, women lost 0.5 pounds, and body fat went down by this much as well. Vegetarians had triple the estrogens in their stool, meaning they were eliminating them more effectively, leading to between 15 and 20% lower blood estrogen levels. Lower fiber intake also means more constipation.

A large-scale study led by researchers at the Harvard School of Public Health found breast cancer risk to be 12 to 19% lower in women who get adequate daily dietary fiber during their early twenties. Eating a high-fiber diet during adolescence, according to one study, was associated with a 24% lower risk of developing breast cancer before menopause, due to lower overall exposure to estrogen, while a low-fiber diet has been associated with numerous diseases. While a diet high in fiber inhibits the reabsorption of certain forms of estrogen, thus decreasing circulating levels, here's the caveat—it takes a healthy microbiome for this to work. The good news is that fiber also helps to feed healthy gut flora.

Six to eight servings of veggies and one to two servings of fruit each day will also give you the fiber you need each day to keep your bowels moving and gut flora healthy.

Rainbow Veggies

Eat a rainbow! Nutrients and phytochemicals including resveratrol, polyphenols, and catechins, to name a few, have been shown to be able to modify genetic risk factors, improve detoxification, and repair DNA and cellular and tissue damage that has already occurred. Think about it this way: Each of the important phytochemicals we need comes in an array of colors and is part of what makes fruits, vegetables, and herbs color-rich, for example, proanthocyanidins make berries dark blue-purple. Looking at the deficits by color of fruits and vegetables that are absent in the diet gives us an indication of just how low we are in these phytochemicals. A study, published as *America's Phytonutrient Report*, found that Americans are falling short in every color category of phytonutrients:

- 69% fall short in green
- 78% fall short in red
- 86% fall short in white
- 88% fall short in purple/blue
- 79% fall short in yellow/orange

Berries and Other Fruits

More than any other fruit, berries pack a powerful punch when it comes to providing you with a rich array of polyphenols destined to help your liver do its important work of detoxification, your blood sugar stay healthy, your cells heal from the effects of environmental toxins, and your microbiome get a major dose of food fertilization. People who eat berries daily live longer and have less diabetes and better health, and berries are superfoods for your hormones. They can be eaten fresh in season, frozen when not, in parfaits, chia seed pudding, smoothies, salads, or just on their own—my favorite way! Ideally eat some every day.

Of course, all fruits are incredibly healthy;

Greens and Your Thyroid

If you have Hashimoto's, you may have heard that you need to avoid veggies in the Brassicaceae family. These veggies contain a thyroid-suppressing compound, as do millet, soy, and cassava, to name a few foods. However, the risk with greens appears to be associated with eating them raw in large quantities, or if you have Hashimoto's *and* iodine deficiency. Daily intake of moderate amounts of these vegetables cooked is not a problem. Fermenting these vegetables (i.e., eating cabbage as sauerkraut rather than raw) may also inhibit their ability to slow thyroid function. More on thyroid health and your hormones in Chapter 7.

some just have a much higher sugar content, so this category of fruits should be eaten a bit more sparingly. Optimally, eat fresh organic fruit, in season, or frozen if you can't get fresh sources.

Fermented Foods

Fermented foods are a traditional part of almost every culture on the planet, and their importance for the health of your microbiome can't be overstated. We'll be spending a lot of time exploring the microbiome together in the next couple of chapters. While organic yogurt and kefir are terrific options for getting fermented foods into your diet, since we're passing on the animal dairy for now, here are the foods we'll include:

- Coconut yogurt
- Sauerkraut
- Pickled veggies
- Kimchi
- Chickpea and rice miso

I'll show you how to introduce them to your diet in the meal plans in Part Four.

Nutritional Supplements— Do You Need a Daily Dose?

Food is your most important source of nutrition, and supplements are just that— supplements to real food. But even if you're doing your best to get a healthy dose of fruits and veggies, which can be hard enough in a super busy life, there are challenges in our modern food system that can undermine your best efforts at hormone balance. Additionally, certain medical conditions and medications

---

What About Personal Food Triggers?

The Hormone Intelligence Diet naturally eliminates most common food triggers, and this plan will also improve gut health and reduce inflammation, hopefully allowing you to enjoy a wider range of foods. However, if you find foods in the menu that you don't tolerate, swap them for another recipe in a similar category (i.e., an entrée, side veg) in the Hormone Intelligence Kitchen (starting on page 327).

---

can prevent you from getting the nutrition you need. Metformin, prescribed for PCOS, depletes calcium and B12, birth control pills deplete B6, magnesium zinc, and acid blockers like Prilosec can prevent vitamin B12 and calcium absorption. Further, lifestyle factors can additionally deplete your nutrients, for example, stress depletes magnesium, B vitamins, and vitamin C.

Nutrient supplementation can buffer what you're not getting in your diet and can play an important role in the prevention and treatment of PMS, fibroids, endometriosis, fertility problems, and overall ovarian and uterine health.

Here are just a few examples from the research:

- Magnesium, vitamin D, and chromium are all needed to regulate blood sugar; insufficiencies are associated with elevated blood glucose, insulin resistance, PCOS, and diabetes.

- In vitamin-D-deficient women with PCOS, vitamin D supplementation improved ovarian reserve, normalized AMH levels, and improved healthy follicle formation.

- Low vitamin B6 has been found in women with PMS; depression, miscarriage, prenatal nausea, low calcium with PMS, and low magnesium levels have been linked to menstrual cramps and their severity.

- Low vitamin C, vitamin E, and selenium are correlated with higher likelihood of having endometriosis, and the lower the levels of these nutrients, the worse the severity of the symptoms/condition.

- Low ascorbic acid (vitamin C) is associated with reduced ovarian function and progesterone levels, consistent with a study that found that when women were supplemented with ascorbic acid, their progesterone levels rose, their luteal phases lengthened, and their pregnancy rates increased.

- There's a strong relationship between low phytonutrient, phytochemical, and fatty acid intake and endometriosis. For example, women with endometriosis have low zinc levels; zinc influences inflammation and immunity, which seem to be at the core of development of endometriosis lesions.

- Women with low B12 or low folate have an increased risk of recurrent miscarriage, as do women with hypothyroidism and PCOS, all of which are influenced by nutritional status. Low vitamin E levels are connected with an increased risk of anovulation.

- Low vitamin B6 has been found in women with miscarriage and prenatal nausea and vomiting.

- Vitamin D plays a role in helping women conceive after IVF. High homocysteine blood levels are associated with low folate / folic acid levels, low luteal phase progesterone, and a 33% increase in the likelihood of anovulation.

The Hormone Intelligence Diet is specifically designed to provide these nutrients and bridge the phytonutrient gap. The "Daily Dose" supplements (see page 131) give you a jump start, replenishing low nutrient stores and optimizing your nutritional status, helping you to feel more like yourself, more quickly. I recommend four "daily doses" as an insurance plan for getting all your vitamins, minerals, and essential fats. You can find more information and proper dosage in the Botanical and Supplement Quick Reference Guide on pages 372–81.

A plant-based, whole-food multivitamin provides a general baseline for bridging the phytonutrient gap. Look for a multivitamin that doesn't contain sugar, artificial dyes, or additives and contains B-complex with methylfolate B12, zinc, selenium, and iodine. Here are just a few examples of the importance of these nutrients:

- **Methylfolate:** Supports detoxification of environmental toxins and endogenously produced hormones, essential for ovulation and fertility.

- **Selenium:** Supports detoxification by increasing glutathione, one of your body's most important detoxification compounds. It also reduces anxiety and depression, supports healthy thyroid function, and may reduce elevated thyroid antibodies.

- **Iodine:** Is essential for healthy ovulation and progesterone levels, prevention of ovarian cysts, thyroid hormone production; it plays a role in estrogen detoxification and helps to prevent fibrocystic breasts and cyclic breast pain. Due to a combination of these actions, iodine may play an important role in preventing PCOS, fibroids, heavy periods, and menstrual irregularities, as well as breast cancer.

- **Zinc:** Nourishes the ovaries, promotes ovulation, helps with cycle regularity, cycle symptoms, and fertility. It plays a role in the prevention and treatment of endometriosis, PCOS, PMS, menstrual cramps, fibroids, and pelvic pain, and it supports fertility. It's essential for the synthesis of thyroid hormone, is necessary for the health of your gut lining, and plays a role in preventing and treating depression; it may help regulate cortisol by reducing the brain's activation to stress and trauma.

- **Vitamin D3:** Take 2,000 units/day or up to 4,000 units/day for three months if your testing shows that your blood level is low or you have elevated blood sugar or insulin resistance.

- **Magnesium Glycinate or Citrate (the latter if you have constipation):** Take 500 mg/day. Magnesium is a cofactor in hormone production, meaning without magnesium you can't make estrogen, progesterone, thyroid hormone, and others. It's responsible for helping regular insulin and cortisol, and with these, blood sugar, cravings, stress, and anxiety. It helps improve sleep and has been shown to prevent and reduce PMS and menstrual cramps. It's essential for women with PMS, PCOS, and thyroid and adrenal problems, and magnesium citrate is an effective treatment for constipation.

- **EPA/DHA (fish or algae derived):** Take a standard dose of about 850 EPA / 200 DHA 1–2x/day (or the dose recommended in your Advanced Protocol, if following one). You'll learn much more about the importance of these essential fatty acids in this chapter.

You'll find much more information about specific nutrients for reversing root cause imbalances in Part Two, and as part of the targeted symptom and condition treatments in the Advanced Protocols in Part Three.

The Hormone Intelligence Diet at a Glance

Protein

Enjoy 1 serving of protein with every meal.

Fish

Up to 3 servings of fish/week

1 serving = 4–6 ounces (the size of a checkbook)

All fish should be high-quality, EFA-rich, low-mercury fish; see pages 116–17 for more information on choosing fish, or stick to this list:

- Anchovies
- Halibut, Alaskan, small
- Salmon
- Tilapia
- Wild Alaskan sardines

Poultry

No more than 3 servings of poultry/week

Should be free range, grain fed, antibiotic free, hormone free, and ideally organic

1 serving = 4–6 ounces (the size of a checkbook)

- Chicken, skinless white breast
- Turkey, skinless white breast (free range, antibiotic free)

Eggs

Up to 10 eggs/week

Should be free range, grain fed, antibiotic free, hormone free, and ideally organic

Legumes

At least 2 servings/week

1 serving = ½ cup cooked

- Black beans
- Chickpeas (garbanzo beans)
- Lentils
- Tempeh
- Tofu
- White beans (cannellini or northern)

Seeds

3–4 servings/week

1 serving = ¼ cup seeds = 1 tbsp. seed butter

Seeds should be raw or lightly toasted and unsalted.

- Chia seeds
- Flaxseeds
- Hemp seeds
- Pumpkin seeds
- Sesame seeds
- Sunflower seeds
- Tahini (sesame seed paste)

Nuts

3–4 servings/week

1 serving = ¼ cup nuts = 1 tbsp. nut butter

Nuts should be raw or lightly toasted and unsalted.

- Almonds
- Cashews
- Pecans

The Hormone Intelligence Diet at a Glance *(continued)*

- Pine nuts
- Walnuts

Optionally: Beef

No more than 1 serving of beef/week

Should be grass fed, antibiotic free, and hormone free, ideally organic if possible

1 serving = 4 ounces (the size of a deck of cards)

- Beef (grass fed, antibiotic free)

Slow Carbs

2 servings/day

1 grain + 1 energy vegetable
or 2 energy vegetables

- Brown rice
- Brown rice noodles
- Buckwheat (kasha)
- Millet
- Oats (rolled and steel-cut)
- Quinoa
- Red, pink, or black rice
- Wild rice

Fats

Incorporate one of the below into every meal (optimal).

- 1–2 tbsp. olive oil (extra virgin) (up to 4 tbsp./day)
- ½ avocado

- At one meal daily you can swap for 1 tbsp. coconut oil, ghee, avocado oil, walnut oil, flaxseed oil, or grapeseed oil

Vegetables

6–8 servings/day

Leafy Green Veggies

2 servings/day

1 serving = 1 cup (uncooked)

- Bok choy
- Broccoli
- Broccoli rabe (rapini)
- Broccoli sprouts
- Cabbage (all varieties)
- Cauliflower
- Collard greens
- Kale
- Napa cabbage

Rainbow Veggies

4 servings/day

1 serving = 1 cup for lettuces (uncooked) = ½ cup all others (uncooked)

Aim for a wide variety of colors each week.

- Arugula
- Asparagus
- Bell pepper (all colors)
- Carrot
- Celery
- Chard (all colors)
- Cucumber

The Hormone Intelligence Diet at a Glance *(continued)*

- Dandelion greens
- Endive
- Fennel
- Green beans (fresh or frozen)
- Leeks
- Lettuce (all varieties)
- Mushrooms (all varieties)
- Mustard greens
- Olives
- Onions
- Peas
- Peppers
- Sea vegetables (all varieties)
- Snow peas (fresh or frozen)
- Spinach
- Sprouts
- Tomato
- Watercress
- Zucchini

"Energy" Veggies

1–2 servings/day

1 serving = ½ cup potato = ½ cup squash

- Beets
- Parsnips
- Potato (russet, red skin, fingerling)
- Sweet potato
- Squash (delicata, pumpkin, acorn, spaghetti, butternut)

Fruit

Up to 2 servings/day. Either 1 serving of berries + 1 serving of another fruit from the list below or 2 servings of berries

Berries

1 serving = 1 cup of berries

- Blackberries (fresh or frozen)
- Blueberries (fresh or frozen)
- Raspberries (fresh or frozen)
- Strawberries (fresh or frozen)

Other Fruits

1 serving = 1 piece of fruit (i.e., an apple, a kiwi) or ½ cup of fruit (i.e., cherries)

- Apple (all varieties)
- Apricot
- Banana
- Cherries (fresh or frozen)
- Coconut
- Cranberries
- Figs (fresh)
- Kiwi
- Mango (fresh or frozen)
- Nectarine
- Orange
- Peach (fresh or frozen)
- Pear
- Plum
- Pomegranate
- Tangerine

You may also use 1–4 tbsp. of fresh juice daily in salad dressings, water, infusions, etc.

- Lemon
- Lime
- Grapefruit

The Hormone Intelligence Diet at a Glance *(continued)*

Fermented Foods

2–4 tbsp. of fermented foods/day

- Chickpea and rice miso
- Coconut yogurt
- Kimchi
- Pickled veggies
- Sauerkraut

Herbs and Spices

Aim to include at least 3 herbs and spices in your cooking daily.

- Basil
- Cardamom
- Chives
- Cinnamon
- Cumin
- Curry
- Dill
- Garlic
- Ginger
- Oregano
- Thyme
- Turmeric
- Za'atar

Beverages

Aim for 2 quarts of fluids/day. Water is best, but you can enjoy the following additionally:

- Carbonated water (plain or flavored; unsweetened; no artificial ingredients)
- Green tea

- Herbal tea
- Low-sodium organic bone or vegetable broth
- Water with lemon

Daily Dose Supplements

Every woman should take the four supplements listed below, as well as any additional supplements you discover in the next chapters and in your Hormone Intelligence Advanced Protocol, as needed.

See supplement chart on page 372–81 for detailed descriptions.

- A multivitamin
- Fish oil or algae-based (vegan) EFA
- Magnesium
- Vitamin D

Remember, Say No to These

- All refined sugar and products that contain it
- Artificial ingredients, including artificial sweeteners
- Coffee, soda, alcohol
- Dairy products
- Gluten-containing foods
- Processed meats
- Processed oils and trans fats
- Ultra-processed "foods," processed meats, and "simple carbs"

Set Yourself Up for Success

As you now see, I'm not exaggerating when I say that what you eat—or don't—has a profound effect on your hormonal health. But the last thing I want to sound like is Chicken Little saying "the sky is falling," and making you freaked out about food, or the Food Grinch saying "you can't have this or that." In fact, I want you to love food, use food to love your hormones back to health, and love your body again. If you're reading this and your alarm bells are going off, thinking, *Uh-oh, am I going to have to give up everything I love to eat?*, I promise the plan you're going to start on is not one of deprivation and guilt—and it's not about dieting, either! I want your life to be totally joyful, relaxed, and absolutely delicious.

But you picked up this book because your hormones are hurting—and to truly feel like your most awesome self, and to not be dogged by hormonal imbalances, you've got to stick with the plan.

Here are some tips to make the Hormone Intelligence Diet work for you:

- **Prep for the plan.** Give yourself two days before you officially start with day 1 of the program to get your head in the right place, get your kitchen set up, your pantry cleaned out, and some shopping done.

- **Set an intention.** Start each day with an intention for how you want to feel that day, envisioning yourself breezing through the day sticking with your plan like a superhero. Imagine exactly how it will feel when you're successful in your day. Can you see it?

- **Have a support posse.** Get a friend on board or create a small posse to join you and amplify your success, and your fun.

- **Power-start your day, e-ver-y day.** Eat breakfast within an hour of waking to keep your energy steady through the morning, maintain your focus and clarity, and avoid blood sugar crashes that send you heading for a sugar fix. Breakfast should always include protein and a healthy fat.

- **Listen to your body.** Are you hungry, or are you thirsty? Why can't you keep your eyes off that orange sitting on the counter? Why does salmon sound so good today? The healthier your hormone signaling becomes, the more you'll be able to listen to what your body wants from you in the kitchen every day. When you begin to notice your body asking you for certain foods, more water, a supplement—listen!

Should You Snack?

Allowing four to five hours between meals, and at least fourteen hours overnight without eating, can be tremendously beneficial for your blood sugar, cortisol, microbiome, and cellular healing—thus your hormone balance. Avoid snacking, that's ideal. But if you have a wicked fast metabolism, or blood sugar that tends to bottom out if you don't eat, then yes, please do have a snack. Just make it a Hormone Intelligence healthy one; you can find some options in the Hormone Intelligence Kitchen in Part Four. Once you've been at balancing your blood sugar for a couple of weeks, those energy crashes usually stop.

Cycle Sense Eating

One of the ways to support your cycle, emotions, moods, and cravings is to anticipate the hormonal shifts that are natural to even a healthy cycle with the right foods. Keep these recommendations in mind as you plan out your meals each week, modifying them for where you are in your cycle and how you might best support your body.

Cycle Phase	Emphasize
Follicular Phase	Make up for menstrual blood loss with red meat, dark meat poultry, or iron-rich vegetarian options like dried apricots, leafy greens, lentils, and raisins. Nourish healthy estrogen levels with plenty of leafy greens, flaxseed, and fiber-rich foods.
Ovulation	Just before, during, and in the days immediately after ovulation, your lighter appetite might be satisfied with simpler, lighter meals and plentiful salads; make sure to include seeds, berries, fish, and eggs to send you into the next phase of your cycle with low inflammation.
Luteal Phase / Premenstrually	Increase your healthy carbs, especially whole grains to keep cravings at bay and support mood. Warm up your diet with soups, steamed vegetables, and nourishing foods that are also easy on your digestive system, especially if you get bloating or loose stools, but emphasize fiber if you get constipated. As you get closer to your period, if you don't feel like cooking much, prepare simple, one-pot meals like stir-fries and Goddess Bowls with healthy whole grains and lots of steamed veggies, and enjoy some fish. Indulge in some dark chocolate to boost mood. Take fish oil, calcium and magnesium, and ginger for the five days before your moon time is due to keep your mood steadier and also prevent cramps. Remember to skip the added salt during this time to avoid bloating, and instead enjoy potassium-rich veggies and fruits.
On Your Flow	Keep up your premenstrual foods. A small amount of red meat is appropriate if you tend to lose a lot of blood with your period, or have some lentils or red beans if you're vegan. Quinoa is rich in iron, protein, and magnesium, so are a nice choice, too. Dark chocolate and healthy treats are also healthy indulgences if you're feeling like you need a little something sweet. Include ginger in your cooking, enjoy a turmeric chai latte (page 369), or sip ginger or mint tea to help with cramps or digestive symptoms.

- **Eat at consistent times.** Try having meals at the same time every day, and don't eat late at night.

- **Don't get "hangry."** A wee bit of hunger or an appetite by the time you're ready for your meal is healthy for reducing inflammation, improving metabolism, and supporting a healthy microbiome. But don't ever let yourself get overly hungry to the point of having low blood sugar symptoms or being "hangry," because this is a major hit to your cortisol and hormones. When you do have a meal, eat to be satisfied, not to be full.

- **When in doubt, eat dark chocolate.** Dark chocolate is a fermented plant food rich in polyphenols. Women who include a couple of ounces in their daily diet tend to be slimmer, have lower blood pressure, less depression, and *fewer cravings*. A few squares are a great healthy indulgence, and a sure craving buster. For added pleasure, dip it in some almond butter, enjoy with a serving of Frozen Banana

The Food-Mood-Symptom Journal

Studies show that just the act of tracking what we eat can lead to much healthier food choices and outcomes. Learning how foods make you feel, also does this. I highly recommend keeping a food journal for three days before you start your Hormone Intelligence Diet, then for one day a week, if you have time, over the next six weeks. You'll gain insight into:

- Food habits and patterns you might not even realize you have
- How various foods make you feel (physically and emotionally)
- Any trouble spots you encounter throughout your day (i.e., the 3 p.m. crash)

Here's a sample; download a blank template at avivaromm.com/hormone-intelligence -resources.

Time/Meal	Foods/Beverages Eaten	How I Feel	Good Elimination (a.k.a. went to the bathroom)
Breakfast 8 a.m.			
Lunch			
Dinner			
Other (i.e., snacks)			

While you don't have to write down the answers to each of these questions, pay attention to them as you're keeping the journal so they become second nature:

Before I ate _____ (these foods) I felt _____.

After I ate _____ (these foods) I felt _____.

Examples are:

- Before I ate that bowl of ice cream I felt hungry, tired, bored.
- Before I ate that apple with nut butter I felt mindful, proud of myself for going for a healthy snack.
- After I ate that croissant I felt bloated, gassy, blue.
- After I ate that salmon/greens/buttered sweet potato meal I felt calm and satisfied.

It takes a little work to remember to food journal, but the benefits can be significant.

Soft Serve, or the Almond Butter Cup Smoothie.

And here are some tips to troubleshoot "when life happens":

- **Stuck at work, getting hungry, 4 p.m. energy dip?** Keep a no-crash emergency snack stash (see page 155) with you to prevent low blood sugar and the inevitable sugar or carb binge—especially when your coworker's Hershey's Kisses bowl is sitting on her desk, calling you over.

- **Dine out wisely.** Eating just one meal out weekly translates to a two-pound weight gain each year; and the average American adult eats out five times per week. Restaurants know that we love to get a big bang for our buck, and increasing portion size doesn't add much to a restaurant's overhead, so we get served supersize portions. To preempt overeating, or regretting your food choices, have a healthy snack before you go out, and stick to the lighter items on the menu.

- **When everyone is having drinks.** Eat before you drink alcohol or at least while you're drinking; otherwise you'll end up smashed and famished, with no control over what you eventually scarf down to sop up the alcohol and set yourself straight. Sip slowly and sip smart: order simple drinks that are gluten free, cut with still or sparkling water, and ask that they have no simple sugar added. Wine spritzers, vodka with lemon and sparkling water, or gin and tonic are examples. Or stick to red wine, no more than one glass, and sip slowly.

- **Work a full-time job and often short on time to shop and cook?** Cooking at home dramatically improves weight loss and health, doesn't have to cost more, and can be done creatively so that you learn to save time. It's also incredibly satisfying to prepare and eat a delicious meal, and if you plan ahead, you'll have leftovers to make the next day's lunch easy and healthy. It's also a sure way to drop some unwanted pounds.

- **Be a weekend warrior.** It's the weekend, you're out with your besties, you've put in a long week, and you deserve a reward. Enjoy one, but trade your usual "fuck it, it's the weekend" food splurge with a Healthy Indulgence from Part Four.

Slipped Off the Plan? Don't Say "F-It!" Just Reboot!

So many women throw in the towel or say "Screw it, I've messed up, no point now." Don't quit—just keep going. There is no failure. You don't have to start over from the beginning. Pick up where you left off. Yes, sometimes the going gets tough, and sometimes we slip up. It's what we do with it that counts: stand up tall and keep going!

out of survival mode

THE STRESS-HORMONE CONNECTION

The body says what words cannot.
—**Martha Graham**

Have you ever done a happy dance when an appointment or date got canceled, knowing you now had the unexpected time to yourself? Does having a cold—or even menstrual cramps—give you a much-needed excuse to curl up on the sofa and do nothing? When was the last time you took a break just because you needed—or (gasp!) wanted—to?

I hear the strain all the time—women telling me they're maxed out, stressed out, living on fumes. I've yet to see a woman who put stress near the top of her symptom list. The nearly relentless pressures most women are under include: home, work, money, kids, "to-do" lists—plus the inner pressure to be perfect, eat the perfect diet, do yoga, get the promotion, be the best mom on the block. It's mind-boggling.

Add to these the hidden stress of income disparities, the experience of racism, caring for older parents or a sick family member, hidden workplace stressors including harassment, and it's no wonder women are feeling the burn—or more accurately, the burnout!

In fact, women actually do have more stressful lives than men. We shoulder more daily work; even in the many households in which women who are the primary "breadwinners" (even with stay-at-home partners!), women still bear the greatest burden for household and childrearing tasks. Women also do more "emotional labor"—the job of keeping everyone else happy. We're much more likely than men to be asked—and say yes—to volunteer or take on extra responsibilities at work, our kid's school, and in our family, than men. As

Hormone Intelligence: The Stress-Hormone Connection

- Learn how stress (and HPA axis disruption) impacts hormone health and acts as a root cause of gynecologic problems.
- Identify where stress is hanging out in your life.
- Create a daily relaxation practice that you'll love from the many options in this chapter, and even try a new one each day.
- Prioritize what's important to you and learn to stop energy "leaks."

the icing on the cake, we internalize that we're supposed to "lean in" so we can have it all and do it all. Even when we know intellectually that this isn't possible, we may feel guilty for not meeting those unrealistic expectations.

We have an incredible capacity to push ourselves to meet our often enormous daily demands. But often, we're doing so at the expense of the rest and reset aspects of life. We stop listening to the needs and messages of our bodies. We put our health on the back burner while taking care of everyone else. And we "self-reward" in ways that usually ultimately make us feel worse—the glass or three of wine, the cookie binge, the extra couple of hours we stay up at night (often surfing the internet, leaving us feeling "compare and despair") just to have a minute alone at the end of the day.

According to a 2016 study published in the *Journal of Brain & Behavior*, women are twice as likely to suffer from stress, including severe stress, and anxiety as men. It's not just that we *feel* we're under more stress, we are—and changes seen on MRIs comparing women's responses to stress and men's prove it. The American Psychological Association (APA) reports that *women top the charts in all stress-related statistics, including having more physical symptoms* such as headaches, irritable bowel syndrome, and depression, for example.

This chapter is designed to get you off the hamster wheel of stress. It's going to show you how to (finally!) get out of survival mode and keep your cup replenished—because as you're about to learn, running on empty has an impact on your hormone health.

What Is Stress, Really?

Stress literally means a strain or pressure that causes something to bend out of shape. I know you feel me on that! But it's more than an emotional state, it's a series of physiologic responses, called *the stress response*, that occur as a result of any number of triggers, properly called *stressors*, that threaten your sense of security or safety—whether consciously, unconsciously, or biologically. Let's take a deeper look.

Your Stress Response

The **stress response** is orchestrated by one of the axes I mentioned early on in the book (page 29): The hypothalamic-pituitary-adrenal (HPA) axis. It starts in two little almond-size regions of your brain called the *amygdala*, your own natural surveillance system. They pick up on even tiny triggers—sights, sounds, smells, feelings—and if any seem like a threat to your safety, they send an automatic relay to your "emergency response central"—your *hypothalamus*. So if you smell smoke, your brain will immediately get you to scan your environment for a fire. If you see an obvious, unthreatening source, your brain calms down, but if you can't rule out a fire—or there is one—your brain goes into alarm mode and you spring into action, either fighting the fire with your handy fire extinguisher or running.

This chain of events begins when your hypothalamus detects danger and produces *CRH* (corticotropin-releasing hormone), which in turn alerts your *pituitary* gland that something's up and help is needing to get mobilized. Consider it the 911 center of your brain dispatching emergency services, which happen to primarily hang out in your *adrenals* in the form of a hormone called *cortisol* and the neurotransmitter *adrenaline* (a.k.a. *epinephrine*). These are then dispatched much like the police, fire department, and an ambulance—all at once—throughout your body to protect you from whatever the danger might be.

So imagine this. You're watching a *National Geographic* special about African animals. Gazelles are comfortably drinking at a watering hole on a golden plain in Africa when along comes a pride of hungry lions and a chase begins. The gazelles go into *survival mode* and run. They're pumping out adrenaline, the first responder in the stress response. Adrenaline fuels the "fight or flight" you're familiar with: your back gets tight as if you're ready to spring or run, your heart beats faster, your breathing changes, and you become hypervigilant to danger. In the process, your blood vessels constrict and your cardiac and respiratory rates increase.

After a few minutes, if the danger persists, cortisol kicks in, mobilizing blood sugar to your muscles to provide fuel so you can run from or fight the danger. Insulin production also revs up to deal with that extra blood sugar so it doesn't linger when the danger's over and cause inflammatory damage. Cortisol gets your immune system ready to protect your boundaries, like the National Guard, against infection that could occur if you got injured, and it changes the way your brain works so that you're reacting on automatic pilot rather than using your willpower and higher thinking; you need to be instinctual during a crisis, not thinking about your taxes or to-do list! The lions pursue, and eventually catch one of the older, sicker, or slower gazelles. But then what happens? The remaining gazelles go right back to the watering hole as if nothing happened. They go from red alert back down to it's all okay. This is called *stress resolution*. And it all happened in a matter of minutes.

The ability to respond and adapt to stress and still stay healthy is known as *allostasis*, a term that means that we're extremely resilient to stress. The stress response is ingeniously orchestrated, if you think about it. So why, if it works so well to protect us, does stress cause so many problems? The answer is that when the stress response is activated day in and day out, adrenaline and cortisol go from friends to overstaying houseguests—and your health and hormones pay the price. And for most women, chronically activated it is!

Stuck in the "On" Position

The stress response is a beautiful thing. While cortisol has gotten a bad reputation as the "stress hormone," it should be called the *survival hormone* because we can't live without it. It keeps our blood pressure, blood sugar, inflammation, and energy balanced and plays a major role in maintaining healthy immunity, willpower, focus, and memory. It is the music that keeps almost every cell in your body hummin' in time to the right beat, as you'll learn in the next chapter when we talk about circadian rhythm.

Cortisol gives us serious survival advantages: a little bit of stress keeps you on your toes should danger present, and it stimulates problem solving, focus, and immunity. It makes us feel excited and alive, and it helps us to grow. But the stress response was meant to be a short-lived response. You get away from danger and the response calms right down in a matter of minutes—hours at the most. It was never meant to be stuck in the "On" position. But for most of us, that's the situation. And that's where our hormone problems get started.

Modern living causes us to get too much of a good thing and so we experience chronic activation of the stress response without enough time and relaxation for resolution, to the point that we get stuck in survival mode. The very system designed to protect us backfires and leads to a host of consequences, sometimes small symptoms, sometimes diagnosable conditions.

The Wear and Tear of It

At the heart of our modern hormone epidemic is a modern problem called *allostatic load*, the physical *wear and tear* that happens as a result of repeated or chronic stress. A sustained high cortisol level wears at muscle and bone; slows healing time; impairs digestion, metabolism, and cognitive function; interferes with healthy endocrine function, and impairs immunity. It can disrupt your sleep, digestion and microbiome, and blood sugar; can cause you to have food cravings (especially for fat/sugar/salt/carbs) and to gain or have trouble losing weight; and can result in that root of all root causes—inflammation. Because all your endocrine system is interconnected to your nervous and immune systems, when the HPA axis is on alert, it puts the brakes on ovarian and thyroid function. Even relatively short stretches of stress can impact your sex hormones and cycles. And it doesn't stop there: the latest research on stress shows powerful links to irregular periods, menstrual pain, PMS, endometriosis, fertility challenges, PCOS, and more.

Under Pressure: The Stress-Hormone Connection

When your stress response gets activated, your body diverts energy away from what Stanford University evolutionary biologist Robert Sapolsky, author of *Why Zebras Don't Get Ulcers*, politely calls "optimistic activities"—meaning sex and reproduction. Your body is actually trying to do you the favor of protecting

Should I Get My Cortisol Tested?

If you're experiencing stress symptoms, you don't have to get tested to "prove" it. But if you're unsure whether stress is causing symptoms, you can get a 24-hour salivary or a serum cortisol test. Some integrative or functional medicine doctors also test for DHEA, progesterone, testosterone, and insulin, which provide information on the impact of stress on your sex hormones and metabolism.

you from getting pregnant when times are hard or resources are scarce.

Your brain is the link between what's going on in your external world and your ovaries (and thyroid). But I want to be clear about something: talking about the impact of stress on your health, hormones, or any related hormone or gynecologic condition does not mean it's in your head! I'm emphasizing this because the term *hysteria*, which is derived from the Greek word for "uterus," *hysterikos*, was a medical diagnosis that was used for centuries, and well into the twentieth century, as a diagnosis to dismiss women who presented with almost any of the hormonal and gynecologic conditions in this book. Stress creates a very real physical impact on our health and hormones.

Gonadotropin-releasing hormone (GnRH) is a hormone produced by your hypothalamus that starts the relay of messages that stimulate ovulation and your cycles. High cortisol levels, as well as some other chemicals that your body ramps up when you're stressed, suppress GnRH. But that's not all cortisol does. In further attempts to prevent you from ovulating, it also inhibits pituitary FSH and LH production. But let's say you do manage to produce enough FSH and LH to reach your ovaries. Cortisol has that covered, too, making your ovaries more resistant to these hormones, and also blocking maturation of your ovarian follicles. And there's still more: cortisol blocks your progesterone receptors, so even if you do ovulate, you don't reap the benefits of progesterone throughout your brain and body. As a result of yet another domino effect in your endocrine system, your estrogen and progesterone levels decline, your menstrual cycles go all wonky, and you don't ovulate regularly or at all. Out goes ovulation, regular cycles, and your sex drive—all the functions that have to do with baby-making.

Chronic stress is now recognized as having such a big impact on our hormone health that it's considered an endocrine disruptor, much like other environmental toxins that I'll talk more about in Chapter 10. Subtle hormonal symptoms like irregular periods, increased cramps, or breast tenderness—the kind we're told are just normal so don't pay them any mind—can be important early signs that you're under too much stress.

Menstrual Cycle Problems and PMS

Stress can have a significant impact on your menstrual cycle. Women under high stress may be twice as likely to have painful periods. Research found high levels of stress during the first half of your cycle of the previous month had a greater association with dysmenorrhea than at other times of the cycle. In a study of 166 female college students, stress was found to dramatically increase menstrual cycle length to 43 days or longer, while women who report high levels of perceived stress due to common factors such as starting a new job, getting married, or having major family responsibilities are twice as likely to experience long menstrual cycles. Chronically elevated cortisol can cause irregular or skipped periods, lack of ovulation, and **hypothalamic amenorrhea**, which I told you about in Chapter 4. One study found that women with hypothalamic amenorrhea (HA) had twice the cortisol levels of women without HA in a comparison group. It's the body's way of protecting you from getting pregnant in a high-stress environment when your brain may perceive that the environment isn't safe or adequate resources aren't available for you to have a baby. Undereating and overexercising are two very common activities with a direct link to HA and anovulation.

Stress-Sleep-Pain

Stress has also been found to increase pain perception, and stress causes interrupted sleep, which has also been found to worsen our sense of pain. Either one of these factors—or both in combination—can cause or worsen premenstrual sleep problems and menstrual pain. A 2010 study published in the *Journal of Women's Health* showed that stress worsens PMS symptoms. Women who reported feeling stressed two weeks before starting their period were 2 to 4 times more likely to report moderate to severe symptoms compared to women who reported no signs of stress.

Stress and PCOS

A chronically activated stress response is a recipe for blood sugar problems and insulin resistance—a key underlying factor in PCOS for at least 70% of women with this condition. Additionally, when we're stressed, we eat more sugar and carbs. Elevated insulin triggers your ovaries to produce more testosterone. Further, under stress, your adrenal glands increase DHEA, DHEAS, and androstenedione production, because these hormones help to buffer the brain from the impact of cortisol. When elevated they also contribute to PCOS and its symptoms. It gets even more complicated; for yet unknown reasons, possibly genetic or due to intrauterine factors that set us up for PCOS even before birth, women with PCOS are more sensitive

Trauma—A Hidden Cause of Stress

There are a million microaggressions that women experience that affect our safety, body image, and self-efficacy, and act as a chronic low- or high-level HPA axis trigger, impacting our hormone health. Sexual trauma has been associated with increased risk of chronic pelvic pain, painful sex, vaginismus, chronic vaginitis, and gastrointestinal disorders like IBS or chronic constipation. Intimate partner violence (IPV) is associated with a greater rate of depression, pelvic pain, menstrual disorders, pain with sex, bowel symptoms, and sleep problems.

Women who have experienced sexual harassment have a higher prevalence of poor sleep and high blood pressure, and sexual assault is associated with a higher prevalence of depressed mood, anxiety, and poor sleep. IPV has been linked to a wide range of chronic conditions: asthma, diabetes, cardiovascular disorders, chronic pain, autoimmune conditions, depression, anxiety, PTSD, eating disorders, substance-use disorders, pelvic pain, menstrual disorders, headaches, difficulty sleeping, palpitations, gastrointestinal symptoms, and fibromyalgia. Sexual and physical abuse may alter neuroendocrine immune processes, leading to a higher risk for endometriosis, and one study found that women in abusive relationships were more likely to have a higher level of pain with endometriosis.

After all, where do we store our trauma and life's pain but in our bodies? What harms our psyches—our souls—reverberates through our whole being. It's been said, "the body keeps the score." While there's no easy solution to healing the impact of trauma in our lives, as we work together to restore resilience to your stress response system and create a loving relationship with your body, my hope is that this program will become a supportive part of your healing journey.

to the effects of cortisol, so these reactions are all exaggerated. As if that's not enough, due to alterations in response to other important hormones, like leptin, which controls appetite and satiety, women with PCOS are also more susceptible to cravings and binge eating and have a tougher time losing weight—a vicious cycle. Getting out of chronic stress to reset the brain-ovary and adrenal-ovary connections are important secrets to halting PCOS.

Stress and Endometriosis

Endometriosis is a condition in which the immune system is altered, and displaced endometrial tissue is abnormally inflammatory. Chronic overactivation of the stress response causes a domino effect of immune dysregulation and inflammation, which can aggravate—or may even be one of the contributing causes of—endometriosis. Chronic stress also causes increased pain perception, and researchers now believe that this phenomenon plays a role in nerve fiber changes that are associated with endometriosis pain.

Not Tonight, Honey . . . Sex and Libido

Stress is at the top of the list of factors that can reduce your sex drive. It's like a foot stepping on your brain's sexual arousal brake, literally called your *sexual inhibition system*. It's the counterpart to your brain's sexual accelerator, or "gas pedal"—technically called the *sexual excitation system*, which is designed to notice all the sexually relevant stimuli in your environment and get you excited. In other words, stress just makes you notice all the reasons you *don't* feel in the mood. Typical stressors that hit the sex brake are exhaustion and overwhelm, irritability, unhappy body self-image, financial, family, and other life stressors, negative perceptions about your partner (which are on overdrive when we're tired and stressed), and here's one—stress about worry-

ing about not feeling like having sex, or about sex itself. Like other aspects of stress, cortisol is at the heart of libido suppression—part and parcel of that whole inhibition of reproduction thing that happens. Recognizing that this is normal when you're under stress—which most people are—can be the first step to rekindling your sexual desire. This chapter will help you unwind from stress and that alone can help you to reawaken your desire—and I've got additional tips for you in Chapter 17. I also highly recommend the book *Come as You Are* by Emily Nagoski.

Stress and Fertility

Stress is an underappreciated contributor to fertility challenges, particularly because it can cause hypothalamic amenorrhea. Stress is also an almost inevitable result of going through months of trying to get pregnant; most women find conventional fertility treatment emotionally and mentally trying.

The Food-Stress-Hormone Connection

If you're chronically stressed it's likely that chocolate, ice cream, cookies, or a couple of glasses of wine at night have become a routine you're having trouble shaking. Sugar and fat are the molecules that get burned up rapidly to fuel the stress response. Your brain practically ensures that when you are under constant stress, you'll go for sugary, fatty, and salty foods by releasing a flood of feel-good nervous system chemicals such as serotonin and dopamine that calm your nervous system with every bite as they also bring cortisol back into normal range. That's why they are called "comfort foods"—they are comforting your nervous system.

This comfort comes at a price. We become addicted to the foods that are bringing comfort, and since these are typically sugary and fatty foods, we eat more of them, causing us to pack on belly fat and VAT, or visceral adipose tissue, a type of hidden abdominal fat that produces inflammatory cytokines that wreak havoc on the entire body—and your hormones. Further, so many of us feel the constant pressure to be thinner or eat "cleaner." But being underweight—or undernourished—is one of the most common causes of anovulation.

From a survival perspective, your brain may just be your body's most important organ to protect. And one of the things your brain needs for not just survival, but functioning, is a steady supply of energy. Low energy, which happens when your blood sugar gets low, triggers your brain to go into DEFCON 1—survival mode gets activated. In one study, a 40% calorie restriction in women led to a heightened stress response, which caused women to stop cycling, increased hormonal masculinization, and led to an overall negative impact on reproductive function. You need ample body fat to make hormones; it takes having about 20% body fat to maintain regular ovulation and menstruation. Chronically low calorie intake and low blood sugar are stressors, causing your body to ramp up cortisol production, which then makes you store weight (it does this in part by suppressing thyroid function).

The problem is, your brain doesn't register the difference between a very low-calorie diet so you can fit into your wedding dress, and an actual famine. Limited calorie intake (or overexercise, or both) puts you at risk of low estrogen levels and hypothalamic amenorrhea, and with it, cessation of ovulation (which leads to low progesterone levels), long menstrual cycles, skipped periods, fertility problems, and ultimately, muscle loss and bone loss (which can lead to osteoporosis). This can be the result of getting too little energy from healthy fats and carbohydrates in your daily meals due to dieting, anything that causes sudden weight loss (crash dieting, fasting, illness), overexercising (which can, believe it or not, even include too much yoga!), anorexia nervosa, athletic training, or "orthorexia"—the restrictive eating problem I discussed on page 101.

While the amount of weight loss, underweight, and exercise that's enough to tip you into irregular cycles varies from woman to woman, weighing 10% below what's considered a normal range for your height can interfere with ovulation.

Stress and Your Thyroid: A Special Connection

I'd like to introduce you to one of your most important regulatory glands: your thyroid. This butterfly-shaped gland in the front of your neck is the thermostat regulating the energy for your entire body. It also controls everything from your mood to your menstrual cycles to your metabolism—and about a thousand other biological functions. Like your adrenals (HPA axis) and ovaries (HPO axis), your thyroid activity happens in an axis connecting your brain and thyroid: the hypothalamic-pituitary-thyroid (HPT) axis.

When you're under prolonged chronic stress, your adrenal system tells your body to conserve, rather than spend too much energy. Your thyroid slows down, too. Even if you produce enough active thyroid hormone, cortisol blocks your body from activating it and letting your cells use it. It's like a warning system that protects you from overusing precious energy reserves. In a next-level effort to prevent you from expending energy, your thyroid puts a lid on your ovarian function, because ovulation is a very energy-intensive process. It's one of the main ways that all thyroid-hormone connections get activated.

High estrogen levels, whether due to endocrine disruptors from the environment, estrogen in birth control or other medications, or your own hormone imbalances, can also block thyroid function. Elevated estrogen levels lead to an increase of thyroid-binding globulin (TBG), which binds circulating thyroid hormone, making it unable to do its job, and giving you symptoms of a slow-functioning thyroid even when your thyroid is perfectly healthy (this is important because it might also be missed on thyroid tests unless TBG and SHBG are also checked).

Your Thyroid, Your Ovaries, Your Hormones

Thyroid function is intimately involved in healthy ovarian function, sex hormone production, your cycles, and fertility, so when things aren't so great in your thyroid function, it shows up in your cycles and symptoms. For example, a slow-functioning thyroid, the most common form of thyroid problem for women, has also been linked to:

- Irregular, missed, more frequent (in hyperthyroidism), and heavier periods

- Anovulation

- PCOS

- Ovarian cysts, which may be recurrent and painful

- Endometriosis (Hashimoto's thyroiditis was 6.5 times more common in women with endometriosis)

- Subfertility

- Depression, as well as problems with memory and concentration

How Do You Know If You Have a Thyroid Problem?

If you have an underactive thyroid (hypothyroidism, Hashimoto's), in addition to the hormone and gynecologic problems above, you may experience:

- Fatigue, constipation

- Dry skin

- Brain fog or trouble concentrating

- Depression

- Anxiety

- Hair loss

- Joint and muscle aches (even carpal tunnel syndrome and tendonitis!)

- Generalized swelling

- Cold intolerance (or you always feel a little cold)

- Dry skin

- Low heart rate

If you have an overactive thyroid, you might experience a rapid heartbeat, anxiety, insomnia, insatiable appetite, diarrhea, and weight loss. The most common symptoms of hypothyroidism are also among those that are the most likely to be chalked up by doctors to "just stress," so women can go for years with a missed diagnosis—leaving many feeling confused, blaming themselves, feeling like they're doing something wrong or aren't doing enough to have more energy and feel better. They're driving themselves crazy dieting but can't lose weight, beating themselves up for not being happier, and suffering from the grief of fertility problems and miscarriages—all because of a problem for which there's easy detection and treatment.

With thyroid, test, don't guess. Most doctors don't routinely check a full panel of thyroid tests, so they miss a thyroid diagnosis, leaving millions of women without answers and suffering with symptoms and health consequences. Your thyroid uses iodine to produce T4, which is converted to T3 in your liver, and your thyroid also directly produces small amounts of T3. T3 does most of the thyroid's heavy lifting throughout your body.

Here's what I order in a complete thyroid panel:

- TSH
- Free T3
- Free T4
- Thyroid peroxidase antibodies (TPOAb)
- Thyroglobulin antibodies (TgAb)
- Reverse T3
- Iodine

Self-Assessment: Is Stress Affecting Your Hormones?

If you find yourself nodding your head to more than a couple of the symptoms below, it's likely that stress is playing more than a small role in your hormonal imbalances and gynecologic symptoms. While the recommendations in this chapter are for everyone, they may be especially important for you.

- ☐ Difficulty falling asleep, interrupted sleep, or waking up too early
- ☐ Feeling "tired but wired"
- ☐ Feeling tired or anxious in the morning, even after a full night's sleep
- ☐ Chronic overwhelm, fatigue, burnout
- ☐ Anxiety or depression
- ☐ An energy slump around 3–4 p.m.
- ☐ Needing coffee to start the day; sometimes need another cup in the afternoon
- ☐ Craving chocolate, sweets, salty foods
- ☐ Feeling chronically stressed, irritable, overworked, or overwhelmed
- ☐ Jumping at loud noises
- ☐ Low willpower
- ☐ Low (or no) sex drive

- ☐ Regularly having "blood sugar crashes"
- ☐ Brain fog
- ☐ Extra weight around your middle
- ☐ Finding yourself frequently self-critical or critical of others
- ☐ Eating to calm stress
- ☐ Looking more wrinkly than you think you should
- ☐ Catching every cold and "bug" going around
- ☐ Having trouble relaxing or having fun
- ☐ Back, neck, shoulder, jaw, or other muscle tightness or pain
- ☐ You're using cigarettes, alcohol, other substances, or shopping, to relax
- ☐ You're the primary income provider and you do most of the domestic work

I sometimes also order SHBG and TBG if I suspect that there's a link between elevated estrogen and a thyroid problem, but these are not part of my routine thyroid panel. If you suspect a thyroid problem, see your primary care provider to get a proper diagnosis.

Thyroid TLC

The core plan in this book is helpful for supporting your thyroid health. However, thyroid support may also require taking thyroid hormone medication, which as one of my patients described it, is like putting jumper cables on an engine that needs charging—it gets your thyroid revved up again! Because so many women come to me with thyroid problems I wrote a whole book about it: *The Adrenal Thyroid Revolution*, which I'm sure you'll enjoy.

The supplements below, taken singly or in combination, can help to improve thyroid health and function and are recommended if you have hypothyroidism. These include:

- **Vitamin D3**, which tends to be lower in women with hypothyroidism.

- **Selenium**, a mineral that the body turns into the powerful antioxidant glutathione, which protects the thyroid from inflammation and can reduce thyroid-attacking antibodies. Selenium is also critical in forming the most active form of thyroid hormone (FT3), which does most of the heavy lifting.

- **Zinc**, an important nutrient for nourishing your thyroid and producing enough active thyroid hormone. It may also improve stress-related thyroid problems.

- **Inositol**, which used in combination with selenium can help to reduce thyroid-attacking antibodies—and also to improve thyroid function.

- **Ashwagandha, an herbal adaptogen** (see more on page 157), has been shown to increase active thyroid hormone levels and also reduce cortisol—a win-win in stress-related thyroid problems.

If you're on thyroid medication, work with your medical provider because if your thyroid health starts to improve, you might end up needing less medication—a good thing—but you want to check so you're not overmedicating. You can find more information and proper dosage in the Botanical and Supplement Quick Reference Guide on pages 372–81.

Healing the Stress-Hormone Pathway

I'm not saying that when you start to address stress in your life, life is suddenly going to be a breeze, or that you're going to magically have hours of free time in your schedule to practice self-care. What I am saying is that we have to take a radical, proactive stand in favor of our health by getting out of a chronic stress mindset and into one that intentionally invites inner calm and a slower, more rhythmic, natural pace of life, regardless of your life's circumstances. It's about making the inner changes that help you start to reclaim your life, personal freedom, and empowerment. You create a life in which self-care becomes nonnegotiable, even if for just a short time each day, and a longer time each week. Healing your life to reduce expendable stressors, and nourishing calm and resilience, has a powerful and lasting ripple effect. If you want to bring hormone health back into your life, and reverse a major root cause of gynecologic problems, reducing stress has got to be a commitment. And take this to heart: self-care is not selfish—it's self-preservation!

Following is my stepwise approach for getting your brain and ovaries realigned and clearing as much noise off your HPA axis—hormone channels—as possible. Read through each section and pick a new practice to incorporate each day, or every three days if you prefer. Remember, this is not just a short-term plan, it's a lifestyle—so the goal is to make your new self-awareness and self-care a part of your hormone-healthy life!

Step 1: Pay Attention to Your Inner Landscape

How do you want to feel? This is an important question I ask my patients, and one I encourage you to ask yourself at the start and end of each day. And as a follow-up, check in with how you actually do feel. We often get so busy that we're disconnected from how we feel, other than the symptoms that dog us, and most of us were never taught that we have any measure of control over our inner landscape. Paying attention to how you feel—becoming aware of the earliest signs that your stress response is getting activated—is the first step to getting—and staying—out of survival mode.

To do this, practice becoming more aware of the sensations and messages you're getting from your body and your mind, throughout the day and before you go to sleep. Signs that your stress response is activated include: tense shoulders, shallow or rapid breathing, racing heart, digestive symptoms. Our thoughts and thought patterns are also indicative: increased anxiety, worry, ruminating, negative thoughts, and overwhelm are signs that your stress response has ramped up a notch—or

ten! If you're feeling maxed or exhausted from juggling too much, are finding yourself anxious, overwhelmed, or depressed, this is not some failing on your part; these are also messages telling you loudly and clearly it's time to step back, take stock of what's on your plate, and reprioritize.

Once you learn to recognize when you're in the grip of stress (or distress!), you can respond quickly with a relaxation response practice rather than react with a prolonged stress response. I can't overstate the importance of taking a stand against a culture that demands ever more of us, in favor of our own health and well-being. The feelings and thoughts associated with being stressed out are your inner GPS telling you that you're overwhelmed. Learning to get aligned with your inner GPS is going to get your hormone inner guidance system back on track! Turning off chronic stress is hard—after all, it's addictive. Life doesn't just turn itself off for an hour while a red carpet rolls itself out to your essential-oil bath. We have to be committed to getting off the hamster wheel.

What can you do to stay more in touch with your body and purposefully use your sense of *interoception*—a lesser-known sense that helps you understand and feel what's going on inside your body? A therapist colleague I know calls it "dropping in," getting out of our heads, which we tend to spend a lot of time in, and remembering to check in with our physical selves and sensations. To do this, pause periodically throughout the day to deliberately get quiet, and notice *how you feel*. What are the sensations going on in your body right now? Are you breathing deeply? Clenching your jaw? Your pelvic muscles? Is your posture upright? Are you knitting your brow?

To truly *know* our own bodies, we have to pay attention—which means turning off a lot of the distractions life seems filled with these days, from Netflix to your cell phone to your Amazon shopping cart, and the 24-hour anxiety-inducing news cycles—to look within, to hear the quiet and stillness that also reduce stress hormones and inflammation and start to allow the body to heal.

I call the language of the body *BodySpeak*. BodySpeak awareness creates time for checking into yourself and creating mindful centeredness. As a result, you make better choices and become more aware of:

- How you feel when you eat various foods (both your mood when eating them and how the foods affect how you feel afterward)

- Emotions associated with your lifestyle habits—which feel good to you and which don't

- How you feel in your various relationships and in social and professional settings

- Where in your body you hold stress

- How you feel during different phases of your cycle

Practices that help you cultivate more inner calm and resilience include:

- Meditation

- Breathing practices

- Yoga

- Dance

- Tai chi

- Getting a massage

- Relaxing in a bath

- Eating mindfully

- Anything that brings more comfortable, relaxed, fluid awareness to you and ease in your body

How to Meditate (Even If You Don't Love Sitting Still)

I don't love sitting still for an hour in meditation, not even for thirty minutes! But I value the importance of meditation in so many aspects of health. So I practice my all-time favorite meditation called the *Quickie* (not what you think!) that you can do anywhere, anytime, even while driving (with your eyes open, of course!), for practically instant relaxation results.

Here's how to do it: Wherever you are, sitting or standing, get comfortable and take a few deep breaths in through your nose and out through your mouth. If you are sitting, close your eyes. On the next inhalation, which you will do to the count of four, say to yourself "I am" and on the exhale to a count of eight, say to yourself "at peace." Repeat this cycle of inhalations and exhalations four times.

It can be done in as short as a minute, or you can repeat it for longer. It's remarkably effective at taking you from feeling like you're heading into a big emotional earthquake back to inner peace and calm, cutting through irritability in a flash. It's the perfect antidote to grocery-checkout-line impatience or road rage and can be done in a meeting or job interview or when your partner or kids are driving you nuts. It's also one of my favorite sleep-inducing techniques, so remember that when you get to the next chapter!

In addition, pay attention to your normal daily body signals and respond to them rather than put them off. When you need to eat, then eat; drink, then drink; go to the bathroom, stretch, nap, get outside—do it. Paying attention to the common body signals will make you more aware of your BodySpeak.

Step 2: Manage Your Energy

The next practice is to match your outer landscape to *how you want to feel.* Take inventory of the areas of your life that are sapping your energy, causing you overwhelm, or throwing you into survival mode. What are the biggest sources of stress in your life, the biggest energy drains? Now make a plan for how you're going to eliminate or at least minimize them. This might mean saying no to some things

you've taken on, rethinking how you approach your work-life ratio, taking more time for self-care so you can have the resilience to cope with what's on your plate, or rethinking your economics to want less of what you don't need and earn more so you can have what you do need.

Here are some of the ways I recommend shifting your priorities, simplifying your life, and plugging energy drains.

Pick your priorities, shorten your to-do list, and stick with it. Most of us live with the (awful) illusion that we're never doing or giving enough, that we always have to do more, be more, give more. Many of our workplaces reinforce that—if you don't stay later than the next person, you don't get the promotion or raise. It's great to have high expectations

Pick Your Priorities

If overwhelm is your middle name, take 5 minutes to ask yourself these questions to clarify your bigger life priorities, and then each day, ask yourself these questions to help prioritize your day:

- What are the 5 most important things/people/projects/activities to me right now?

- What do I *really* want to do / take on right now? (Be ruthlessly honest with yourself on this one, and ask yourself *why*—it might help you shorten your list.)

- What can I let go of that I don't have to do, don't want to do, and that's causing me pressure?

- What can I realistically get done without undue pressure? (Hint: Calculate the amount of time you *think* a project will take, then increase that by 30%—that's how much we tend to underestimate how long tasks will take.)

When you identify your priorities, stick to those until they are complete and only then add a new one; outsource whatever your finances allow you to (and what might surprise you is that hiring someone to do a task for you might free up time for you to be creative—and you can monetize that time and make *more* money, or you're just happier and more relaxed). If you forget and start to take on too much or get overwhelmed, revisit this practice until doing less and sticking with your priorities become second nature.

of yourself, and lovely to give and give. But where does it end if you become depleted in the long run and then have nothing left to give. That's when health suffers, too. It also feels great to check things off your checklist—but if you have too many things on it, it becomes impossible to do that, leaving you feeling overwhelmed, unable to relax, disappointed in yourself, and worried that you're disappointing others. Having a more realistic to-do list, with clear priorities, can allow you to have a new level of ease and a sense of accomplishment at the end of each day!

If it's not a hell yes, it's a no. I truly live by this principle. Life inevitably hands us a parade of invitations, offers, and requests we feel we should say yes to. In the moment, some of those things might even feel exciting. But pretty soon, we end up with too many events, cakes to bake, presentations to give, parties to go to. Like buyer's remorse, we experience YES remorse, end up overwhelmed and stressed, and wish we had said no (or we bail and feel guilty). Try this: learn to say yes to only those things that you truly think about in advance, assess your time and energy level for doing, and check in with whether these are "on brand" with your personal priorities for a more chill life. You do have to get good at saying, "Let me think about that before I say yes," or, "No thanks" (with no explanation needed). It may be uncomfortable at first, but I promise you, the relief you'll feel with less on your plate—priceless.

Fix your energy leaks. We all know that person—the one you see in the grocery store or the hallway at work or whose number appears on your caller ID—the one you try to avoid because somehow, after talking with them, even for five minutes, you feel exhausted, bad about yourself, or like you want to take a shower or a nap.

Some people, for whatever reason, drain our

> ### Repair Energy Leaks
>
> Take a few minutes to reflect on what's draining your energy and jot down what you can do differently about this. It's a good practice to do at the end of each week, and look at what you're going to shift for the following week.

energy. So do some situations—relationships you know that aren't serving you, a job you've outgrown, a boss who is emotionally or verbally abusive, even a family member or friend who lacks boundaries. While I don't recommend just shutting people out of our lives unless there's a good reason for it, learning to avoid or set boundaries with energy-draining people, and making bolder decisions to change a situation that is draining you, can help you repair energy leaks. And what about things you just don't need to do that you're saying yes to? Remember, don't say yes when you want to say no!

Practice soft power. Women are truly "boss," but fitting into male-dominated power structures, and the male executive stereotype that has dominated most workplaces for decades, isn't consistent with how women's nervous systems work. One of the ways we can check our inner landscape is to catch when we're feeling like we have to lead and live like men—and remind ourselves that feminine power is equally powerful, and that we're more wired to connect and cooperate. Whatever your role is at work, make sure that you're leading others, especially other women who are juggling the same busy lives and dealing with the shit you are, with soft power. It's what creates the revolution that changes the whole game.

Make your life easier. I'm all for home-cooked meals and handcrafted holiday gifts, but let's be real: there's just so much time in a day and we can't be and do everything. Identify those time-intensive special things you LOVE doing, or feel you'd somehow lose your identity if you didn't do; keep those on your priority list and simplify (or outsource) everything else. Be merciless about making your life simpler. Think of all the ways you could spend your time if you weren't spending it exhausted.

Quiet your inner critic and reframe. One more thing about making your life easier: we have to stop criticizing ourselves. The world demands enough of us already without us dumping on ourselves, yet most women have an inner critic chattering in the background all day long—and sometimes well into the night. We beat ourselves up for not doing enough all day long—whether it was at work, what you ate, not pushing hard enough in your Pilates class, or not doing enough for your kids. Recognize self-criticism for what it is—old and unhelpful messaging that got programmed into you at some point in your life, reinforced by a culture that demands ever more of us, yet tells us we're never doing enough. Let it go. No more beating yourself up about your body, health, hormones, diet, hair, nose, teeth, accomplishments, income, relationship status, your home, or anything else. Crush that critical self-chatter with kindness; some positive self-reinforcement never hurts. Every time that inner critic pushes her noisy little comments into your thoughts, let her know you're good and don't need her help. Instead, channel your best friend—what would she say to you about how you did today? Take a few minutes each night before bed and think of something you felt proud of that day. Revel in that. Eventually, this practice will teach that inner critic to quiet down and leave you in peace. It's an important part of this plan—because I don't want you judging yourself along the way (or ever)!

Step 3: Make "Relaxed" a Way of Life

Just as we have a stress response, there is a flip side to that coin: the **relaxation response**, the antidote to the impacts of stress on your health and hormones. This section is going to help you develop a regular "stress decompression" practice by building your relaxation response tool kit. Relaxation techniques such as meditation, mindfulness, and active stress reduction help to let your adrenals know that you are safe—and this allows your system to recalibrate to a lower stress state, including pumping out fewer stress hormones. It can even help you reverse stress-driven damage. As a longtime yoga-practicing, journal-toting, nature-loving hippie, I've personally been overjoyed in recent years to see so many of what used to be considered "fringe" and "woo-woo" practices be backed by solid science showing their effectiveness for a wide range of health conditions, including hormone problems. For example, solid studies demonstrate the benefits of yoga and meditation for preventing and also reducing menstrual

---

How to Simplify

List three areas of your life that feel overwhelming, unnecessarily hard, or complicated. What are two things you can do to simplify each of those areas? Example: Area that's hard: Cooking for my family feels hard but I want us all to eat healthy. Solution: Plan meals and shop weekly, or subscribe to a meal prep and delivery service for three days of the week.

pain, PMS, and endometriosis pain and for improving fertility, including increasing conception rates even with assisted fertility.

Give yourself permission to pause, regularly. Ralph Waldo Emerson said, "Guard your own spare moments. They are like uncut diamonds." We all need PERMISSION TO PAUSE, regularly. Sadly, few of us have "spare moments," so we have to create them intentionally because they truly are invaluable when it comes to restoring your nervous system. Too often we don't, and we end up irritable and spent, replacing a bottle of wine and a box of cookies for rest and self-care. Downtime is the "off" we need to balance the constant "on" of our HPA axis.

Women are especially bad at taking time for ourselves. Mothers are even worse. We are so trained to keep going in the face of no sleep, emotional exhaustion, and constant external demands that we forget we have a right to be "human beings" and not just "human doings."

Having trouble hitting the pause button? Ask yourself these five questions:

- If I took some time for myself, what would be the best thing that could happen?

- The worst thing?

- How much time do I need, realistically, and how often, to feel recharged?

- How am I going to create this time?

- And what would I like to do with the time?

I think you'll realize that the world will not stop spinning on its axis if you put down a few of the balls you're spinning in the air, to replenish yourself.

Don't stressercize . . . but do move. Exercise is a huge stress reliever—and so important for your body, mind, and mood. Whether you're trying to get pregnant, get better sleep,

or reduce metabolic imbalances and improve PCOS, exercise is indispensable. It improves most health parameters, and not only has sitting too much been found to cause inflammation, it keeps our pelvic and abdominal organs all bunched up all day, compressed on each other, and prevents us from getting healthy pelvic circulation.

However, overexercising, a common problem for women, is an especially significant cause of hypothalamic amenorrhea, made even worse if you don't consume enough energy (calories) to keep up with what you're burning off. What's the sweet spot? At least thirty minutes of some form of gentle to moderate movement every day, for example, walking, dancing, gardening, yoga, running around with your kids; with about an hour of a more rigorous workout three to four times a week—ideally a combination of cardio, weights, and stretching. You can mix it up any way you like; the important thing is to get SOME movement in every day so you're not sedentary. If you're thinking, *Nice idea, Dr. Aviva, but I've got a desk job*—don't let that be an excuse! You can still get your "steps" in (and the latest science shows that even just four thousand steps a day is very beneficial). Consider a standing desk, stretch in your office, take your meetings on the move, get out for a vigorous walk at lunch, or do fifteen minutes of stairs if your office building has them.

Get a daily dose of vitamin P. That is—pleasure! It's an essential nutrient that reduces stress hormones and inflammation, boosts immunity, relieves depression, reduces pain, improves satisfaction, improves mood chemicals, and improves memory and focus. Figure out what makes you happy—truly happy—and do more of that, even if you have to schedule it in.

Get with your girlfriends. The reality is that maintaining a healthy social life is no easy feat because our responsibilities keep us overscheduled. But studies show that when we connect with each other, our progesterone levels increase, improving our feelings of calm; giving us better sleep, all the benefits of cycle regularity, and optimal fertility; and helping with our overall sense of well-being. It happens through a hormone called oxytocin—a neuropeptide synthesized in the hypothalamus that gives us courage and helps us to be more sensitive to others—which gets released when we reach out to and connect with peeps we love. And it works reciprocally; being there for a friend also bumps up our "love hormone." So make time for phone or online chats, group dinners, a cup of tea on the weekend, or a playdate that allows the moms to connect too.

Become a tree hugger. Okay, you don't *actu-* *ally* have to hug trees (though it is quite nice), but spending time in nature is relaxing for a reason: it helps lower cortisol levels and activates the parasympathetic nervous system, promoting relaxation and getting us out of our "fight or flight" response. Forest bathing—literally just spending time in the woods on a regular basis, ideally several hours at a time—can even restore healthier immune system functioning, including some of the immune alterations associated with endometriosis, with lasting results.

Step 4: Keep Your Battery Charged (a.k.a., Your Blood Sugar Balanced)

It's midday, you're feeling shaky, losing your concentration, maybe even a little light-headed.

My Top-10 Permission-to-Pause List

1. Do something—anything—in nature: Take a walk alone or with a pal but try walking in silence, lie in the grass and stare up at the sky (find creatures in the clouds), work in your garden if you have one.

2. Take a hot bath or a long shower—make it feel like a spa with some lovely essential-oil scents (lavender is relaxing, rose is calming, mint invigorating, amber or sandalwood grounding and sensual).

3. Have a cup of tea and read a book or write in your journal.

4. Rock it out in a solo dance party. Crank up your tunes; break a sweat.

5. Watch a favorite movie without ever once opening up the computer to check email or other social media.

6. Turn off all electronics and meditate for 10 minutes, do yoga for 30 minutes, or take a nap for 45 minutes.

7. Prepare a special, wonderful meal each week and eat slowly, deliberately, with perfect attention to just the experience of the meal.

8. Hop on the phone with your best friend.

9. Make art. Or love.

10. Get a massage.

Quick Snack / Emergency Food Stash

- A small container of almonds or walnuts, or individual nut butter packets
- Organic turkey or salmon jerky (if you eat meat)
- Hard-boiled eggs
- Unsweetened trail mix or gluten-free granola
- Hummus and veggies or gluten-free crackers
- Quick turkey roll-ups or another type of lettuce wrap
- A small container of unsweetened coconut yogurt with some nuts and seeds, a handful of unsweetened trail mix, or fresh berries tossed in

You suddenly realize you haven't eaten since this morning. Okay, you've eaten a little bit, but just coffee and a muffin—but not real food. Most of us know the feeling; the blood sugar crash, or "food emergency," is super common—and, when it's a recurring theme, takes a major toll on the adrenal stress system. That's because your brain is DEPENDENT on a steady supply of glucose to keep it happily humming, and low blood sugar triggers your stress response to get mobilized and sends you in search of quick energy. So what do we do? Grab the muffin, candy bar, or bag of chips. Most of us are eating on the fly—and forget to regularly check our inner battery—not noticing it's low until the alarm is going off.

Keeping your blood sugar steady keeps your brain out of survival mode. It's also my top-tier solution for getting and staying free of sugar and other cravings. So you've got to "feed your head." Regularly. With protein, high-quality fats, and carbs from whole grains and veggies. The Mediterranean diet, upon which eating for Hormone Intelligence is based, has been shown to reduce HPA-axis stress—largely because it's so effective at helping women to maintain blood sugar balance. So you're already on your way!

My top tips for keeping your blood sugar steady are:

- Start your day with a power breakfast.
- Eat some form of healthy protein at each meal.
- Make sure to get enough healthy fats into your meals.
- Don't skip meals.
- Commit to those two servings of slow carbs a day.
- If you haven't cut back on caffeine, now's the time.
- Keep a healthy emergency stash of high-protein snacks on hand.

Step 5: Leverage Your Cycle Sense

Remember to leverage cycle sense as part of staying in a healthy, less-stress mind-set. Knowing that you're more or less susceptible or resilient to stress at certain phases of your menstrual cycle can help you prepare for and respond more effectively during those times. During your follicular phase, close to ovulation, you might feel more energetic, and in the mood to say YES to life—and everything that comes your way. So enjoy being more active and starting a new project; just be cautious not to overextend or start too many new projects during this time. Conversely, as you get into the days or week leading up to your period, even natural drops in estrogen and progesterone, along with lower levels of serotonin, can cause your mood to be low or lead you to feel more overwhelmed, irritable, or anxious. Instead of wondering what's wrong with you, reframe your mind-set to "How can I work with this?" If you have premenstrual or period symptoms, try to designate some time for self-care just before or during the first couple of days of your period; any practice you find relaxing and replenishing can improve your menstrual experience.

Step 6: Use Adaptogens and Nutrients to Reset Your Stress Response

By supporting your stress response system, you can improve communication between your hypothalamus, ovaries, and thyroid—getting optimal functioning back online. Here are my favorite herbs and supplements for doing this. You don't have to take all of them. A good multivitamin with B-complex and magnesium will provide what you need for daily nervous system support. You can find more information and proper dosage in the Botanical and Supplement Quick Reference Guide on pages 372–81.

Magnesium: Called "the calming mineral," and one that most of us are deficient in, magnesium is an important daily supplement for hundreds of important reactions in our bodies, including blood sugar and insulin regulation,

bone health, mood, detoxification in the liver, and muscle relaxation.

Phosphatidyl Serine: A compound similar to a dietary fat and found widely in the brain and nervous system, PS reduces excess cortisol and adrenaline release under stress. It has many adaptogen-like effects: improving mood, physical energy, and cognitive function, including enhancing memory, attention, and information processing speed, while also improving exercise capacity.

Vitamin C (Ascorbic Acid): Found abundantly in the adrenal cortex where it plays an important anti-inflammatory role protecting the adrenals, vitamin C is depleted by stress. Supplementation helps to normalize cortisol and replenishes the adrenal glands.

Zinc: It may help regulate cortisol by reducing the brain's activation to stress and trauma and is effective in preventing and treating depression.

A Probiotic: Exciting research on the gut-brain connection shows that beneficial gut flora relieve anxiety and depression, reduce inflammation, and reduce HPA-axis overstimulation. The strains to use include *Lactobacillus* and *Bifidobacterium* species, specifically *Bifidobacterium infantis* and *B. longum*.

Adaptogens: Herbs for Stress Resilience

Adaptogens are a special class of herbal medicines that have been used in traditional Chinese and Ayurvedic medicine for centuries to promote a sense of well-being. They're used to restore health, vitality, immunity, and stamina and to promote longevity, and the science behind them is impressive.

The term *adaptogen* refers to the unique

ability of these herbs to help you adapt to the stress in your life. They do this by "normalizing" or "regulating" the adrenal stress response. An important caution, however: Adaptogens are not meant to be used to keep you pushing harder and for longer. They're not a substitute for sleep, meditation, time in nature, time with friends, or good food. While adaptogens may give you the extra support you need for those occasional times when you just can't hit the pause button, the real goal is to address the underlying issues that are keeping you in survival mode. My favorites follow.

Ashwagandha: With over 4,000 years of traditional use in India, ashwagandha has been found helpful in healing stress and related symptoms including deep exhaustion, sleep, anxiety, and memory. Cortisol levels can be reduced by as much as 30% in otherwise healthy but stressed people, which is significantly larger than with many other supplements. It is also very helpful if musculoskeletal aches and pains are keeping you up at night or have started to appear as a result of exhaustion. Contrary to popular misinformation, this herb is considered safe for women with Hashimoto's. It is a nightshade but is not usually considered troublesome for those avoiding them.

Reishi Mushroom: Reishi is highly regarded in Chinese medicine for its ability to nourish and support adrenal function. It calms the nervous system and can be taken before bed for deeper, relaxing, and restorative sleep. It is a powerful herb for your immune system, so if you're getting sick a lot because of stress, or never get sick and then crash on your first day of vacation, this might be a great choice for you. It may also help reduce PCOS or androgen-triggered hair loss.

Holy Basil: Holy or "sacred" basil calms the mind and spirit and promotes longevity. This herb, called *tulsi* in Ayurveda, is used to improve energy and relieve fatigue, and it elevates the mood, especially providing relief from mild depression. While this herb is related to common basil, that is not a substitute.

Rhodiola: Helps promote a calm emotional state and supports strong mental performance, optimal immune function, and hormonal balance. It improves mental and physical stamina, improves sleep, and reduces stress, "burnout," and irritability. It boosts the immune system, decreases the frequency of colds and infections, and reduces inflammation, and may help reduce stress headaches.

Shatavari: Considered the "queen of herbs" in Ayurvedic medicine, shatavari is beloved

Dark Chocolate

While I definitely don't want you to overdo the caffeine, small amounts of chocolate are the exception. In one study, eating 1.4 ounces (40 grams) of dark chocolate every day, half in the morning, half in the afternoon, for two weeks reduced levels of stress hormones in people feeling highly stressed, and eating dark chocolate daily reduced stress hormone levels in those who had high anxiety levels. It also reduces insulin resistance, improves brain function and health, increases serotonin, and helps prevent cravings—giving you a "treat" to look forward to—and it has been shown to help with weight reduction! So overall, dark chocolate, in moderation of course, increases health and happiness.

as one of the most powerful rejuvenating tonics for women. It is nourishing and calming, as well as hormonally balancing; it is used for irritability and many hormonal imbalances affecting the mood, for example, emotional symptoms of PMS and menopause.

Maca: The Quechua people of Peru consider maca a food that promotes mental acuity, physical vitality, endurance, and stamina. Maca reduces anxiety and depression and is rich in essential amino acids, iodine, iron, and magnesium, as well as sterols that may possess a wide range of activities that support adrenal and hormone function. Bonus: it's known to boost libido, too! You can try maca in in the Women's Bliss Bites on page 366.

Curcumin: An extract from turmeric, a spice that has been used in Indian cooking for thousands of years, curcumin has now been found helpful in resetting HPA-axis–driven anxiety and depression and is a fabulous anti-inflammatory.

While you can experience benefits from adaptogens in just a couple of weeks or less, be patient and give these herbs 6 to 12 weeks to get started, and stick with them for up to 6 months (or longer)—it can take some time to calm and soothe your stress system, especially if you've been in stress overdrive for a while.

More Connections Ahead!

When we're tired, stressed, and overwhelmed, we need to give ourselves what might seem impossible—time to restore, heal, and replenish. We need permission to pause. If you can learn to hit the reset button when you need to, the benefits will be many: greater longevity, inner peace, better relationships, a healthier, more vital body and mind—and happier hormones. And if the idea of relaxing gets your achievement brain into a panic attack, don't worry; you'll also be more productive, not less! One of the most important ways we pause, heal, and replenish is through sleep. Let's look at how sleep affects your hormone health and what you can do to get your z's on.

it's about time

RESET YOUR BODY CLOCK TO SYNC YOUR HORMONES

If we surrendered to earth's intelligence,
we could rise up rooted, like trees.
—**Rainer Maria Rilke**

Do you start your day jumping out of bed bright and sunny, ready to take on the day? Or are you more likely to hit the snooze button and pull the covers over your head? Do you wake up groggy or have a groggy slump in the middle of the afternoon, when you start craving some sugar or caffeine? Do you lie awake staring at the ceiling at night, or wake in the middle of the night, tossing and turning, and worrying about not just life, but how tired you're going to be tomorrow?

A whole lot of us are living our lives completely out of sync with natural daily rhythms: we're staying up too late trying to squeeze out the last bit of work we need to get done because our jobs might depend on it (and if not, our internal-pressuring perfectionist compels us to), or we're grabbing some late hours just to have some quiet time to ourselves after the kids

have gone to bed or work is done. As a result, we're zipping through our days with a harried inner landscape and not getting enough sleep to replenish us; we're spending too little time in nature, and we're exposed to artificial lighting for so much time each day that our primal biological rhythms aren't so sure whether it's day or night! Over time, irregular sleep hours, lost sleep, and even sleeping in the setting of unnatural light, sound, and temperatures can lead to desynchronization of our internal clocks—a phenomenon called *chronodisruption*. But those inner clocks are what keep our hormones ticking along to our innate inner blueprint.

Our ancestors naturally lived in harmony with nature's rhythms and cycles, and since ancient times, the cycles of the moon and women's cycles have been tied together in myth, religion, and healing practices. The terms *menstruation* and *menses* come from Latin and Greek words meaning "moon" (*mene*) and "month" (*menses*), while menstruation is referred to as "the moon" in any number of languages, from French to Mandingo. Circatrigintan (yeah, I can't pronounce that either) cycles refer to those that occur in monthly rhythms. The most common of these are menstruation and the lunar cycle.

How much sleep do we need to live the most basic of healthy lives? No less than seven hours every night (and no more than nine hours; requiring or getting too much sleep is not good for your health either). A lot of women are getting by on less than this recommended amount at least several nights a week, if not nightly.

While it's not scientifically true that we cycle with the moon, nor do we actually sync our cycles with the women we live with—both common and fun myths that seem true because statistically sometimes our cycles do sync up with the new or full moon, or our flat mates or best friends—menstrual cycles are something women have experienced since the beginning of time. This powerfully connects us as something we all do have in common, and even if you are no longer cycling, you're still part of the club. The connection between women and nature, and natural rhythms, however, is not simply a romantic notion. Our deepest, most innate, ancient biology is rooted in the rhythms of nature, and our hormonal cycles depend on tightly orchestrated internal events that take their cues from nature. Our cells are still looking for those ancient cues—but instead are getting very different signals—and those "wrong" signals make a dominant contribution to our modern hidden hormone epidemic.

Chronobiology: The Rhythms That Guide Our Cycles

The hormone epidemic we're facing is, in part, a reflection of life out of balance—with nature, with daily rhythms, with ourselves. To restore balance, we have to return to nature's rhythms, particularly the circadian rhythm. Amazingly, it's something that can happen in just a matter of weeks, and I'm going to show you exactly how.

Timing Is Everything: Meet Your Circadian Rhythm

You have a central internal clock, located in an area of your hypothalamus called the *suprachiasmatic nucleus* (SCN). The SCN coordinates your body's functions around a twenty-four-hour clock, the **circadian rhythm** (*circa* means "around," *diem* means "day"), coinciding with

---

Hormone Intelligence: Reset Your Body Clock

- Reset your morning and evening routines and learn how to pace your day for better energy.
- Learn how to eat for a healthier circadian rhythm.
- Enjoy the evening wind-down as a new part of your nighttime routine.
- Get the best tips for falling asleep more easily, sleeping restfully through the night, and waking up refreshed every morning.

the twenty-four-hour rotation of our planet around the sun. It evolved so that functions and behaviors most appropriate for daytime—for example, being awake when there's natural light, eating, digesting, eliminating, and being immunologically primed to neutralize the viruses and bacteria we're more likely to encounter while we're awake—and those that occur at night—for example, sleep and higher levels of cellular repair and detoxification—occur respectively during the daytime or nighttime hours.

Circadian rhythm disruption is an important and often overlooked "missing link" between nature and human biology—and one that conventional medicine completely misses when considering the influences on health and chronic disease. It's so significant that there's now an entire scientific field called *chronobiology* (one of the most fascinating to me!) that studies the links between natural rhythms, health, and disease. Scientists studying one particular aspect of this—the molecular mechanisms controlling the circadian rhythm—won the 2017 Nobel Prize in Medicine!

Tick, Tock, Peripheral Clocks

In addition to this central master clock, every organ and cell in your body—from your brain, heart, liver, spleen, your fat cells, and adrenal glands, to specific immune tissues and cells, to your ovaries, fallopian tubes, and uterus—has its own individual circadian-synced clock. These are known as *peripheral clocks*, and their timing and functioning are specific to the optimal timing for the actions of those organs and cells to occur. As such, the central clock regulates essential functions including hunger, nutrient absorption from food, intestinal motility, immunity, growth, sleep, metabolism, body temperature, and, apropos to what's brought us together in this book, your hormones. This harmonization between our organ systems and our circadian rhythm is called *entrainment*; our life rhythms are also meant to be entrained to our circadian clock. Undisrupted, our internal clock runs with exquisite precision, synced up to its biggest cues: daily exposure to cycles of light and dark, which respectively trigger two important hormonal regulatory signals—cortisol and melatonin—as well as the timing of when you eat, sleep, and eliminate, and the cyclicity of your hormones.

To keep your functions coordinated, however, they all must remain synchronized, or "entrained," to your central clock. The whole system works like an orchestra: your SCN is the conductor and your peripheral clocks are the musicians. If your central clock gets off track, then your peripheral clocks can lose their timing. It's like an orchestra that's trying to play without a conductor—all the instruments will be out of rhythm. From an ancestral perspective, this wouldn't be good! Think of it this way—your ancestors wouldn't have wanted to go in search of dinner or have to go poop in the middle of the night as this might have meant venturing out of a warm safe cave or hut to possibly face a hungry nocturnal predator!

It Goes Both Ways

The relationships between these peripheral clocks and your central clock are bidirectional, meaning that disturbances in the central clock can disrupt the peripheral clock and alter its function, and vice versa—disruption in any of your body's ecosystems can alter peripheral clock timing and disrupt your entire circadian rhythm, impacting any (or every) other system in your body. For example, chronic inflammation leads to the production of cytokines and other immune factors that upset circadian rhythm, and cross talk between imbalances in gut microbiota and your central circadian clock can unfavorably alter its rhythm.

Hormone Intelligence simultaneously helps you to reset your circadian rhythm while also getting to the bottom of the root causes that disrupt it—the same ones that upset hormone balance.

Living Jet-Lagged

If you've ever experienced jet lag, you've experienced the acute impact of your circadian rhythm being out of sync. Your mind feels foggy, you're tired but can't seem to get normal hours of sleep, you crave sugar, you may wake up at 4 a.m. ready for a meal, and your digestive system is often too far ahead or too far behind where you need it to be, making you constipated—or your bowels wake you at weird hours! Jet lag is an example of an acute disruption in your circadian rhythm. But you don't have to travel internationally to experience jet lag. Most of us now live with some degree of what is essentially, modern jet lag—our lives are chronically out of sync with natural rhythms.

A poll by the National Sleep Foundation found that 43% of participants said that they rarely or never get a good night's sleep, and 63% of Americans say their sleep needs are not being met during the week. Reductions in sleep duration have become common due to the socioeconomic demands of modern society. Sleep time has decreased by nearly two hours in the US in the past couple of decades; nearly a third of Americans get six hours of sleep or less per night. Many don't even try to get into bed before midnight, using those late hours to try to relax after an evening in which work bleeds into home time, or not even leaving work until well into the dinner hours. Who's getting the least sleep? Women. Sleep disruptions are much more common in women, with reports of insomnia occurring 1.5–2 times more frequently than in men, and sleep disturbances are often worse in the premenstrual part of our cycles. And statistically, working moms have it the worst.

Cortisol and Melatonin: Your Central Clock Messengers

If your SCN is the conductor, and your peripheral clocks the musicians, cortisol, which I introduced to you in the previous chapter, and melatonin, are the musical notes that guide which instruments are playing which notes,

The Circadian Rhythm

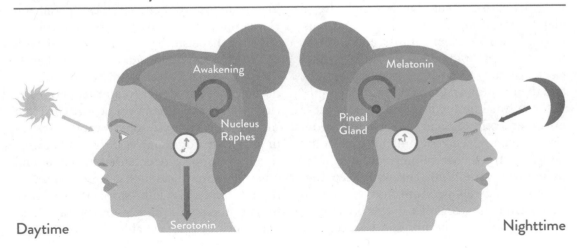

Daytime — Awakening, Nucleus Raphes, Serotonin

Nighttime — Melatonin, Pineal Gland

at which time. Melatonin is a neurohormone, meaning it affects both your nervous and your endocrine systems. Produced in the pineal gland of your brain like cortisol, it follows a diurnal pattern, with alternating twelve-hour peaks and valleys. As such, they are both intimately involved in maintaining your circadian rhythm and are central in orchestrating the various functions that happen under their watch. They are also profoundly interrelated, having opposing twelve-hour rhythms. The neurons in the Nucleus Raphes produce most of our serotonin, are highly active when we're awake, and like the pineal gland, also regulate circadian rhythm.

Cortisol is highest in the morning, when it gives you a natural surge of energy for waking up (the cortisol awakening response or CAR), boosts your immune system, and keeps inflammation in check, among its numerous actions. Cortisol wanes over the course of the day and into the evening, until around midnight when it's at its lowest. As cortisol declines and the evening sets in, melatonin, which was suppressed by daylight and by the presence of daytime levels of cortisol, begins to increase. Under its healing, restorative influence, we enter into a phase of rest and repair while we sleep—the parasympathetic nervous system takes over your inner landscape. Thus, I think of melatonin as the healing queen of sleep.

Melatonin has numerous powerful therapeutic effects. In addition to ensuring that we get sleepy in the evening and have a restful night, melatonin:

- Reduces inflammation and repairs many of the damaging effects of oxidative stress

- Supports ovarian function, ovulation, and the health of the ovum

- Helps to regulate the circadian rhythm inherent in the gut microbiome

- Helps preserve the integrity of your gut lining, protecting against leaky gut

- Reduces the pain response

- Clears daily toxins we naturally accumulate in our brain through a network called *glymphatic cells*

The Circadian-Hormone Connection: A Whole New Meaning to "Biological Clock"

From your brain down to your ovaries and uterus, your female hormonal physiology is deeply entrained to your circadian timing system. The pulsatile secretion of GnRH, that hypothalamic hormone that gets puberty rolling and sets the pace for ovarian hormone production for the next forty years of your life, isn't random—it's dialed in to your circadian rhythm. So is the LH surge that triggers ovulation; in a large number of women it predictably occurs during nighttime sleep. FSH is also influenced by sleep and circadian rhythm: women who get less than eight hours of sleep secrete 20% less FSH compared with women who sleep longer.

The uterus and ovaries have circadian clock genes that synchronize their clocks to the SCN using estrogen, which, like melatonin and cortisol, has a diurnal rhythm. Circadian clocks in the ovary may play a role in the timing of ovulation. Disruption of the clock in ovarian cells or *desynchrony* between ovarian clocks and circadian pacemakers elsewhere in the body may contribute to the onset and progression of a number of gynecologic problems. Loss of circadian rhythm affects ovarian hormone production, affecting ovulation, progesterone, estrogen, and testosterone levels, as well as fertility. Thus, women appear to be particularly susceptible to desynchronization in our circadian rhythms. Other hormones that influence our female hormones, including thyroid-stimulating hormone (TSH) and prolactin, cycle with a twenty-four-hour rhythmicity and are also sensitive to sleep-wake state. Further, all the ecosystems upon which hormone balance depend—metabolism and blood sugar balance, nutrient absorption from your food, the health of your microbiome, regular elimination, immune health and inflammation control, even liver detoxification—require a healthy, synced circadian rhythm.

Shift Work and Your Hormones

One in five employees in the US now works nonstandard hours, a rate that has increased substantially over the past couple of decades and that only seems to be getting worse in the digital age. Yet overwhelming evidence now points to harmful impact of shift work, defined as anything outside 9 a.m. to 7 p.m., on women's hormones. Aside from sacrifices to relationships, time with family, and social lives, there's a huge health impact from the circadian misalignment that occurs as a result of night shifts or excessively long work hours, leading to disruption in sleep-wake cycles and eating times. Shift workers are significantly more likely to report menstrual irregularity and longer menstrual cycles than women with "day jobs."

Shift work is associated with fertility problems, increased risk of adverse pregnancy outcomes including miscarriage and preterm birth, and sleep disturbances in women. Flight attendants who worked while they were pregnant were twice as likely to have a miscarriage when compared to flight attendants who did not work during their pregnancy. There also is accumulating evidence that circadian disruption increases the risk of breast cancer in women, due to altered light exposure and reduced melatonin secretion. Women who work the night shift are also more susceptible to depression, weight gain, menstrual cycle irregularities, dysmenorrhea, endometriosis, fertility challenges, diabetes, and even breast cancer. In 2007, night shift work was reclassified from a possible to a probable human carcinogen (class 2A) by the International Agency for Research on Cancer.

You may be thinking, *I don't work the night shift, so none of this applies to me*, but it's not just night shift work—even working more than forty hours per week, including that overflow that you take home, may impact your hormone balance. Working more than a forty-hour workweek has been linked to increased rates of miscarriage, preterm delivery, low-birth-weight babies, and preeclampsia—all sure signs of circadian rhythm disruption and hormone imbalance that can also be affecting you if you're not pregnant. For her 2012 book, *Sleeping with Your Smartphone*, the Harvard Business School professor Leslie Perlow found that of the sixteen hundred managers and professionals she surveyed, 92% reported putting in fifty or more hours of work a week, with a third clocking sixty-five hours or more. And that didn't include commuting time or work taken home at the end of the day or week.

We have hormonal needs that are hard-wired to a much more natural, softer pace of life, more connected to nature's rhythms, and a more feminine, twenty-eight-day infradian cycle, than a more male-driven, twenty-four-hour, testosterone-driven cycle. Yet we feel that we have no choice but to try to match the male-driven cycle—and in doing so, our female cycles get derailed.

Much like stress, circadian rhythm disruption and sleep loss are major hormone disruptors. In the previous chapter, I explained the impact of chronically elevated cortisol on your hormones—and sleep is perhaps our biggest trigger of chronically jacked-up cortisol. Melatonin also has many significant regulatory effects on women's hormonal cycles and reproductive functions, including regulating the pulsatile release of GnRH in the brain, which signals production of estrogen and progesterone, and regulating the timing of the LH surge that leads to ovulation. Thus, low melatonin can reduce ovarian function and ovulation. Further, high levels of melatonin are naturally found in the fluid surrounding a healthy, mature ovum; it's thought that because ovulation is a slightly inflammatory process, the presence of melatonin protects both the corpus luteum and the ovum from inflammatory damage.

The importance of healthy melatonin levels on menstrual regularity, fertility, including in successful assisted reproductive technologies, and pregnancy is evident from a growing body of research in these areas. Studies now show that supplementing with 3 mg of melatonin daily can improve ovarian health and function, restore regular menstrual cycles, improve fertility, delay menopause onset—and improve sleep in the bargain. Low melatonin may also negatively affect thyroid function; supplementation may improve it.

What interferes with melatonin production? Because cortisol suppresses melatonin, any-thing that keeps cortisol production revved up into the evening—that is, stress, exposure to the blue light coming off electronic devices, caffeine, or alcohol—skews the ski slope, and your body's cortisol and melatonin rhythms get disrupted. Because melatonin is produced from serotonin, whose production depends on adequate estrogen levels, low estrogen, which can occur due to being underweight, not getting enough healthy carbs in your diet, or premature or natural menopause, may lead to low melatonin levels.

Hormone Imbalances and Sleep Problems: A Two-Way Street to Desynchronization

Have you ever noticed that you seem to naturally sleep better at some times of the month than at others? For example, it's harder to sleep on those few nights before your period, and maybe your dreams are more vivid?

Sleep and circadian rhythm disruption impact all areas of your hormonal health, and your hormonal changes affect your sleep. Let's take a look at these relationships.

Cycles Out of Sync: Chronodisruption can cause us to lose hormone **cyclicity**—affecting both daily and monthly rhythms. Disruption of clock function anywhere in the HPO axis from chronic circadian disruption is associated with irregular menstrual cycles, increased menstrual pain, changes in length and amount of menstrual bleeding, more fatigue around the period, and greater premenstrual sleep troubles. Not getting enough high-quality sleep can increase the amount of period pain you experience and reduce your ability to cope with it. One study found that having insomnia caused women to report higher levels of more severe dysmenorrhea and greater interference with daily activities due to period pain than women without insomnia. Poor sleep also leads directly to inflammation due to disruption in circadian rhythm and our cortisol cycles, pain perception, immunity, and inflammation.

Declining estrogen and progesterone levels in the week before your period can lead to sleep disruption, and interestingly, PMS is associated with decreased REM (deep) sleep and decreased response to melatonin premenstrually. Period pain can also make sleep more difficult.

Circadian Rhythm, Ovulation, and Fertility: Circadian disruption is associated with altered follicular phase length, changes in the level of FSH secretion, increased risk of fertility problems, and miscarriage. PCOS and endometriosis may be exacerbated by desynchronization between circadian clocks in the hypothalamus, pituitary, ovary, and uterus. Women undergoing fertility treatments who were found to have low ovarian reserve were twenty times more likely to have sleep problems. A recent study found that women who work at night or have irregular shifts, switching between day and night shifts, leading to circadian rhythm disruption, may experience up to a 15% decline in fertility. Shift and night workers had fewer eggs capable of developing into healthy embryos than those who worked regular daytime hours, according to researchers at Harvard University. Similar research that reviewed studies on night shift work from 1969 to the present showed that nearly a third of women who work night shifts have an increased rate of miscarriage, while at least 22% who worked changing shifts had menstrual disruption.

Circadian Rhythm and Endometriosis: Melatonin has a broad spectrum of effects, including as an antioxidant, free radical scavenger,

anti-inflammatory agent, and potential immunoregulator. As such it plays a powerful role in protecting us from tissue damage from oxidative stress. This is significant in endometriosis, where chronic inflammation and immune disruption causes oxidative stress at a local tissue level, increasing inflammation, scarring, adhesions, and pain. Maintaining healthy biorhythms is important in maintaining healthy melatonin levels—and thus preventing and reducing oxidative stress damage. More on using melatonin therapeutically for endometriosis is in the Endometriosis Advanced Protocol.

Circadian Rhythm and PCOS: Women with PCOS are twice as likely to suffer from sleep disturbances due to higher levels of testosterone and lower levels of progesterone. PCOS also leads to a significantly greater risk of sleep apnea. Short or disrupted sleep, conversely, increases prolactin, which can block ovulation and fertility, while leading to stress-induced increases in estrogen and testosterone, which can be associated with a wide variety of symptoms from heavy painful periods to PCOS-like symptoms.

In addition to poor sleep impacting blood sugar, inhibiting ovulation, increasing risk of depression, and affecting weight—both causing weight gain and making it harder to lose weight, PCOS is also a highly inflammatory condition; women with PCOS have been found to have high levels of blood markers of oxidative stress. Further, ovulation is almost always compromised in PCOS. Loss of sleep, chronic overexposure to bright light, and lowered melatonin all appear to play a contributing role in PCOS. Melatonin can play an important role in reducing PCOS-related oxidative stress, while improving ovulation and the health of the ovum, improving conception and pregnancy rates, in women with

PCOS trying to conceive, and may also reduce miscarriage risk.

What's Keeping You Up at Night?

The biggest disrupter to our circadian rhythm can be summed up in two words: disconnected and overstimulated. We're constantly exposed to triggers that keep us revved up and distracted from healthy internal and life rhythms, and we're disconnected from natural external and internal sleep cues. We start our days by checking email on our phones before we even get out of bed in the morning and do a final check before we fall into bed at night. In between we're constantly on the go, reaching for coffee and sugar all day to keep us going, and a glass of wine or two in the evening to help us unwind. Yet too often, restful sleep is as abundant as unicorns! Most of us have trouble shifting our brains into sleep mode at the end of the day, and millions of us have trouble staying asleep even if we do get some z's for a couple of hours.

The most common sleep disruptors are:

- Light pollution
- Screen time, especially before bed
- Bedroom too warm
- Around-the-clock eating
- Stress, worry, depression, and anxiety
- Chronic pain
- Caffeine
- Alcohol
- Nicotine
- Family stress or worries
- A partner who snores

Not sure what's keeping you up at night? Keep a sleep journal. A sleep diary is a helpful tool both to identify the factors that might be

Sleep Apnea

Sleep apnea is a potentially serious sleep disorder in which breathing repeatedly stops and starts. The most common type is obstructive sleep apnea (OSA). While it's generally stereotyped as a problem of overweight people, anyone can have sleep apnea, and as many as 50% of women with PCOS have sleep apnea, regardless of weight. Symptoms include daytime sleepiness, headaches, snoring, waking up from sleep with a gasp for air or realizing you weren't breathing (or someone telling you this happens while you sleep), waking up with a dry mouth, difficulty concentrating or with memory, irritability, difficulty losing weight, and high blood pressure. Untreated, consequences include severe daytime sleepiness and dysfunction, metabolic syndrome, diabetes, heart disease, and liver disease. A sleep study, which can now be done at home, is important for a diagnosis, and treatment is easy with an at-home sleep device.

interfering with your sleep and also to set sleep goals. Download your copy at avivaromm.com /hormone-intelligence-resources to assess your sleep habits and track your sleep progress.

The Hormone Intelligence Solution: Healthier Rhythms, Healthier Hormones

When it comes to resetting your circadian rhythm, timing truly is everything. It doesn't require any fancy foods, crazy diet plans, or complicated dance steps. It does, however, require a commitment to reclaiming some balance in your life. But who doesn't want *that*?

To reconnect to nature's intended rhythms, we have to disconnect from the unnatural rhythms of our culture wherever we can. It takes nothing short of living a revolutionary lifestyle to support and honor your natural ebbs and flows. But, hey, you're here reading this book, which means you've got a little bit of the rebel in you. If you stick with this new routine even for just a few weeks, not only will you be helping to restore hormone balance, you'll find yourself catching up on much needed sleep and feeling more refreshed, energized, and focused, and you'll continue to see cravings fall away.

Sleep is the ultimate pause you need at the end of the day; it's impossible to reset your internal clocks without high-quality sleep—and enough of it. Here's the magic number: you need from seven to nine hours of good sleep every night to reset your natural clock. Especially important is a regular sleep cycle that has you waking and going to bed at roughly the same time each day, preferably waking by about 7 a.m. and getting to bed between 10 and 11 p.m. Good sleep doesn't start the minute you put your head on the pillow. It starts the minute you wake up in the morning. How you start and spend the day also plays a huge role in your circadian rhythm and whether you ultimately get good sleep. And of course, how you sleep sets the tone for how you feel when you wake up and throughout your day. So before I jump into how to get good sleep, we're going to talk about what's known about how to create an ideal day for optimal circadian rhythm, from the time you wake to when you do finally lie down to rest at night. This is an extension of the work you started in the previous chapter, resetting your brain-hormone connections.

Did You Know That . . .

Regularly sleeping with someone who works a night shift or late/irregular hours can disrupt your sleep; in one survey, 34% of women say their partner's sleep/wake schedule interferes with their circadian rhythm. Love may be blind, but it's not deaf; sleeping with a snorer can lead to as many as twenty sleep disruptions in your sleep quality a night, which is perhaps why according to another study, over 40% of American women would rather sleep alone than with a partner.

Until we find that balance between on and off, movement and stillness, expending energy and replenishing it, striving and just being, our hormonal ecosystem is going to be paying the price with irregular cycles, skipped periods, painful cycles, skipped ovulation, low sex drive, and a whole lot of symptoms; and cortisol-driven insulin resistance and chronic inflammation are going to compound the problem, seeding problems like endometriosis, PCOS, and fertility challenges.

For the next six weeks, you're going to start aligning your hormonal blueprint and inner cycles with natural rhythms.

Step 1: Start and Spend the Day in Rhythm

Again, how you start the day has everything to do with how the rest of it goes. Good sleep starts during the day, with a rhythmic flow to the day that leads into a healthy pace at night. But it's amazing how quickly even the best night's sleep can be laid to waste by the morning stress and anxiety. It's an interconnected cycle. Here's how to create more rhythm in your hormones, starting when you wake.

Slow it all down. The first step to creating a healthier daily rhythm is to slow down. Rushing through life is pretty familiar to most of us. But rushing is literally fight-or-flight mode! To realign our brains and nervous system with our innate hormone blueprint, which naturally evolved to a much slower pace of life, we too have to slow down—ideally *before* we feel too stressed. I find that being mindful of my internal landscape as I'm going through my day is much more likely to keep me aligned with a healthy pace of living. That's why the practices in Chapter 7 are an absolutely important part of this week's plan, too.

Morning Practices

Start early and at the same time most days. Try to wake up no later than 7 a.m. You can use an alarm to help you, and don't let yourself keep hitting snooze. As much as you might groan at the idea of becoming a morning person, especially if you fancy being more of a night owl than a lark, the contrast between getting bright light in the morning and then diminishing light in the evening is essential for resetting your circadian rhythm.

Slowly start your day. Even if you're a morning person, the typical morning rush can quickly wipe away the glow. I personally like to get up thirty minutes earlier than I *have* to, so I can have a relaxed, easy start to my day. This gives me time to make the bed (always a plus in my book, because it makes it so much nicer to get into at night), have a healthy morning pace, eat a real breakfast, and connect with my sweetie. Bonus points if you can fit in some morning snuggles, a shared morning walk, or, one of my favorites, a couple's shower (wink, wink)—any of which can give you a nice shot of relaxing, mood-building oxytocin. Or try this: practice five minutes of meditation or deep, intentional relaxing breathing before you get out of bed, and think of one thing you're grateful for and one thing you're looking forward to that day. It's seriously been a life-changer for me!

Stay off your devices. A message from an irritated boss or coworker, a snarky comment on your social media, or comparing and despairing when you see someone's perfect Instagram life—it's enough to shoot anyone's day to hell. So protect your space! Rather than checking your email or texts or hopping on social media before you even get out of bed, wait until you've done your morning self-care routine—and optimally, stay off your electronic devices until your workday officially starts.

Throughout the Day

Let the sunshine in. Bright light in the morning gives your central clock a very important natural wake-up call. Getting thirty minutes of sunlight in your eyes in the morning can regulate your energy, mood, and clarity—and hormones. Natural morning light gives your brain a major boost, supports healthy immunity and reduced inflammation all day long, and also stimulates your digestion and metabolism. Throughout the day, try to get natural light exposure by sitting near a window when you work. If getting up early is tough, or you simply can't get natural light in the morning where you live, try light box therapy instead. It's been found to be effective for treating PMS (and PMDD) and may help to restore ovulatory cycles, and having a morning and late afternoon session may optimize results. Affordable home-use devices are easily found online. You want one that delivers 10,000 LUX.

Take "ultradian breaks." What if I told you that there's a quick, easy way to stay replenished and calm, even in the middle of a crazy workday? This little trick can help you work smarter, not harder, and it's the one thing you can do every day to combat burnout—no matter how busy you are. The secret is to tune in to your ultradian rhythm, which, simply put, is your balance of activity and rest. Ultradian rhythms are short cycles that happen throughout the day, lasting 90 to 120 minutes, in which we have bursts of productivity and focus followed by the need for 15 or so minutes of rest. Creating breaks in your day is simple, and you can start to feel improvements in your stress, energy, focus, and mood almost immediately. It comes down to paying attention to your body and mood. If I'm working on a project and I start to feel distracted and antsy, I don't move past that inner feeling telling me to change the scenery. I use that as a natural signaling mechanism from my body that it's time to get up, shift my focus for fifteen to twenty minutes,

then come back to it. Here are six ways to take an ultradian break:

- Take a bio break (hydrate; go to the restroom).

- Eat something healthy.

- Move your body.

- Connect with a friend or colleagues.

- Get outside—or at least look out the window.

- Take five minutes for meditation or deep breathing.

Step 2: Eat for Circadian Rhythm (and Stress Relief)

Getting your sleep-wake cycle on track is probably the most obvious way to reset your circadian rhythm, but there's another that's also important: when we eat throughout the day and evening. Just as our ancestors used daylight for preparing food—and had food put away safely before nighttime predators started their own hunt for food—we are meant to fuel our body while we're awake and need the energy for our day's tasks, and be in a rest and repair mode while we're asleep. Your central body clock is designed to naturally stimulate your appetite during daylight hours, and each organ in your digestive system also has a clock that is entrained to our central clock, so that, for example, our pancreas is meant to be awake and active, producing insulin at optimal levels, during those daytime hours, and our elimination clock is set so that we typically don't have to go to the loo for a number two in the middle of the night—rather, we ideally have a morning "constitutional."

Diet-induced thermogenesis, or how much calorie-burning power we have, also has a circadian rhythm: it's strongest in the morning, when insulin sensitivity is also the highest, and declines throughout the day. Perhaps this explains the adage to eat breakfast like a king, lunch like a prince, and dinner like a pauper. When we emphasize our greatest calorie consumption earlier in the day, and lighten our food intake progressively, making dinner the lightest meal of the day, we have the easiest time maintaining healthy weight—and losing weight if that's a goal. This effect also appears to be even more significant for women than men.

A growing body of evidence from an emerging research field called *chrononutrition* now shows that when we override natural eating rhythms by skipping a morning meal, eating very late at night, eating erratically, or eating all day long, we're sending signals to our organs at the wrong times of day, upsetting their balance, and also confusing our hunger and satiety signals. Our metabolism takes a hit and we're more likely to have cravings and weight gain. Sleeping less than seven hours a night has been shown to increase our preferences for sweets, and just getting an extra forty-five minutes of sleep each night can reduce your sugar cravings—and consumption—dramatically. When we're not sleeping enough, or well, our digestion feels the impact, too. Microbiota rhythms are also regulated by our meal timing; eating irregularly or too late at night can affect microbial diversity and the metabolic activity of your microbiome.

Eating for circadian rhythm also helps to

Pay Attention to the "3 P.M. Slump"

Once your energy and circadian rhythm are nice and steady, and you've got a healthy sleep groove on, you won't experience afternoon crashes anymore. Seriously. An afternoon slump is usually a sign of one of these causes:

- Poor sleep the night before, leading you to feel tired late in the day, usually because of low cortisol—of course, that's what we're working on in this chapter: don't hit up the coffee and sugar no matter how tired you are; try one of the tips below instead.

- Low blood sugar, usually from not eating enough at lunch, or having a blood sugar crash if your lunch was high in sugar or simple carbs: work on eating more power-packed lunches, skip the sugar and carbs (of course!), and have a high-protein snack; and if you are craving something sweet or caffeinated, this is a good time to have some of that dark chocolate.

- You're dehydrated: have some water or, if you can, have some green juice for an extra burst of energizing minerals.

- You've been sitting for too long: you know what to do!

optimize metabolism and insulin levels, which fluctuate according to natural circadian cycles, and is part of a plan to prevent and reverse inflammation and cravings and bring you to a healthy weight naturally. Aligning when we do and don't eat with natural circadian rhythm can help us to realign our hormonal biology with our internal clocks, and in doing so, also reset our metabolism; support a healthy microbiome; improve our moods, focus, and productivity; and lose weight.

Here are seven principles for doing this:

1. **Eat an energy-packed breakfast.** This means a healthy meal with protein and high-quality fat, to keep your blood sugar steady—and with it your stress low and cortisol healthy. Starting on page 327 I've given you a host of healthy breakfast options to choose from. Research has shown that consuming the majority of our calories at breakfast allows us to not only improve insulin sensitivity, but also reduce high androgen levels and improve ovulation in women with PCOS, and also improve cortisol and inflammation, even if you don't have PCOS.

2. **Eat consistently, but space it out.** Eating on a regular schedule during the daylight hours keeps your peripheral circadian clocks (liver, etc.) in sync with your core circadian rhythm. It's important for your body to have clear times for eating and clear times for digestion. According to one major study looking at the impact of food frequency and timing on circadian rhythm, researchers found that 25% of food is eaten within 1.5 hours of a previous meal—not giving us ample time to digest. However, giving your body time to rest between meals helps to entrain your circadian rhythm. While

you can definitely have a healthy snack if you're hungry, making it a practice to eat more energy-dense meals that keep you satisfied, and snacking less, can be an important part of entraining your circadian rhythm.

3. **Don't shun the carbs.** While a low-carb diet may sound like a weight-loss winner, interestingly, and particularly in women, a *very* low-carb diet increases your cortisol and likelihood of putting on, not taking off, belly fat. In fact, eating a small healthy carbohydrate choice three to five hours before going to sleep has been shown to create a healthier cortisol pattern while improving sleep—a win-win. Healthy choices include a serving of a whole grain, for example, brown rice or quinoa, and/or a serving of sweet potato, winter squash, or potatoes—baked or roasted and cooled almost to room temperature before eating.

4. **The right dinner can help you sleep better.** Eating lighter in the evening, not eating within three hours of going to bed, and including a complex carb at dinner can help you sleep better. If you eat too early in the evening, however, or don't get enough protein or high-quality fat with your meal, low blood sugar may send you in search of an evening snack, keep you up at night, or cause you to wake in the night hungry. The sample meal plans starting on page 334 will show you how to assemble healthful dinners that help you get a good night's sleep and also give you leftovers so you don't have to worry about tomorrow's lunch.

5. **"Fast" overnight.** While there's no food restricting whatsoever on this plan,

allowing your body a nightly period of rest from food is one of the top ways to reset your circadian rhythm. Allowing this time for your body to rest and repair without digesting has been shown to reduce inflammation, improve insulin levels, reduce depression, and also to benefit the health of the gut microbiome. Time-restricted eating (TRE), more commonly called *intermittent fasting*, is the practice of narrowing down the eating window to allow for this rest and repair time. Evidence shows, however, that overly restrictive intermittent fasting isn't optimal for women's hormone balance. In fact, one study showed that blood sugar control worsened in women after three weeks of intermittent fasting with meal skipping, which was not the case in men. But when done properly, it can be incredibly effective for reducing insulin resistance and improving blood sugar balance—beneficial both for healthy cortisol levels and especially for women with PCOS and insulin problems. Just eight to twelve weeks of intermittent fasting has been shown to lower insulin levels by 20–31% and blood sugar levels by 3–6% in individuals with prediabetes. One study also found that eight weeks of intermittent fasting decreased depression and binge eating behaviors while improving body image in overweight adults.

So how can you reap the benefits without risk? The best way is to do a 12:12 meal plan daily. This means that you keep your food intake to twelve hours each day, and then have twelve hours where you don't eat at all—not even snacks. Sound hard to do? It's not—because you'll do most of it while you're sleeping! The trick is to have a twelve-hour food-free window each night. To do this, you'll want to eat dinner early enough in order to maintain your healthy evening cortisol rhythm, and then not eat again until twelve hours after your evening meal ended.

6. **Avoid late-night eating.** Nighttime snacking can disrupt your circadian rhythm. Make it a personal commitment not to eat after dinner; this means making sure to eat enough to fill you at dinner, getting to bed when you're tired rather than using food to keep you awake, and keeping tempting snacks out of your home. If you do go out for the evening, keep your snacks to some nuts or veggie sticks, and if you live with a nighttime snacker, keep your hands busy with some knitting or handwork while you watch your favorite shows. Pregnancy and breastfeeding are exceptions—if you need to eat at night, eat.

7. **Skip the alcohol.** As counterintuitive as this might seem, since alcohol can help you to feel relaxed and even sleepy, research indicates that even a modest dose of alcohol up to an hour before bedtime can reduce melatonin production by nearly 20%. Alcohol has a direct effect on circadian rhythms, diminishing the ability of the master biological clock to respond to the light cues that keep it in sync. Kicking the evening glass of vino and other alcohol-containing beverages is one of the quickest sleep fixes I know. Almost all my patients report that their sleep improved dramatically, particularly their ability to stay asleep and feel refreshed in the morning, when they

stopped drinking alcohol. Grumble now, but you'll thank me later!

Step 3: Exercise for Sleep and Circadian Rhythm

Do you remember being a kid in the summertime? You probably played outside all day and then hit the pillow and slept like a baby at night. Regular physical activity and time in nature help to keep our circadian rhythms cyclic, and together they're a dynamic duo! Like most of the other cells in your body, your skeletal muscle has an extensive network of clock-controlled genes that are entrained to your central clock. Regular physical activity is an important variable in keeping these synced up and improves overall sleep quality, whereas sitting all day can take its toll on your body as well as your body clock and sleep. Exercise also helps to repair your brain cells, and as you've been learning, healthy hormones don't just happen in your lady parts—they start in your brain! So getting any exercise at any time of the day is absolutely fantastic—don't get hung up on doing this "right." But new studies show that exercise timing and types can help you to maximize your exercise benefits and reset your diurnal rhythms. In turn, resetting your circadian rhythm can improve your exercise endurance and strength. So consider these options as you weave movement into your lifestyle.

Morning (before 10 a.m.): Start your day with something aerobic—a brisk walk, five minutes of jumping rope (equivalent to about fifteen minutes of running!) or the 7 Minute Workout (online).

Afternoon (3 p.m. to dinnertime): Most of us think of exercise as a before or after work thing, but afternoon is a fantastic time to get a move on. It gets your blood flowing and is energizing, which can also help you curb caffeine or sugar urges and give you that same second wind you need to get through the rest of the day and your evening—especially if you have a busy after-work life ahead of you. Muscle tone also goes up in the late afternoon and evening—so this is a great time to build muscle and tone. Interestingly, this is the time of day when injury is least likely because strength and coordination are at their peak; so premenstrually, this may be the best time of day to exercise to balance out that natural decrease in muscle repair and increase in pain sensitivity. Afternoon exercise also increases calorie burning and reduces appetite, so if weight loss is one of your goals, for example, with PCOS, then this is an optimal time of day to hit the gym, go for a run, or lift some weights. Then you can have a healthy protein at dinner to support muscle recovery.

Evening (after 7 p.m., earlier in dark winter months): Evening is the best time for movement that helps you reset into a slower pace—so yoga, swimming, dance. If you haven't gotten any cardio in all day, some vigorous movement is important, but keep in mind that vigorous exercise is stimulating and increases cortisol when you want to be supporting its natural decline, while delaying the onset of your melatonin rise—both of which can delay your ability to fall asleep. Nighttime exercise also increases your core temperature, which can impact sleep and your ovulatory rhythm, which depends not only on circadian cycle temperature changes, but on the infradian temperature rhythm that coincides with the menstrual cycle and is superimposed on the daily rhythm. If night is the only time you can fit in some exercise, take extra efforts to wind down and cool down after—with a short meditation, a shower, and so on.

Step 4: Sleep Your Way to Hormone Health

Sleep is the ultimate restorative for all our systems. Good sleep is not just a lifestyle habit, it's a spiritual practice! You have to make it a priority, not just at bedtime, but in the hours before bed. It may take a month or so before you see consistent results if your sleep problem is pretty bad, but it will be well worth it: better sleep makes us happier, healthier, and more relaxed in every way. And when you are happier and more relaxed, you are better for everyone and at everything you do. The following steps, practiced daily, will eventually help you sleep like a dream.

Get a Head Start on Sleep: Reset After Work

Huge shifts can happen in resetting your nighttime cortisol and sleep if you take a mini restorative break between your workday and evening routines. Studies have shown, for example, that nurses who take a fifteen-minute break when they get home from a stressful workday have healthier cortisol rhythms at night. Healthier evening cortisol levels help your weight, hormones, blood sugar, cravings, and sleep. Make it a habit to decompress for fifteen minutes with a favorite activity when you get home from work. Here are some reset ideas:

- Take a long shower.

- Take a brisk walk (double benefit: movement + time in nature).

- Read a chapter of an inspirational book.

- Do fifteen minutes of restorative yoga.

- Put on music and DANCE hard!

Wind Down to a Slower Pace

As the evening advances, start to switch gears into nighttime mode. Here's how:

- **Turn the lights down low.** We're wired so that as it gets dark in the evening, our eyes perceive this, and send a signal to our pineal gland that it's time to dial up the melatonin production, which makes us start to feel sleepy. The continuous presence of bright light, from both artificial street and home lighting and our electronic devices, prevents this from happening, keeping us wired and awake. One of the most important things you can do to reclaim a good night of z's and resync to your circadian rhythm is to harmonize your environment to your brain's natural evolutionary sleep cues by creating natural night at home. Here are three easy steps you can take to do this:

  - At dinnertime, or at least a few hours before your ideal bedtime, begin to dim the lights in your home. Turn off any unnecessary lights, and shift from using overhead lighting to dimmer table and floor lamps. Small lighting shifts in the evening can make a big difference in your sleep. A candlelit dinner is a real plus for setting a peaceful mood while you eat and as you move into your evening routine, and I love Edison light bulbs—they're old-fashioned and modern at the same time, and importantly, the light they give off is softer and more yellowish than typical bulbs.

  - Schedule or manually shift your phone into "night mode," which changes your screen lighting from blue to softer oranges and reds—more like a sunset sky!

  - If you must use your computer (see Digital Detox below), use a program that automatically changes the color of your computer's display to adapt to the time of day, warm at night and like sunlight during the day. Most computers can be set to automatically adjust screen brightness in the evening.

— Also, or alternatively, if you must be on a device in the evening, wear amber-colored blue-light-blocking glasses in the evening, or at least in the couple of hours before bedtime, to encourage melatonin production.

- **Slow your inner landscape.** Enjoy these simple evening rituals, the old-fashioned way! Here are my top suggestions:

  — Read a book. A real book. Made of paper. As in not on a device. A great novel. Or inspiring nonfiction.

  — Meditate, breathe deeply, sleep.

  — Listen to quiet music—but keep your listening device away from your bed so you're not tempted to check email or texts one more time!

  — Skip intense workouts in the evening. Gentle, restorative yoga sequences (see page 261) are a better choice to help you unwind your body and your mind prior to bed. YogaGlo, a fantastic website with a wealth of recorded yoga classes with well-known teachers, offers a selection of yoga classes to help you relax. Do an evening class, then take an aromatherapy bath to help you unwind.

  — Intimate connection is a win for oxytocin release, which is an "antidote" to stress and cortisol, so connecting with your partner or a friend over a cup of tea, playing cards or Scrabble (unless you get competitive like I do!), and having sex can be a win-win for intimacy and relaxation.

- **Soak it up.** A hot aromatherapy bath before bed can relax your mind and your muscles. Add one cup of Epsom salts and five to seven drops of pure lavender essential oil to your tub of hot water. SOAK away your day's troubles. Lavender promotes relaxation and sleep. This can be done nightly just prior to going to bed and is safe for pregnant and nursing mothers, too.

- **Pay attention to your body's cues.** As you've heard me say throughout the book, we're so accustomed to ignoring and overriding our body's natural cues that we don't notice them until the consequences are bonking us on the head! But you're going to change all that by reconnecting to your internal cues that it's time for bed, which might include feeling tired or sleepy, getting irritable or overwhelmed, or perhaps confusing fatigue for hunger that's driving you toward a late-night snack. Honor the fact that you need seven to nine hours of sleep, so you have to get to bed at a time that allows you to meet your sleep needs and still wake up when you need to for work, family, and so on in the morning.

Commit to a One-Hour Digital Detox—Every Night!

I can't tell you how many of my patients come to me at their first visit with sleep problems, and how many are on some kind of electronic device—texting or talking on their cell phones, reading on an iPad or Kindle, checking email or hanging out on Facebook, or watching TV until the last minute before heading off to bed. Most bring their devices into bed and are on them until lights out or beyond. Not. Good. For. Sleep. To reconnect with our sleep cycles, we've got to disconnect from our devices for a set time each evening.

Many of us live "tired and wired"—we're dragging all day and then can't sleep at night. Being "plugged in" to computers, email, and smartphones all day and evening exposes you to electromagnetic waves that potentially interfere with sleep, but also keeps you plugged into the endless "to-do's" that prevent you from ever turning it all off and getting rest. If you are going to improve your sleep, this means powering down for a designated couple of stress-free hours before bed.

Do you check your email before you go to bed? Texts? Instagram? Make it a habit to do a daily digital detox—I promise, your nervous system will thank you. Stay off all electronic devices after 9 p.m. each evening, or at least for a full two hours before going to bed. No cell phone. No email. No Facebook. No computer. Make your sleep space a device-free zone. Keep your chargers anywhere but your bedroom and if you do need to use your phone as an alarm clock, put it on the other side of your bedroom, well out of reach, and make sure all notifications are turned off. (I keep mine off 24/7 so I'm not called to the siren song of my phone—ever.)

Do Your Worrying *Before* Bed

I have my patients keep a pre-sleep journal—any blank notebook will do. One hour before bed they write out all their worries and concerns, as well as their to-do list for the next day. Doing this allows you to go to sleep with a clearer head. Oh, and did I say you can vent in there, too? Never go to sleep angry. If you do, you run the risk of troubled dreams and waking up tired. After you've done your writing, take an aromatherapy bath, read something inspirational, and head to bed.

Turn Your Bedroom into a Sleep Sanctuary

While some lucky ones can fall asleep with a jackhammer going outside their bedroom window (it's mostly just men that can do this, eh?), the rest of us need a somewhat quieter ambiance. Ideally, your bedroom should be a place for sleep, relaxation, and sex. Period.

Here's how to make your bedroom a place of peace and repose:

- **Make your bedroom an electronics-free zone.** Do not allow TV, computers, or other electronics in there—ever. (Small apartment? Get a room divider to separate your sleep and desk area.)

- **Cool it.** That is, check your thermostat. The temperature that encourages the best sleep in most of us is right around 67°F (that's 19.5°C). Hormone bonus: the cooler temperature is a boost to ovulation and fertility and can help prevent hot flashes.

- **Sleep in the dark.** Block streetlight glare in your bedroom. If light is still sneaking in, try a silk sleep mask or eye pillow, which is usually filled with flaxseed or rice, making them weighted enough to put a little bit of rest-inducing pressure on your eyes.

- **Reduce ambient noise.** If there are sounds you can't control, consider headphones, earplugs, or a noise-canceling machine.

- **Invest in a comfortable mattress, pillows, and bedding.** You can't put a price on quality sleep. If you tend to have trouble falling asleep and are sensitive to overstimulation generally, consider a weighted blanket.

- **Paint and decorate your bedroom in restful colors.** Apparently purple and gray are very bad choices, blue is the best, and neutrals and yellows pretty good for supporting calm and sleep.

- **Use good scents.** Scent can deeply calm our brain's primitive stress centers and has been used since ancient times for healing. Lavender is the classic aromatherapy choice for getting more restful sleep. But lavender isn't the only option. A 2002 study found that jasmine scent was very effective at lulling people to sleep, trumping the benefits of even lavender. Studies done in Japan in 2005 and in Germany in 2010 confirmed jasmine's power as a natural sleep aid. Aromatic compounds in jasmine and lavender reduce anxiety, induce relaxation, and act as mild sedatives by increasing your brain's level of the calming neurotransmitter gamma aminobutyric acid (GABA), similar to the way Valium works, but without any of the side effects or addictive potential.

Don't Jet-Lag Yourself on Weekends

It's tempting, after a full workweek, to stay up late on the weekends and then try to catch up from your week of sleep debt by sleeping in. Unfortunately the evidence is in and this just doesn't work. Sleeping late on the weekends is equivalent to giving yourself jet lag. In fact, chronobiologists call this phenomenon **social jet lag**, which an estimated 87% of adults now experience as a result of attempts at weekend sleep compensation. It leads to confusion in your central clock, making it even harder to bounce back from your sleep debt over the weekend, and then trying to reset again on Monday morning compounds your brain's confusion even more. Instead, it's best to try to continue to go to sleep and wake up at the same time every day—including on your days off. If you use an alarm, keep it set to the same time every day, including on weekends and vacations. If you do need to catch up on sleep, there's a better way than sleeping in—it's

If You Have to Work Late or Work Nights

This is a tough situation, because working nights is inherently harder on your circadian rhythm. But there are things you can do to protect yourself:

- Get extra sleep *before* your shift. I know that sounds wonky, but you can sleep bank ahead to store up on rest—it is scientifically proven to help prevent exhaustion and physiologic consequences from missed sleep.
- Eat well on the job. It's so tempting to nosh out at night, but keeping only to nutrient-dense foods overnight can keep your cortisol sane and the unhealthy calories off.
- Stay hydrated with water, but skip the overnight caffeine.
- Make time to decompress when you get home (see above).
- Use adaptogen herbs, especially eleuthero and rhodiola (page 157), which have been shown to offset the stress on body and brain of night shift work.

called *sleep banking*—and one way to do this is to master the art of the power nap.

Step 5: Follow Your Cycle Sense

Period Time (Week 1): Achiness or cramps may make it harder to get a good night of z's. When your period starts, add in the Luna Yoga Flow (see page 261) and take a hot shower with essential oils to help relieve cramps and promote sleep. Take a hot water bottle to bed with you, and position yourself comfortably draped over a body pillow. Orgasm—yes, even during your period—can help relieve cramps and can help you sleep, too.

Follicular Phase (Week 2): Estrogen peaks and has powerful effects on your body temperature regulation, circadian rhythms, and stress reactivity. This lovely hormone can activate your thinking and worries, keeping you staring at the ceiling, waiting for sleep to come. An evening wind-down practice is the perfect antidote; include the relaxing bath or shower, meditation, supportive sleep herbs, journaling, and a good old-fashioned analog book to take to bed with you.

Luteal Phase (Week 3): At first you might sleep like a baby, bathed in all that soothing progesterone; the only downside is progesterone can slow your GI system, aggravating bloating and heartburn if you've been prone to those. In the postovulation luteal phase, body temperature is elevated due to progesterone, but the cyclic rhythms of melatonin and cortisol are slightly blunted, so as you head into your premenstrual week, you might start to notice that it's harder to settle down at night, get to sleep, or stay asleep. Keep that evening wind-down going, and add in relaxing sleep herbs for extra support.

Premenstrual Phase (Week 4): This time of the month is notorious for disrupting our sleep. The higher progesterone and estradiol levels that occur in the late luteal phase correlate with less of the deep REM sleep we need to feel restored. And then as you get close to your period, estrogen plummets. Lower estrogen leads to lower serotonin production and may be associated with increased sensitivity to light, noise, and environmental disturbances in your premenstrual phase. Make sure your bedroom is dark and quiet at night; stay off electronics completely in the evenings, and consider blue-light glasses, which also help prevent migraines. Take your sleep herbs and supplements. Also, check out the pain-relieving recommendations in the Period Advanced Protocol in Chapter 12, and start these a few days before your moon time, including using period cramp prevention remedies, like magnesium and ginger, so that cramps don't keep you up in the days before and when your period starts.

Step 6: Use Sleep Support Supplements and Herbs

Not only do sleep-aid medications not help to reset your circadian rhythm, they pose unique safety hazards for women, and surprisingly, they don't work that well. A study by Best Buy Drugs found that these drugs add just three to thirty-four minutes to total sleep time. Their effectiveness is so limited that as of late 2014 they were no longer considered a first-choice treatment for chronic insomnia by the American Academy of Sleep Medicine (AASM). Even when taken as directed, sleep aids pose risks. OTC sleep aids—such as Advil PM, Sominex, and ZzzQuil can cause daytime drowsiness, confusion, constipation, dry mouth, and problems urinating. Sleeping pills increase dizziness and, with this, falls and fractures. Some sleep medications increase the risk of death 4.6 times over an average observation period of two and a half years compared to death among nonusers, with a greater than threefold increased risk of death even when less than eighteen pills per year are taken.

A study published online in June 2015 by the *American Journal of Public Health* found that people prescribed sleeping pills were around twice as likely to be in car crashes as other people—and because of how women metabolize these drugs, the risks for us are greater. One sleep medication had to be issued with a black box warning because it was associated with over six hundred car accidents in women who had used the drug properly before bed, but in the morning had so much in their system that they were essentially driving as if drunk. The researchers estimated that people taking sleep drugs were as likely to have a car crash as those driving with a blood alcohol level above the legal limit; to address the dangers of next-day drowsiness, the FDA has cut in half the recommended doses for Ambien and Lunesta.

Therefore, when more is needed than just the reset steps I've given you above, or as additional support, I turn to nutritional supplements and herbal remedies, many of which work well and are much safer. You can combine any of these; I've put them in order of my personal preferences in both the nutrient and herb sections below. There are also some wonderful products on the market that include several of these natural remedies in combination. As a rule I recommend you not combining sleep herbs or nutrients with any sleep medications without the supervision of a skilled, licensed integrative medicine practitioner. You can find more information and proper dosage in the Botanical and Supplement Quick Reference Guide on pages 372–81.

Sleep Supplements

Melatonin: If you have trouble specifically with falling asleep, melatonin can be a great choice. It can also be helpful for improving ovarian function in anovulation, fertility challenges, and primary ovarian insufficiency, and peri-menopausal hot flashers may also get some relief and sleep from using this remedy. It can be taken 30 minutes before bedtime, though it's ideal to take melatonin two to three hours before sleep. If taken too close to your evening meal it can keep blood sugar elevated, so allow at least an hour, ideally two, after you've eaten. This is especially important if you have PCOS, insulin resistance, or metabolic syndrome, or are on diabetes medications. Start with the lowest doses and work your way up as needed.

Vitamin B6: Vitamin B6 is necessary for melatonin production; it's also one of the most important supplements we have for preventing and reversing PMS and period problems (see Chapter 12) It can be taken before bed specifically to relieve night waking by reducing nocturnal cortisol spikes.

Vitamin B12: Plays an especially important role in allowing your body to reset its circadian rhythm, possibly also due to its effects on melatonin production, and improves quality of sleep, leading to feeling refreshed when you wake up. I recommend taking it before noon as many people find it slightly stimulating.

Calcium and Magnesium: A combination of calcium and magnesium, or magnesium alone, can promote relaxation and sleep. Magnesium may also help if restless leg syndrome or muscle cramps interfere with your sleep, including during pregnancy.

Glycine: Taking this amino acid one hour prior to sleep can help you fall asleep and sleep more deeply.

(5-HTP): 5-hydroxytryptophan (5-HTP), a product of the amino acid tryptophan, is converted into serotonin in the brain. Serotonin helps to regulate sleep and reduces nighttime awakenings.

Herbs for Sleep

Take any or a combination of these herbs before bed.

Lavender Oil: One of my favorite products for sleep and anxiety, Lavela is a proprietary lavender oil product so look for this brand. (I have no conflict of interest.) It's easy to take—one pill about an hour before bedtime. It's also helpful if you suffer with anxiety that keeps you awake, performance anxiety, or test anxiety. I've even had several patients come off long-term benzodiazepines (you have to work with your doctor to taper off these medications!).

Passionflower: This herb has been used traditionally to promote sleep, and some evidence shows that it can improve sleep quality; thus, it can help you stay asleep and feel more rested when you wake. It is also useful in the treatment of anxiety disorders. There is also some evidence that drinking passionflower tea increases the production of GABA, a brain chemical that works to inhibit other brain chemicals that induce stress, such as glutamate.

California Poppy: California poppy is widely used by herbalists for its gentle sedative effects. It is also a gentle analgesic and muscle relaxant. It is strong and should not be taken during the day or before driving.

Hops: With a long traditional history as a sleep herb, this mildly estrogenic herb is a common beer ingredient and is wonderful for promoting deep sleep. I recommend the tincture (liquid extract) one hour and again thirty minutes before going to sleep. It's too strong for daytime use, should not be taken with alcoholic beverages, and should not be used if you suffer from moderate to severe depression or have a history of estrogen receptor positive breast cancer.

Ashwagandha: With roots in Ayurvedic medicine, this herb is specific for the "tired and wired," and as such not only helps sleep in the short run but helps relieve "adrenal fatigue" and burnout when taken for at least three to six months or longer. It improves cognitive function, immunity, and stress resilience as well.

Cannabis and CBD: Cannabis has been used as a medicinal herb for thousands of years. The need for safer treatments for sleep, pain, and anxiety has led to a resurgence of interest in and research into this plant, and with it, changing laws. As of this writing, thirty states allow for legal medical use, and many states now also allow legal recreational use. Cannabidiol, or CBD, is one of the main cannabinoids, a group of active compounds in the cannabis plant. Because it isn't psychoactive, you don't get high from using CBD, but research does suggest that it can help you to get a good night's sleep, may relieve anxiety, and might help with painful menstrual cramps or pain from endometriosis that could be keeping you up at night. Though CBD is generally quite safe when manufactured and used properly, a 2019 study done on mice did raise concerns about CBD's potential for liver damage. CBD may also interact with other medications you're taking, so speak to your doctor before using it. Remember to use high-quality CBD products. Unfortunately, CBD isn't regulated by the Food and Drug Administration (FDA). As a result, some weak and possibly dangerous products out there are labeled as "CBD." Before you buy CBD do a little research and opt for a CBD product that has been tested by a third party. I strongly recommend against vaping! Product quality and safety are too variable and may pose respiratory risks. Instead I recommend cannabis tincture or CBD oil.

How Will You Know When You've Reset Your Rhythms?

Simple. Your symptoms will improve. You'll feel better. You'll wake up refreshed, in a good mood, ready to face the day, and with energy to match that. You'll have steady energy throughout the day, and when night comes, you'll feel ready for sleep and it will come easily and will be refreshing, taking no more than about ten minutes to settle into a good sleep. You won't crave caffeine, sugar, carbs, or other quick energy foods. Aches and pains will go away, inflammation will go down, and your blood sugar will reach healthy levels and so will your weight. Your mental clarity, focus, and memory will improve; so will your moods. You'll feel much more stress resilient. And you'll notice improvements in your hormones, cycles, and gynecologic symptoms—and if your libido has been low, it might just start to fire up again!

the world within you

THE GUT-HORMONE CONNECTION

Most ancient healing traditions, from Chinese to Ayurvedic to ancient Greek medicine, recognized digestion as central to health, healing, and vitality. The rate at which science is confirming the powerful role our gut health plays in nearly every aspect of our health is mind-blowing. We now know that our digestive system, particularly the small and large intestines, is in a constant dynamic, two-way conversation with our endocrine system. Beyond a doubt, the health of your gut can truly make—or break—your hormone balance, and given that as many as 90% of women experience digestive problems, this is no small root cause to consider.

How is it that gut health is so intrinsic to hormone balance and gynecologic symptoms?

Hormone Intelligence: The Gut-Hormone Connection

- Identify your personal gut imbalances.
- Learn to eat for gut health to support your Hormone Intelligence Diet.
- Learn how to have healthy, regular elimination and why this is important for hormone health.
- Heal your gut, including IBS, leaky gut, and dysbiosis, with a targeted food and supplement plan if digestive symptoms are prominent for you.

Your gut is the garden soil where the roots of hormone health are nurtured. It's fascinating and I'm excited to tell you more!

What's Your Gut Got to Do with It?

In Chapter 3, I showed you how estrogen, progesterone, and prostaglandins affect your digestion throughout your menstrual cycle. In this chapter you'll learn how to restore your gut balance using strategies that I've found instrumental for making periods more regular and easier, reversing PCOS, healing endometriosis symptoms, and optimizing fertility (both naturally and when assisted reproductive technology is needed), while helping you get rid of bloating, acne, sugar cravings, mood swings, and a whole host of gut-hormone-pathway-related symptoms. Most of this action takes place in your intestines, so this will be our focus.

A Semipermeable Membrane: Your Intestinal Lining

The intestines are a long, continuous tube running from the stomach to the anus. Your small intestine is about twenty feet long, an inch in diameter, and extends from the end of your stomach to where it joins with your large intestine. The large intestine is about five feet long, three inches in diameter, and the last portion is the rectum. The colon absorbs water from wastes, creating stool. As stool enters the rectum, nerves there create the urge to have a bowel movement. The inner surface of your intestinal lining is far denser than you might imagine. Stretched out, it would cover the floor of about a 10 × 20-foot living room (or half a badminton court, according to the geeky scientists who measure this stuff!). How is this possible?

The small intestine is not a flat surface but consists of millions of tiny fingerlike projections like those you'd see on a sea anemone, which stick out into the tube of your small intestine (the lumen) and massively increase the surface area. The villi are covered with cells that are in turn covered in microvilli, which provide an enormous surface area for nutrient absorption, and through their wavelike motions also help move the wastes to your colon.

Throughout much of the intestine, the surface layer cells are made up of a single layer of cells called *enterocytes*. These, too, interface with the inside tube of the intestine, forming its lining. On the surface of this lining is a rich mucus coating that protects these cells by creating a physical barrier, a healthy pH, protecting the lining from inflammation and supplying your microbiome with important nutrients that help it to thrive. This physical barrier is meant to allow peaceful coexistence with your intestinal guests—the trillions of bacteria, yeasts, and other organisms that live in there—without triggering a massive immune reaction to them, while providing a selectively permeable barrier that lets the nutrition you need from your food (which some of those organisms even help to manufacture) into your body. This physical barrier keeps what's in the tube (food breakdown particles, bacteria and other organisms, a variety of protein fragments from these organisms, and anything else you ingest such as medications) from reaching what's beneath it, because if that layer is breached, havoc can result.

That's because in the layer beneath the enterocytes you find one of the important parts of your immune system. It turns out that about 70% of the body's immune system, and the largest repository of lymph tissue, is located just below the gut lining, in lymphatic tissue called *gut-associated lymphoid tissue (GALT)*, and in the small intestine, additionally, *Peyer's patches*. Your body does a marvelous job being highly selective about what gets across the inner layer to the GALT—and what doesn't—using a series of "gates" called *tight junctions* between the enterocytes, serving a bit like border-crossing guards looking for the right passports that signal "sure, you can pass," or not.

Leaky Gut

When the integrity of the gut lining is breached, which can happen due to inflammation, damage to the enterocyte layer, certain medications, stress, or foods that trigger the tight junctions to "leak," the ability to maintain a discrete border crossing station is disrupted and the intestinal lining becomes more permeable. This is technically called *intestinal hyperpermeability*, or more commonly *leaky gut*. Leaky gut allows food particles, fragments of bacteria and other organisms, and other small intestinal waste products that are hanging out in your gut waiting to be eliminated instead to cross into the immune-system-rich layer of your intestinal lining. When this happens, an immune reaction is triggered in the GALT or other lymph tissue, or those particles get into your bloodstream. One major systemic situation that can arise is endotoxemia. This is when specific fragments from the outer coats (called *lipopolysaccharides* or *LPS*) of certain bacteria translocate across that leaky barrier and into your general circulation.

When any of these migrate across the inner protective barrier of your gut and into your circulation, the body recognizes them as foreign invaders—just like it would any bacteria, virus, or foreign body—and begins to mount an attack. Immune cells are dispatched to neutralize the invaders and inflammation goes rampant. LPS are toxic to your body, creating endotoxemia. These changes, in turn, lead to inflammation. Proteins and other particles

from your food can also alert the immune system to send out the troops to neutralize them, which can inadvertently start to target your own cells—which is one proven trigger of autoimmune disease.

Both inflammation and endotoxemia spell big, often chronic, and seemingly unrelated systemic problems in the form of inflammatory reactions and immune system overstimulation. Leaky gut can be a "silent" condition in that it may not show up as digestive symptoms. You might experience the effects of the low-level chronic inflammation it causes systematically—including hormone problems. As you'll soon learn, this is now considered to be one of the possible causes of endometriosis, but it is also associated with the same insulin resistance that we see with PCOS, and the inflammation we see with period pain and PMS. Additionally, the presence of LPS in the blood has been found to alter circadian rhythm, as does chronic inflammation.

Your Own Secret Garden: The Microbiome

In addition to the multifaceted protective, nutrient-extracting, and immune-regulating roles of the intestinal lining, your digestive system has another important microecosystem at work, keeping you healthy and your hormones happy—your **microbiome**. This little universe is made up of trillions of microorganisms—beneficial species of friendly bacteria, viruses, and yeasts—collectively called the *human intestinal microbiome*, sometimes referred to as its own "virtual organ."

There are up to a thousand different species hanging out in there, and these organisms are so abundant they outnumber your own cells ten to one. In fact, 90% of the cells of your body are your microbiome, the majority of which are living in us symbiotically, meaning that they have beneficial interactions with each other and with us. We can't live without them, nor they without us.

A healthy microbiome is made up of a very wide variety of the right types of organisms, in the right amounts, in the right places in our intestines, varying from the small intestinal regions, through the large intestine, and into the colon, which has the greatest abundance of microflora. Each of us has our own microbiome "fingerprint" if you will; the types and organisms that make up your microbiome are highly individual, and for each of us, vary somewhat with diet, lifestyle, and even ethnic background. Because each of us has our own normal, there's a limit to the value of most microbiome testing kits commercially available at this time.

There isn't much going on in your body—and mind—that isn't influenced by the composition of your microbiome. Remember how important those phytochemicals in Chapter 6 are for your health? It takes enzymes specifically produced by a healthy microbiome for those plant-based chemicals to be bioavailable. Without a healthy microbiome you can eat fruits and veggies all day long and not make use of them for your health! And while the liver is the major player in the detoxification of everything from our hormones and the breakdown products from our foods to environmental triggers, your gut microbiome isn't just playing second fiddle. It's right on up there in importance. Many of the environmental exposures we get happen through food; those chemicals that are poorly absorbed after we ingest them are swept into the small intestine, and guess what starts to break them down? Yup—your microbiome! The microbiome also plays a critical role in their elimination, too.

Your microbiome affects your immune balance in ways that are now known to trigger all manner of immune system problems, including endometriosis, Hashimoto's, and more.

The Gut-Brain Axis

It keeps getting more interesting! There's a powerful connection between what goes on in your intestines and your brain—called the gut-brain axis—a constant bidirectional communication pathway between your gut and your brain. If you've ever had butterflies in your stomach or had to run to the bathroom a bunch of times before taking a test or going into a job interview, you know firsthand that acute stress messes with your gut.

That's because your brain has a direct connection to what goes on in your gut. In fact, the gut has been called "the second brain" because of this connection, and this is pretty accurate. Your gut lining is home to a network of approximately one hundred million neurons that are embedded in it and communicates using over thirty-five neurotransmitters; in fact, 95% of your serotonin is found in the intestines. This enteric nervous system, or "second brain," channels about 95% of the information coming through your gut, along one of your body's largest nerves, the vagus nerve, which goes from the gut to the brain. It may be that many of the emotions you experience don't originate in your brain, as it's long been assumed, but reflect the state of what's going on in your gut.

Stress alters your gastrointestinal motility and leads to loose stools, constipation, gas, and IBS; it also damages your gut lining, causing or worsening leaky gut. Stress reduces the number and diversity of beneficial bacteria and "feeds" the harmful bacteria, allowing them to dominate. Stress also impacts our food choices, and the very foods we crave when we're tired or "in a mood" are the ones that tend to be the least beneficial for the health of good gut flora. The sum of this can also be development of endotoxemia, in which, as mentioned earlier, particles of bacteria in your gut called lipopolysaccharides (LPS) enter into your circulation through that leaky gut and can lead to gynecologic conditions like endometriosis, and also autoimmune conditions, including Hashimoto's thyroiditis.

Beneficial species of gut flora also get in on the act. For example, some gut bacteria produce butyrate, a short-chain fatty acid (SCFA) that keeps the intestinal lining healthy and intact, protecting you from infection and inflammation, and helps to prevent anxiety and depression. When the microbiome or the intestinal lining is perturbed, butyrate production drops, explaining in part why microbiome disturbances have been linked to depression and anxiety. Leaky gut adds inflammation to the soup causing "brainflammation," which estimates suggest is a root cause of about 30% of cases of depression.

The connection between mind, mood, and microbiome is so strong that there's now a whole area of research going on in "psychobiotics"—studying the potential for using probiotics for mental health problems. The number of studies demonstrating the connection between what's going on in our gut and anxiety, depression, and cognitive function is phenomenal to say the least. For example, in one highly publicized study at UCLA, researchers found that simply adding a cup of yogurt to the diet twice daily for four weeks led to substantial reductions in anxiety in the twenty-five women in the study group. The researchers concluded that the probiotic organisms in the yogurt favorably changed the intestinal microbiomes of the study participants, which changed their brain chemistry. Your microbiome influences brain signaling that can cause or contribute to PMS, anxiety, and depression. Healthy, higher levels of an important beneficial organism called Bifidobacterium are associated with more favorable lower cortisol levels, linked to less stress, less anxiety, and better emotional resilience and sleep.

Another study done in 2015 found that among forty-five individuals given a prebiotic, a carbohydrate that feeds healthy gut flora, there was reduction in cortisol, stress, and anxiety, with a shift in thinking from negative to more positive thoughts. Both gut dysbiosis and leaky gut have been found to activate the HPA axis, resulting in a chronically triggered stress response, but also, get this, increased perceptions of abdominal pain.

Sleep not only plays an obvious role in our moods and stress levels, but our gut microbiome is highly sensitive to circadian rhythm disruption; less sleep means more dysbiosis. Reduced sleep time and, specifically, decreased melatonin, can contribute to leaky gut and intestinal inflammation. They can also cause alterations in gut microorganisms. Poor sleep has been found to increase firmicutes in the gut, an organism specifically associated with weight gain and metabolic syndrome. In one interesting study, when intestinal microbiota samples from individuals who had been experiencing jet lag for twenty-four hours were transplanted into mice, the mice began to show weight gain and decreased glucose tolerance. In addition, poorer food choices like sugar and quick carbs that we eat to compensate for fatigue also feed the wrong kind of gut microbes, worsening dysbiosis and our symptoms. Interestingly, as yet one more example of "it's all connected," we now also know that an altered microbiome affects our sleep timing and quality.

So your microbiome has this profound impact on nutrient absorption, detoxification, even your moods, appetite, food cravings, and mental function, and when out of balance, it can lead to inflammation, obesity and diabetes, hormonal problems, anxiety, depression, and brain fog. The interfaces between your gut, immune, and nervous system govern inflammation, and with it your moods, weight, insulin sensitivity, sleep, pain levels—and what brings you to this book, your hormones. It's so central to hormone balance, in fact, that a special branch of your microbiome is devoted solely to regulating your estrogen balance.

Meet Your Estrobolome

To understand how your gut influences estrogen levels, it's important to know how this hormone makes its way into your digestive system. Estrogen is produced in your ovaries, and to a lesser extent, your fat cells and adrenals. It then circulates in your bloodstream throughout your body, from your brain to your heart, bones, uterus, and the millions of cells that have estrogen receptors, doing all the amazing things that estrogen does. At the end of its journey, estrogen makes its way to your liver, where it is broken down, inactivated, and packaged up for elimination. Packaged estrogen is mixed with bile, secreted into the intestines, and meant to be excreted in your stool. When estrogen is in your intestines, it meets a very special microbiome, the **estrobolome**, whose entire job is regulating estrogen levels.

These bacteria contain special genes that are specifically capable of regulating how much estrogen is eliminated or reabsorbed and recirculated into your body. They do this by producing an enzyme called *beta-glucuronidase* that breaks down estrogens into their active forms and regulates how much estrogen is reabsorbed via a process called *enterohepatic circulation*. Bacteria in your estrobolome are also little manufacturing centers, able to make estrogen from plants in our diet. They do this by converting compounds called *lignans*, found in vegetables, legumes, and in especially high amounts in flaxseeds, into estrogen-like compounds called *phytoestrogens* (plant estrogens), which the body couldn't make use of if the bacteria didn't act on them. Phytoestrogens are incredibly important; when your estrogen levels are high, they can block the receptors and protect you from the risks of excess estrogen exposure, yet when estrogen is low, they can provide enough to keep your estrogen levels supported.

When your estrobolome, along with the rest of your gut microbiome, is healthy and well nourished, you have a huge advantage for hormone health. But when things get imbalanced, a problem called *dysbiosis*, things can get wonky. But before we get there, let's talk about your second brain.

Dysbiosis: Trouble in the Garden

One of the most important keys to a healthy microbiome, in addition to what's thriving in there, is microbial diversity. Comparative studies looking at the limited number of people still living close to ancestral ways of life have shown that their microbial diversity far outstrips that of the rest of us living modern, industrialized lives. With decreased diversity comes an increase in diseases of all kinds, and most notably, chronic diseases, which are largely absent among people living more traditionally. One amazing and well-studied example of this is the Hadza people, who live the same traditional hunter-gatherer life they have since time immemorial, with a diet that rotates with what's available seasonally, with a wide diversity of foods, including those that have soil organisms remaining on them, and with a whopping 100 to 150 grams of fiber daily. They are healthier and have vastly more diverse microbiomes.

Basically, you want your gut to be like an

ideal Amazon rainforest—lushly filled with an abundance of symbiotically thriving life-forms. Instead, for too many of us, the situation is a bit more like deforestation—reduced diversity, stripped soil, and loss of species resilience, some even going extinct as a result. And much like the planet relies on the rainforests for oxygen, your body relies on your microbiome for, well, nearly everything! Indeed, for many of us, healthy gut flora has become an endangered species. So it's time for a little personal ecological restoration. As Justin Sonnenburg, a microbiologist at Stanford University who has studied the Hadza, says, "The further away people's diets are from a Western diet, the greater the variety of microbes they tend to have in their guts. And that includes bacteria that are missing from American guts."

When the type or number of bacteria gets messed up, when you lose diversity of the types of bacteria, fungi, and viruses, your gut can no longer perform its hormone-regulating functions properly. The technical name for disruption in your gut microbiome is **intestinal dysbiosis**. It can result in an overgrowth of unfriendly species, loss of helpful species, and a lot of health problems.

The most common and obvious symptoms of gut dysbiosis (which you can use as a gut health self-check list!) include digestive symptoms such as the following:

- Bloating
- Chronic constipation
- Fatigue after meals
- Gas
- IBS
- Loose stools

Here are other common symptoms that may show up, even without obvious digestive symptoms:

- Brain fog
- Chronic anxiety or depression
- Chronic yeast and other fungal infection
- General fatigue
- Intolerance of sugar, sometimes even including fruit, carbs/grains, or alcohol (feeling tired, moody, puffy, or other symptoms within 1 to 12 hours after having one of these)
- Sugar or carb cravings

Dysbiosis can also show up without any obvious digestive symptoms and still cause gynecologic problems and hormone symptoms, including a long list of women's health problems. Here's just a partial inventory of the women's conditions associated with dysbiosis (which you can also use as a gut health self-check list!):

- Acne
- Anxiety
- Bladder infections
- Breast and endometrial cancers
- Chronic pelvic pain
- Cyclic breast symptoms (cysts, tenderness)
- Depression
- Endometriosis
- Estrogen—high or low
- Hashimoto's
- Infertility
- Insomnia
- Insulin resistance
- Interstitial cystitis
- Miscarriage

- Obesity
- PCOS
- Period pain
- PMS
- Premenstrual digestive symptoms
- Recurrent vaginal infections
- Stress
- Sugar cravings

Some are a result of chronic inflammation, for example, insulin resistance, obesity, PCOS, period pain, PMS, anxiety, and depression; some are due to the immune system going haywire or not properly regulating itself, for example, endometriosis, and sometimes even turning on itself, as in the case of Hashimoto's and other autoimmune conditions. Some, including PCOS, endometriosis, and PMS are also due to estrobolome disruption.

The Goldilocks Factor: Estrogen and Your Estrobolome

When your estrobolome is properly functioning because your gut has the right type and diversity of microorganisms, it hums along smoothly, absorbing and excreting the right balance of estrogens so that you enjoy healthy hormone balance. If dysbiosis causes your estrobolome bacteria to overgrow, you may produce or reabsorb too much estrogen, which also happens to be a slightly more problematic form of estrogen. Remember, too much estrogen creates all kinds of noise in your endocrine system and can lead to heavy, painful periods; it's also a trigger to endometriosis, fibroids, and mood swings and can increase the risks of endometrial and breast cancers. Do you recall I told you that alcohol also increases estrogen

levels? One way it seems to do this is by altering your estrobolome!

On the other hand, low microbial diversity can cause your estrobolome to poorly convert and absorb your own estrogen, and also produce lower levels of beta-glucuronidase so that you can't utilize those potentially protective plant-based estrogens. This can lead you to have low estrogen levels—a problem for your sleep, moods, vaginal health, bones, heart, and brain as you edge into perimenopause and your levels are already on the natural decline. Speaking of vaginal health and your microbiome, this is something we should chat more about.

Vaginal Ecology: Your Vagina Has a Microbiome, Too

You also have an amazing mini ecosystem right in your very own vagina. Like your gut, skin, and many other parts of your body, your vagina has its own unique microbial environment—the vaginal microbiome. Your overall health affects the health of your vaginal ecology, and your vaginal ecology in turn affects your overall health—you and your microbiome create your internal ecosystem, and your external, day-to-day world influences this. The ecosystem of organisms that live in your vagina keep it, and you, healthy. The health of the vaginal flora is also dependent on the health of the gut flora. Like in garden soil, healthy microorganisms keep down the "bad bacteria" and other bugs in the soil that can harm the plant's roots, damaging the whole plant.

But like other forms of dysbiosis, vaginal dysbiosis can lead to major problems affecting your hormonal health and lady parts. Vaginal dysbiosis has now been found in women with PCOS and is particularly associated with elevated androgens (i.e., testosterone).

It also appears that these changes make us more susceptible to the inflammatory effects of several environmental toxins and increase a woman's risk of developing endometriosis. Vaginal dysbiosis may also play a role in chronic pelvic pain, due to chronic inflammation in the uterus and pelvis. Gut and vaginal dysbiosis have been directly linked to implantation problems, as well as to recurrent miscarriage. The wrong kind of gut flora can prevent conception, has been shown to reduce or even prevent IVF and embryo transfer effectiveness, can increase miscarriage risk, and can lead to preterm birth when you do get pregnant. Getting your gut health in order is one of the first, most important steps to healing.

The Gut-Hormone Connection

So how does this connect to the hormone and gynecologic troubles women are commonly experiencing? Let me show you, because it will help you more thoroughly understand the "why" of this pillar of Hormone Intelligence and can help you commit to a healthy gut as part of your overall hormone balance and healing.

Endometriosis: Major research shows that dysbiosis is involved in the onset and progression of endometriosis. Women with endometriosis have higher amounts of dysbiosis overall, as well as a greater amount of activity in the estrobolome leading to higher estrogen levels that stimulate endometriosis growth. Leaky gut is also on the short list as a cause: women with endometriosis have four to six times higher amounts of LPS and gram-negative bacteria, which cause immune system misfiring, in their blood, vagina, and peritoneal cavity. Abnormal levels of inflammatory cytokines and immune cell activation in the peritoneal cavity are, in turn, major

hallmarks in the pathogenesis of endometriosis, so gut dysbiosis itself creates a potentially self-perpetuating system causing or contributing to endometriosis. When LPS come into contact with the ovaries, the resultant local inflammation can result in suppressed progesterone production, demonstrated by the fact that women with higher levels of LPS in the blood have elevated markers of inflammation in fluid inside the ovary (follicular IL-6) and correspondingly low progesterone levels. The combination of LPS in large amounts and high estrogen is considered yet another level of problem—a perfect storm for developing endometriosis. The gut-endometriosis connection may also explain why so many women with endometriosis have IBS, bloating, and digestive problems, previously thought to be solely due to bowel adhesions but more likely due to a combination of factors including adhesions, but also leaky gut, dysbiosis, and stress, a phenomenon called *endo belly.*

Upward of 90% of women with endometriosis suffer with digestive problems. *Endo belly* refers to the often severe, chronic, painful bloating that is very common in women with endometriosis. As with IBS, which was for decades discounted as "in women's heads," most doctors have denied women's experience of endo belly, chalking this symptom up to IBS. Studies have found a strong correlation between endometriosis symptoms and IBS symptoms; in one study, 79% of women who had been previously diagnosed with IBS were eventually diagnosed with endometriosis. It's possible that this was an initial misdiagnosis, the fact that endometriosis can cause bowel adhesions that slow motility and alter digestion, or that both share dysbiosis as a root cause.

PCOS: Gut dysbiosis may be a significant factor in the shifts in ovarian function and testosterone levels that cause PCOS and its symptoms. Recent studies have identified significantly less gut microbial diversity in women with PCOS compared to those who do not have this condition. Vaginal dysbiosis has also been found in women with PCOS and is particularly associated with elevated androgens (i.e., testosterone). Altered gut microbiota in PCOS women may promote increased androgen biosynthesis through lowered beta-glucuronidase activity. Further, the type and diversity of bacteria in our gut have a causal effect on both insulin resistance and obesity, which is particularly relevant for women with PCOS, especially those that are struggling with their weight, food cravings, and binge eating, and also with depression—through the gut-mood connection. The connection becomes even more intriguing: experimental fecal microbial transplant has been found to improve fertility and decrease androgen levels in an animal model of PCOS. Finally, leaky gut and dysbiosis both lead to chronic stimulation of the immune system, leading to chronic inflammation, and have been connected as a root cause of insulin resistance, a major risk for PCOS.

Fertility: In the vagina, the good flora keeps the vaginal environment at ovulation at the right pH and sugar level to support the passage of the sperm and thus facilitate conception. When the good flora aren't hanging around in adequate numbers, the not-so-good guys that can contribute to or cause fertility problems become out of control. The wrong kind of gut flora can prevent conception, has been shown to reduce or even prevent IVF and embryo transfer effectiveness, can increase miscarriage risk, and can lead to preterm birth when you do get pregnant. Gut and vaginal dysbiosis are directly linked to implantation problems, as well as to recurrent miscarriage. When those good flora aren't hanging around in enough numbers and variety, inflammatory signaling results,

and also organisms like BV, which interfere with fertility and even IVF, can take over the neighborhood. Add to this the fact that the gut microbiota is the conductor, coordinating the communication between the immune, neuroendocrine (think serotonin, dopamine, adrenaline, melatonin, and oxytocin), and endocrine systems. When this communication isn't happening smoothly, any of the hormone symptoms and gyn conditions we're talking about in this book can result, with some of the big ones related to disruptions in this triad including PMS, especially mood swings and food cravings, sleep problems, endometriosis, and fertility challenges, as well as insulin resistance and resultant PCOS in many women.

The Gut-Period Connection

PMS: Because your microbiome is so intimately tied to your estrogen levels, it can have a profound influence on your menstrual cycles, particularly premenstrual symptoms including cravings, bloating, loose stools, migraines (the relationship to estrogen levels was discussed on page 75), how much you bleed, and how much pain you have. The mood-mind-gut connection is also something to consider with premenstrual mood swings, anxiety, and depression. Natural premenstrual shifts in our appetite and cravings may also make us likely to "feed" problematic gut bugs with sugar and alcohol, and if either dysbiosis or hormone imbalance is present, or both are, we're more likely to have those cravings. Period bloating is probably the most obvious gut-hormone connection there is! It's estimated that close to 70% of women experience bloating.

Heavy, Painful Periods, and Then Some: Too

much estrogen from a disrupted estrobolome is associated with heavy periods; even endometrial cancer, fertility challenges, and miscarriage have been linked to dysbiosis, and it also affects breast health.

Cravings (or My Microbiome Made Me Eat It): This may sound crazy, but whether you love chocolate or don't crave it at all, whether you go for kale or cake, may be a factor of what's going on in your gut microbial community! Your gut microbiome has the ability to manipulate you into eating certain foods that specific organisms there need to survive and thrive. It does this in two ways—it creates cravings for foods that they specifically need for their own growth by making our brain register those foods as tastier and more appealing, and they produce toxins that make us feel unwell and alter our mood, through affecting various neurotransmitter levels, until we eat the foods that satisfy them. They literally hijack the messages going from the gut to the brain along the vagus nerve. Hormones in the gut and your brain communicate, telling each other how much energy you need to extract from your food, when you're hungry, and how much you need to eat, and they can even dictate food cravings. There's just no end to the interconnectedness of the human body!

Breast Pain: Increased estrogen due to dysbiosis can lead directly to cyclic breast pain. It's also recently been discovered that your intestinal microbiome affects the microbiome of tissue at distant sites, including your vaginal and breast tissue. To do so, it uses hormonal intermediates, metabolites, and immunologic messengers to communicate. For example, the intestinal microbiome is able to communicate with the distinct microbiome found in your breast tissue, and alterations in breast tissue microbiome are associated with breast cancer. They are talking to each other and talking with your hormone-signaling pathways! One area of tremendous influence is with our vaginal ecosystem.

Pain: New studies are pointing to a hidden root cause of pain that may help us move away from the rather high-stakes pain medications that have become the prescriptions du jour for period pain, endometrial pain, and chronic pelvic pain—namely, opioids. In fact, an imbalanced microbiome appears to increase sensitivity to visceral pain, the very type of pain associated with these common gynecologic conditions. Like so many others, this connection travels the communication pathway between the gut and the brain. Further, the connection between sleep and pain is significant; pain can make it much harder to fall asleep and stay asleep.

Thyroid Function: Friendly gut microorganisms are also partially responsible for the conversion of the less active thyroid hormone, T4, into its active form, T3. When this isn't happening effectively, your thyroid might be perfectly healthy, but your body gets the message that you have hypothyroidism, which can also affect overall hormone levels, as well as your metabolism, energy, mind, sleep, and mood. Leaky gut is also a risk factor for developing Hashimoto's, which, in turn, can lead to significant hormone and menstrual cycle disruption.

Weight Struggles: Different gut flora use energy in different ways—some, especially in the strain called *Firmicutes*, are able to extract a lot of calories from food, meaning that if you're loaded up with this type, you're going to get loaded up with more calories and get fatter. In contrast, *Bacteroides*, another species, doesn't guzzle up the calories—so when you have a preponderance of these guys, you're apt to be leaner. The case for this was made strong when it was shown that fecal transplants (yes, harvesting and transferring poop) from lean mice into obese mice made the fat mice lose weight. Guess what? The same thing has been shown in humans, along with a reduction in insulin resistance.

What Disrupts Gut Balance?

So what gets our guts in such a mess? Fundamental changes in how we live in our culture have drastically altered our gut health. And the reality is that almost everyone living in the modern Western world has some amount of gut disruption going on, the likelihood even more if you have hormone conditions.

Gut health starts at birth, when our microbiome is supposed to be "seeded" by exposure to our mom's microbiome as we pass through the vaginal canal. But because of our 34% cesarean section rate, which causes us to bypass that healthy dose of our mom's local organisms, many of us missed out on that initial beneficial inoculation. Breastfeeding then further increases microbiome health and diversity, but many of us were bottle-fed formula.

Our early childhood environment then plays a crucial role in the formation of our microbiome. Growing up in the country or spending lots of time outdoors getting dirty, having a safe environment, and a pet or farm animals, all play a protective role, while stress, antibiotic exposure, and a diet that's low in a wide diversity of nutrients, fiber, and healthy fats all negatively impact that microbiome.

As adults, the factors that influence our gut health then begin to compound and include:

- Ultra-processed foods

- Diets high in saturated fats and PUFAs

- Artificial sweeteners

- Alcohol

- Stress, history of trauma (the latter strongly linked to irritable bowel syndrome in women)

- Circadian rhythm disruption

- Lack of exercise

- Environmental toxins including herbicides, pesticides, and heavy metals

- Certain medications (especially "the Big Five" described later in this chapter)

- Gluten and other food triggers for some women

- Antibiotic use and other medications (explained on page 201)

Woman Wise: Soft Belly Meditation

In Eastern traditions our bellies are considered a seat of power. But for most women, they are a source of tension. We hold them in, try to flatten them, make them disappear; we freak about looking bloated. A lot of women hate on their bellies, apologize for them. How can we reframe to core, power, center, gut knowing, intuition, trust, soft? Try soft belly breathing, adjusting the Quickie Meditation from Chapter 7 (on page 149) and emphasizing breathing deeply into your belly with each inhale, relaxing your belly fully with each exhale, and saying "soft belly" to yourself as you do.

This regular onslaught of gut-damaging factors has added insults here and there, for example, the antibiotic for the urinary tract infection, the ibuprofen every month for period pain, or the wine binge with that breakup. These seemingly unrelated habits and life exposures can add up to gut trouble, and it doesn't take much to do some major disrupting.

The Hormone Intelligence Solution: Gut Health for Every Woman

I want you to experience the power of fabulous digestion on your health, from when food first enters your mouth, all the way through to your elimination. This allows you to get the maximum nutrition out of your food, keep your hormones happy and healthy, and enjoy the feeling of good gut health—no more bloating, constipation, loose stools, gas, or other digestive misery. Your gut has a remarkable ability for self-repair—and rather quickly. And it's not too complex. You have to remove what's triggering inflammation or leaky gut or disrupting your microbiome; replace or replenish the nutrients your body needs to restore gut lining integrity and nourish a healthy microbiome; reseed your microbiome; and if necessary, add additional support for repairing the intestinal lining.

And here's the exciting thing: you're already well on your way! All the steps you're taking in your six weeks on this plan: eating healing foods, reducing stress, and getting better sleep are already helping to heal your gut (and restore your vaginal ecology). Additionally, you might find tremendous improvement and relief from IBS, reflux, Crohn's disease, or ulcerative colitis in the process.

Step 1: Eat for Gut Health
Your diet has the power to make a more significant impact on your gut health than almost any other intervention. In fact, you can make a significant impact on your microbiome in just three days of shifting your diet. Hormone Intelligence eating provides you with the most important ingredients you need to heal leaky gut and restore your microbiome, simply by removing the most common food triggers and providing your body with the missing nutrients your body has been craving. Here are some especially important foods and nutrients to emphasize.

Nourish the Soil
These top-tier nutrients, found in foods in the Hormone Intelligence Diet, are especially nourishing to your gut lining.

- **Vitamin A and Beta-Carotene:** These nutrients are supplied through eggs; leafy green vegetables; orange and yellow vegetables including carrots, broccoli, spinach, cantaloupe, sweet potatoes, and winter squash; tomato products; and apricots.

- **Essential Fatty Acids:** Omega-3 fatty acids (DHA/EPA) can be obtained from eating fatty (cold water) fish on a regular basis, but if you don't eat fish, or can't eat it at least three times each week, then supplement with EFAs.

- **Butyrate:** Butter is a sacred food to many people, and I'm sure my grandmother's wrinkle-free skin into her eighties had something to do with this amazing source of healthy fats. Butyrate is a fatty acid found in grass-fed butter and ghee ("clarified butter") and is particularly healing to the intestinal lining while providing important nourishment for your healthy gut microbes. This is one of the main reasons ghee, in moderation, is a welcome part of this plan.

- **L-Glutamine:** This amino acid supports gut health and helps to heal intestinal hyperpermeability but tightens gap junctions. Food sources include turkey, eggs, almonds, tofu, and tempeh.

- **Zinc-Rich Foods:** These foods are not as prevalent in the food plan for this program, but oysters contain more zinc per serving than any other food, and poultry and red meat are also rich sources. Beans and nuts also contain zinc, but in lesser amounts; your multivitamin will provide the balance you need.

Eat More Plants

A high-fiber diet has been linked to a reduced risk of digestive conditions like IBS. Plants in your diet are especially important when it comes to a much more hormone-favorable microbiome. They provide ample amounts of fiber, the nutrients so important for gut lining integrity, and prebiotics. Eight to ten servings of veggies and fruit, a portion of whole grain, and a small amount of legumes in your diet will automatically bump up your fiber intake. You can additionally add 2 tablespoons of flaxseed or psyllium seeds to your smoothies, green juice, parfait bowls, Goddess Bowls, greens, or salads for about 14 g of additional fiber daily. And see the Gingery Lemon Green Juice on page 363—it packs in three servings of fruits/veggies in one delicious glassful.

Enjoy healthy fats. Healthy fats do it again! This time they prevent inflammation in the gut lining while providing important food for your microbiome. Keep making foods high in beneficial omega-3 fatty acids, including fatty fish (like salmon, mackerel, and sardines), flaxseed, chia seeds, and walnuts, a regular part of your hormone-healthy diet.

Diversity is everything. As in life, diversity is key to a healthy culture—in this case, your microbial culture! Organic agriculture has taught us that when we grow the same crops over and over in the same soil, we deplete the nutrients and also the natural microbiota of that soil. Healthy soil requires that we plant a diversity of crops in rotation. Similarly, when it comes to gut health, variety isn't just the spice of life; it's what gut health is made of. Your body needs a wide diversity of foods, especially plant foods, to truly thrive. Eating that rainbow provides this diversity of micro-nutrients and phytochemicals your gut needs to cool inflammation, restore the integrity of the lining, and nourish a happy, healthy microbiome.

Learn to use culinary herbs and spices. In addition to the great flavors they impart, culinary herbs and spices like ginger, turmeric, basil, rosemary, cumin, cinnamon, cardamom, and thyme are powerful for our health. They act as antimicrobials, preventing the overgrowth of harmful bacteria in our gut. They are powerful antioxidants, reduce inflammation, improve blood sugar and insulin sensitivity, and even help keep our weight healthy by boosting metabolism—even in small amounts.

Healthy flora need prebiotic-rich foods. Prebiotics are specific starches or fibers (though not all starches and fibers are prebiotics) that serve as food for healthy gut flora. A healthy gut requires healthy gut food. But there's more to the story. Remember in the last chapter I talked about the gut–circadian rhythm connection? In one study, forty-five healthy volunteers received prebiotic supplements daily for three weeks, or placebo. At the end of this time, the morning cortisol response was significantly better in those taking the prebiotic, more proof that a healthy gut can also promote healthy circadian rhythm and improve your overall HPA axis response.

Prebiotic-rich foods in the Hormone Intelligence Diet include:

- Vegetables: Jerusalem artichokes, chicory, garlic, onion, leeks, shallots, spring onion, asparagus, beetroot, fennel bulb, green peas, snow peas, savoy cabbage

- Nuts and seeds: cashews, pistachio nuts

- Fruit: grapefruit, berries

- Resistant starches, a form of carbohydrate that is not broken down into sugar in the small intestine, act as "fertilizer" for your microbiome. These are found in legumes (chickpeas, lentils, kidney beans) and some whole grains, for example, brown rice and oats.

To increase your daily intake, include prebiotic supplements or foods as part of your diet, as well as resistant starch. The Hormone Intelligence Diet provides this for you. As with dietary fibers, some gas or bloating can result initially when you increase the amount of prebiotic foods in your diet. So start with small amounts and allow your gut to adapt.

Eat probiotic foods. Probiotic-rich foods are not only delicious and a part of most traditional diets around the world, naturally fermented foods are an important part of rebuilding a healthy microbiome, improving natural detoxication and elimination, restoring immune system health and reducing inflammation, making weight loss easier, improving mood and mental clarity, and reducing stress.

If you think gut health may be of particular concern to you, make sure to try a few of the recipes from the Gut Support Menu, one of the sample weekly meal plans in Part Four, and try to include at least one serving daily of:

- Coconut yogurt or coconut kefir

- Water- or brine-cured olives

- Lacto-fermented sour dill pickles

- Kimchi (get one that isn't too spicy)

- Sauerkraut

- Pickled vegetables

All these can be purchased at a natural grocery store, and many can be made at home.

Seed your microbiome by taking a probiotic supplement. Probiotics are microorganisms (helpful bacteria and yeasts) that help support various aspects of overall health. Probiotics seem to have an ever-expanding list of superpowers and this may be especially true when it comes to probiotics for women. While research is still young and emerging when it comes to the cause-and-effect relationship between taking a probiotic and specific hormone imbalances and gyn conditions, there are some impressive studies showing use of probiotics can lead to:

- Reduced insulin resistance

- Improvements in fertility, better assisted fertility outcomes, and healthier pregnancies

- Fewer urinary tract and vaginal infections, including BV and group B strep (important for women in labor)

- Improved HPA axis function, reduced stress, and improved resilience

- Reductions in anxiety and depression, which may trickle over to improved premenstrual mood

- Better sleep, healthier circadian rhythm, and breaking the cycle of stress causing sleep problems

- Clearing up IBS, constipation, bloating, and diarrhea

- Achieving a healthier weight; improved weight loss

- Several clinical studies have shown that taking a probiotic can reduce stress, improve sleep quality, and improve memory

Does everyone need to supplement with a probiotic? Not at all, if your diet is rich in lacto-fermented foods and you enjoy gut and hormonal health. But if for some reason you don't enjoy or tolerate fermented foods, you're working to repair your gut, or you have a condition that is known to be benefited by a probiotic supplement, this is a simple way to enhance your healing process.

Step 2: Practice Mealtime Mindfulness

Have you ever eaten a whole meal and not remembered what you just ate or realized you never tasted it? This happens when we've been eating and multitasking. Mindful eating means giving your meal your full attention. Mindful eating can help you to eat "the right" amount and improves digestion because it puts your nervous system into what is called the "rest-and-digest" mode, the opposite of the fight-or-flight response.

Here are some daily practices that can help you to create calm before and while you eat. Mindful eating is the practice of slowing down while you eat; appreciating, not worrying

How to Select a Probiotic

Your probiotic supplement should contain at least 10 billion colony-forming units (CFUs) of a variety of *Lactobacillus* and *Bifidobacterium* species to help restore the normal balance of flora in your gut and repair your gut barrier function. I recommend taking supplements daily for a couple of months, then back down to a few days each week if you feel you're continuing to find them helpful. If a probiotic causes you gassiness or bloating, start with a lower dose and treat bacterial overgrowth.

Unfortunately, the probiotic product market is a bit of a Wild West. Most probiotics do not undergo testing and approval. Manufacturers are responsible for making sure they're safe before they're marketed and that any claims made on the label are true, but there's no guarantee that what's on the label is actually in the product, or that the types of bacteria listed on a label are effective for the condition you're taking them for. Scientific and consumer watchdog company product reviews continue to turn up a consistent finding: most of the products on the market don't contain the strains or number of organisms they claim to, and products touting live cultures don't always pan out to have live cultures. So what you see might not be what you get. I discuss more about choosing reliable brands at avivaromm.com.

about what you're eating; paying attention to the tastes, aromas, and textures of your foods; and noticing how you feel in your body as you eat. Studies show that increasing our awareness in this way while we eat can improve GI symptoms, including those associated with IBS. If the practice—or even idea—of mindful eating is new to you, pick one meal a week to practice it at. Here are some tips for getting started. Pick one and see how it feels:

- **Savor your meal.** Set your kitchen timer to twenty-five minutes, and take that entire time to enjoy your meal. More relaxed eating has been shown to improve digestion. This is an amazing practice for any meal; if you can do it at lunch instead of a "keyboard" lunch, it can reset your afternoon work experience and focus!

- **Start each meal with one minute of silence and gratitude.**

- **Practice *hara hachi bu*.** This means eating until you're 80% full, rather than stuffed all the way.

- **Turn off distractions.** This means the TV, your cell phone, your computer, and so on. As the Buddhist saying goes, "When you walk, walk; when you eat, eat."

- **Chew your food.** Good digestion starts in your mouth, literally, with the digestive enzymes that are released when you chew and that begin to ready the rest of your GI system, including the parts that happen in your brain and food processing hormones. So take smaller bites than usual, and chew, chew, chew your food.

- **Eat with joy.** So many women have told me that as they are sitting in front of their plate, they are worrying how fat their food is going to make them feel or whether they're eating the wrong foods for their health, or in some way or another beating themselves up with a long history of internalized negative food messaging.

Step 3: Get Going

Poop. Kids love to talk about it. We all should, because "taking out the trash" is a necessary part of hormone balance, detoxification, and reducing inflammation. Having a regular, easy to eliminate, daily BM will allow your body to get rid of toxins and improve your gut health. Is there a way to know my poop is healthy? Sure is!

Here are the characteristics of healthy elimination. Healthy poops are:

- A daily (once or twice) occurrence

- Easy to pass: painless, no straining required, and shouldn't take more than ten to fifteen minutes

- Soft to firm in texture; not too hard, not too loose

- Medium to dark brown in color

- Not foul-smelling

- Passed in one single piece or a few smaller pieces

If you're still not sure what healthy poops look like, you can check out the Bristol Poop Scale online; it's a very helpful graphic.

Having Trouble Going? Here's Some Help

If you're still not having a bowel movement at least once daily, most days, here's what you can do:

Realign your circadian rhythm. Better sleep and a more regular lifestyle can improve bowel regularity; conversely, disrupted sleep can literally jet-lag your microbiome, impairing their function and encouraging overgrowth of less favorable sorts.

Make pooping a habit. So often we're in a rush that we just don't sit on the pot, sometimes even ignoring the urge; then by the time you get to work or wherever you're going, perhaps you're too embarrassed to go number 2 in the public loo—this is a super common inhibition leading to chronic constipation. Because by the time you're feeling full or blocked up, you've told your body to squash that urge, and now it's hard to go. So make time every day, ideally at the same time of day, to sit and shit!

Try squatty potty time. Yes, that's right. If you're a nimble yoga-chick, get your feet right up there on the bowl. Not so flexible and balanced? Invest in a Squatty Potty (no, I don't have stock in those!). It's the physiologic way to go and can even overcome pooping problems due to pelvic floor dysfunction.

Move more. If you're not moving regularly, it's likely that neither are your bowels. Further, studies of the microbiota of active versus sedentary women have revealed a higher abundance of health-promoting bacterial species in active women, including *Bifidobacterium* species, which are also associated with healthier weight. Two studies have also shown that exercise alone can change the composition of microbes in the gut—and this in turn can keep your bowels moving regularly. How much exercise is optimal for healthy elimination? Three days per week, sixty minutes at a time.

Fiber up. Fiber helps you to lose weight; it fills you up, decreases unhealthy cholesterol, and improves the detoxification of hormones from your digestive system. Additionally, not only do flaxseed and psyllium increase BM frequency and quality, but psyllium intake improves gut microbiome quality in favor of species that produce the gut-healthy, inflammation-reducing, mood-improving short-chain fatty acid (SCFA) butyrate, and even more so when taken for constipation.

Sometimes not pooping happens for reasons beyond your diet or microbiome. For example, pelvic floor dysfunction due to nerve damage or pelvic organ prolapse postbirth, especially if you've had a large baby, pushed for an extended amount of time, or had a forceps delivery, can slow your bowels down. History of genital herpes is now also known to be a cause of constipation because it affects the nerve plexus in your bowels as well. In these cases, working with a pelvic floor physical therapist can give you a major bathroom breakthrough!

Step 4: Have a Gut-Healthy Lifestyle

Stress less; sleep more. In the previous chapters I highlighted the importance of reducing stress and improving your circadian rhythm. In a nutshell, a healthy gut means less stress and better sleep, and vice versa. So if you haven't made these a part of your lifestyle yet, now's the time to make sure you're on the relaxation and good sleep train. Your gut also depends on it.

Poop Rx

- Magnesium citrate, 400 to 600 mg before bed nightly.
- A probiotic containing *Lactobacillus* and *Bifidobacterium* strains each morning.
- Herbal bitters can help move things along in your digestive system.
- A combination of senna and mint tea taken before bed can help you get a move on in the morning.
- Triphala herbal blend provides gentle herbal laxative support.

Be a dirty girl. When was the last time you played outside? Got dirty? Ate a cucumber off the vine—yes, with some dirt still on it? Most of us live completely devoid of contact with the earth. Yet outdoor play, gardening, or any activity that brings you into contact with soil, plant life, and pets or animals that spend time outdoors, will increase your opportunity for exposure to microbial diversity. A recent study found that athletes who make frequent contact with natural grass, soil, and mud have greater gut microbial diversity than those who don't. The double benefit is that this activity can bring you into plant-rich environments (like a forest) where you'll inhale natural phytoncides, aromatic chemicals secreted from trees that reduce stress and improve immune function.

Step 5: Avoid Unnecessary Pharmaceuticals

Most medications have unintended consequences, and when it comes to antibiotics, proton pump inhibitors, NSAIDs, and acetaminophen, the consequences are damage to your gut ecosystem and infrastructure. To protect both our health and our planet, we have to reduce the number of pharmaceuticals we use. The best way to do this, of course, is by staying healthy and needing fewer medications. But we also need to begin "thinking beyond drugs" and return to more natural approaches to healing. Whenever possible, I recommend **removing "the Big Five."** Speak with your primary provider before going off prescription medications, but these are the big culprits to try to avoid for a healthy gut.

- **Antibiotics:** Of all medications, antibiotics can wreak havoc on the microbiome. Yet over 70% of those prescribed in the US are medically unnecessary, and by the time we're thirty years old, the average American has had thirty courses of antibiotics. Even just one round of antibiotics can wipe out an entire species of your gut flora—permanently. So take antibiotics only when truly necessary, and try alternatives (with your health care provider's blessing) for mild infections. It's not just the antibiotics we take as medications that affect our gut. More than 50% of the antibiotics produced in the US end up in the meat we eat, used to fatten animals faster—so remember to keep all the meat in your diet antibiotic free! Also, take care to avoid antimicrobial

The Power of Flaxseeds

Flaxseeds help you to feel full, eat less, and lose weight; they improve your bowel health and regularity because they feed good gut flora and act as a gentle bulk laxative; and they help to balance your hormones. In supporting good gut flora, flaxseeds help your body eliminate harmful estrogens you may have produced or picked up from the environment, which not only keeps you in better hormonal health, but may prevent breast cancer. They also improve blood sugar, reduce inflammation, and bring down cholesterol. Soluble fiber such as the lignans found in flaxseeds also increases sex-hormone-binding globulin (SHBG), decreasing the amount of available active estrogen, as estrogen bound to SHBG is rendered inactive. I recommend 1 to 2 tablespoons of freshly ground seeds added to your whole grain cereal or morning shake or on top of your salad daily. Just don't heat the flaxseeds.

Gut Imbalances and Healing Rx at a Glance

You can find more information and proper dosage in the Botanical and Supplement Quick Reference Guide on pages 372–81.

Gut Pattern	Most Common Symptoms	Why It Happens	Specific Foods	Specific Supplements
Dysbiosis	Gas Bloating Fatigue after meals Fatigue in general Brain fog IBS Chronic constipation Chronic or recurrent yeast and other fungal infections Sugar or carb cravings Chronic anxiety or depression	Antibiotics Lack of variety in the diet Low dietary fiber History of gut infection Stress Inflammation in the gut lining	Completely avoid sugar, keep grains to the minimum recommended Fermented veggies (sauerkraut, kimchi) Coconut yogurt or kefir	Prebiotics (inulin, chicory fiber, fructo-oligosaccharides [FOS], and galacto-oligosaccharides [GOS]). Probiotics Essential oils including thyme or oregano oil
Constipation	BM < once/day Feeling of incomplete BM Difficulty passing stools	Dysbiosis Low-fiber diet Stress	High-fiber diet with abundant leafy greens, squashes, and sweet potatoes Flaxseeds, chia seeds Increase dietary fiber with leafy green vegetables	Magnesium citrate Senna & mint tea Triphala herbal blend
Leaky Gut	Food intolerances/sensitivities Seasonal allergies Eczema, skin rashes, acne, or other chronic skin problems Autoimmune condition Tired all the time Chronic fatigue syndrome or fibromyalgia Anxiety, depression, or erratic moods Yeast (Candida) overgrowth or SIBO (small intestinal bacterial overgrowth) Can't lose weight in spite of an excellent diet Joints ache and swell Trouble concentrating, trouble with your memory, or other cognitive changes	Antibiotics Stress Dysbiosis Medications (i.e. ibuprofen) Food intolerances (i.e. gluten) Alcohol	Pay specific attention to food triggers Turmeric in smoothies; teas made of licorice and marshmallow root herbs	L-glutamine DGL licorice Turmeric Marshmallow root Zinc carnosine Melatonin
IBS	Bloating Constipation or loose stools Undigested food in stools Fat in stools Endometriosis or "endo belly"	Stress History of trauma Endometriosis Dietary triggers	Hormone Intelligence Diet	Ginger tea, tincture, or capsules Anise or fennel seed tea or tincture Probiotics

products like hand sanitizers; they, too, can breed antibiotic resistance. A lot of household products, including dish and body soaps, contain them. Swap for cleaner cleaning products, like those I discuss in the next chapter.

- **Nonsteroidal Anti-inflammatory Drugs (NSAIDs):** Medications in this category include ibuprofen, Aleve, Motrin, and many of those familiar to women with menstrual cramps, headaches, migraines, and chronic pain. Their ubiquitous use makes them seem benign, but they aren't. Even five continuous days of use can lead to gastrointestinal (GI) bleeding, and many chronic users have chronic inflammation of the GI tract—a major cause of leaky gut, chronic inflammation, and potential autoimmune disease. Further, a 2015 study found that just 10 days of using an NSAID medication (i.e., naproxen or diclofenac, the same class of drugs as ibuprofen) reduced ovulation and decreased progesterone levels, leading to temporarily reduced fertility.

- **Proton Pump Inhibitors (PPIs):** These medications, including Prilosec, Prevacid, and Nexium, to name a few, are used for the treatment of acid reflux (GERD). In addition to interfering with vitamin B12 absorption, which increases risks of depression, detoxification problems (due to interference with methylation, which we'll talk about in the next chapter), PPIs can increase the growth of bacteria in the small intestine, causing small intestinal bacterial overgrowth (SIBO), which can contribute to digestive symptoms and problems with nutrient absorption.

- **Tylenol:** Acetaminophen damages the delicate lining of the stomach, which can lead to gastrointestinal bleeding and problems with the absorption of nutrients needed for gut health. It is one of the leading causes of liver damage in the US annually. It depletes the most important detoxifier we have in our bodies—glutathione.

- **The Pill:** There are many reasons to reconsider the Pill (see Chapter 10). One of these is that estrogen-based contraceptive pills have been associated with inciting or aggravating autoimmune bowel diseases, especially Crohn's disease, due to increasing intestinal permeability.

Step 6: Next-Level Supplements for Gut Health

The steps I've just shared with you are universally important for gut and hormone health. But if you have definite gut symptoms, or think that your gut might be a bigger root problem for you, you'll want to next-level your plan.

The herbs and nutrients listed in the chart on the opposite page are the most effective for restoring a healthy gut lining and microbiome, as well as some for addressing IBS. Try one or a combination from the categories relevant to you. They can be taken for up to six months. See doses and precautions in the Botanical and Supplement Quick Reference Guide on pages 372–81.

How Long Does Gut Healing Take?

There's no hard and fast science on how long it takes to restore the microbiome or heal a leaky gut. What we do know is that when it comes to the microbiome, it can be fast. Studies have shown that even after just a few days on a healthy diet with high-quality fats, ample amounts of fiber, and plenty of phyto-nutrients, we can see colonies bouncing back to health, abundance, and diversity. If you do have symptoms of dysbiosis (see the accompanying gut pattern table on page 202), in my experience, it takes about six weeks on the recommended supplements plus dietary and lifestyle changes to restore microbiome balance and see dramatic gut symptom resolution.

With leaky gut, depending on severity, you want to give it six weeks to even a year. If you're comfortable continuing on your own with supplements, that's reasonable—follow the guidelines laid out earlier in the program and do not exceed the doses on any products. Otherwise, it's important to see an integrative health practitioner for guidance.

The best gauge that things are moving in the right direction is an improvement in your symptoms or how you feel generally. Even in my medical practice, I don't always do much gut testing because between the questionnaires and the tried-and-true approaches I've shared with you in this program and observing for symptom improvement, that's usually enough. You can repeat the gut symptoms questionnaires as a gauge. If symptoms haven't improved, either you need more time on the plan, or it's another root cause into which a deeper dive is needed. Or seek the personalized guidance of someone with experience in integrative or functional nutrition and medicine.

Follow Your Gut from Now On!

As you're moving toward healing PMS, PCOS, or endometriosis, improving your fertility, or overcoming anxiety, depression, or insomnia—all of which you might never before have associated with your digestive system—remember why a healthy gut is so important now and is part of your overall Hormone Intelligence lifestyle. While every woman is unique, and not all women with hormone conditions have gut problems as a root cause, in my experience most women who have hormone conditions do have a gut component—and in my practice, I always treat the gut as part of a patient's hormone solution. If you are struggling with your hormones, I can't overemphasize how important a healthy gut is as part of your overall ecology.

our planet, your body

THE DETOXIFICATION-HORMONE CONNECTION

In nature, nothing exists alone.

—**Rachel Carson**

In the 1960s, biologist Rachel Carson wrote *Silent Spring*, alerting policy makers and the public to what she foresaw as the serious, long-term risks of environmental contamination to biological organisms. She predicted that human health—and the health of much of our planet—would bear the brunt of the "better living through chemistry" model that was rapidly taking over the country, ushering new chemicals into our environment at an unprecedented rate.

Her prescient warnings were largely unheeded then. Now, sixty years later, there are approximately eighty thousand agricultural and industrial chemicals, 90% of which have *never been tested for safety in human health*, and numerous pharmaceuticals in constant circulation in our air, water, soil, home dust, and food supply, causing harm to human, animal, and planetary health. We cannot assume that just because chemicals are in common trade and usage that they have been adequately evaluated for safety by our government nor even that they have been directly approved. Most have not. Since its founding in 1970 the EPA has banned only a few hundred agents in total; instead, most already in use were "grandfathered" into approval without any safety studies and have remained in use since.

While many of these compounds may be harmless, a significant number undoubtedly impact our hormonal and gynecologic health, enough to be considered reproductive toxicants. Disturbingly, the chemical industry is not required, with limited exception, to test most of these for their effects on our reproductive health—or our health in general. Frighteningly, quite a few that have been banned for use in the US remain in use in countries from which we purchase many of our fruits and vegetables, meats, toys, home furnishings, and other items. Thus, they eventually circulate back into our bodies in what has been dubbed "a circle of poison." Further, even the most toxic of chemicals that were banned as much as thirty years ago, DDT for example, remain persistent in the environment for decades, bioaccumulating in the soil, air, and produce, dairy, and meats we consume. *At some point or another, many find residence in our tissues.*

Toxicologists have now proven that the levels at which it was thought these chemicals could cause harm was grossly underestimated. Damage starts to occur at much lower levels. Mere nanoparticles (think less than a teardrop in an Olympic size swimming pool) of many of these chemicals can induce hormone or immune system activity; it doesn't take much to create biochemical chaos. Additionally, many of these environmental chemicals combine with each other in our bodies to form other chemicals that aren't even studied or for that matter yet known. So we're getting a lot of exposure to a lot of things, and we have no idea what they're doing because they've never been tested—or identified! Concerning, too, is that doctors aren't connecting the dots on women's hormone conditions and the exposures we're all getting, and federal regulatory agencies aren't doing the math either.

Knowledge Is Power

Nothing short of a massive industrial overhaul and change in modern consumption patterns will turn the tide on this environmental and chemical tsunami. Yet, even if production of all endocrine disruptors were to cease today or regulations were to become stringent, these chemicals are pernicious and persistent. They last indefinitely in the environment and tend to sequester themselves in the fat tissue of living organisms, sometimes even thousands of miles from where they were initially used. Persistent organic pesticides, for example, that are used in Southern California or Mexico have been found all the way from Antarctica to the Arctic. Because they are highly lipophilic, meaning they love fat, they persist not only in the environment but also in the fat cells of mammals. Dairy products, and sadly, human breast milk, are major repositories and are even used as markers of environmental contamination in various communities.

The fact is, though, industry is not going to do better by us anytime soon. But you can do better for yourself, and if you have a family (or are planning for one), for them, too. I'm going to show you how to be a warrior for your health, allowing you to dramatically reduce your exposures to the toxins contributing to our hidden hormone epidemic. Then I'm going to take it one step further and show you how your marvelous body's internal self-cleaning process works and why it needs your TLC. It will help you to understand why it's so important that we take a stand in our own lives for our personal health by reducing our exposures; if you're in your childbearing years, why reducing exposures now can prevent potential future children from harm; and how practicing Hormone Intelligence is taking a stand for your hormones. Knowledge is power.

We All Bear a Burden

We all bear a burden. *Body Burden* is the term for the amount of environmental chemicals, heavy metals, and other toxins any of us has

Hormone Intelligence: Our Planet, Our Bodies

- Learn where hormone-disrupting chemicals are hiding in your diet, home, and body products—and swap them with hormone-healthier choices.

- Learn how to use specific foods and nutrients to restore, nourish, and enhance the body systems protecting you from environmental toxins and even your own natural hormone by-products.

- Learn which herbs also enhance your body's hormone balance through supporting these systems, and how to incorporate them into your Hormone Intelligence lifestyle.

stored in our body. Most of us have a moderate to even high body burden of any number of toxins at or above levels known to cause adverse health effects, and many of these are affecting our hormones and reproduction.

According to the 2005 US Centers for Disease Control (CDC) biannual *National Report on Human Exposure to Environmental Chemicals*, which provides exposure data for 148 chemicals and their breakdown products in a cross section of twenty-four hundred Americans:

- Over 90% of us have a mixture of pesticides in our bodies.

- Based on measurements of blood, urine, sweat, breast milk, amniotic fluid, placental tissue, fetal serum, and umbilical cord blood, 92.6% of us were contaminated by BPA.

- All these levels are at, or above, current EPA safety standards for daily human exposure levels.

Body burden studies led by the Mount Sinai School of Medicine and the Environmental Working Group (EWG) found 167 different contaminants in the blood and urine of adults and an average of 200 contaminants in umbilical cord blood samples of newborn babies from several different parts of the US. And a study of Asian women in New York who consumed fish as a staple part of the diet (often in sushi) found that at least half of them had mercury levels above what are considered toxic limits by the federal government. We all now carry a stew of synthetic chemicals, heavy metals, and even pharmaceutical contamination in our bloodstreams, cells, and tissues.

Women Bear an Unfair Share

The damages faced by our planet are mirrored in the microcosm of women's bodies. The extent to which we've been living in a toxic soup has been dismissed by government and industry and until recently by most doctors, as fringe science. It is, however, far from fringe. The medical profession is waking up to the extent to which these exposures are affecting our health. For example, the American College of Obstetricians and Gynecologists now recommends that all obstetricians ask women about their potential toxin exposures at their initial prenatal visit. Unfortunately, most still don't.

Women are disproportionately exposed to environmental toxins on a daily basis from our greater use of cosmetics, household cleaning products, feminine hygiene products, hair coloring, and occupationally, whether through the receipts we handle from the grocery store or pharmacy or exposures at work.

A recent study by the EWG found that women are exposed to 186 chemicals a day just from an average twelve or more personal care products; our teenagers are exposed to even more. Studies show that girls and women with the highest level of use of nail polish, deodorant, hair gel, sunscreen, and sun tanning products also have some of the highest blood levels of some of the chemicals in them, including phthalates and parabens. Even though they're low doses, the cumulative effect eventually puts your body out of balance.

Other high-exposure products include shampoo, conditioner, sunscreen, body lotions, perfumes, and antiaging creams. Pregnant women using cosmetics were also found to have significantly elevated blood levels. For over thirty years, triclosan, which was recently banned from use in many household products, was a common ingredient in numerous products handled much more often by women: detergents, soaps, skin cleansers, deodorants, lotions, creams, toothpastes, and dishwashing liquids, and in 2004 it was detected in the urine of nearly 75% of the 2,517 people tested by the CDC.

We also absorb and accumulate more toxins than do men because women have more fatty tissue. Many toxins preferentially bind to fats and get stored in our fat cells. The list of environmental toxins impacting our health is extensive. One particular category is especially important to highlight when it comes to women's hormonal health: endocrine disruptors.

Endocrine-Disrupting Chemicals (EDCs)

Endocrine-disrupting chemicals (EDCs), also called *hormone disruptors*, are chemicals that interfere with the body's endocrine system and produce adverse developmental, reproductive, neurological, and immune effects. EDCs are particularly sneaky because they're readily absorbed and mimic our hormones. But they are *not* our hormones and are found in human tissue at much higher concentrations than "endogenous" (made by your own body) hormones. As a result, they can overstimulate, block, or disrupt the hormone's natural actions by sending mixed messages throughout your endocrine system. Xenoestrogens ("foreign" estrogens) mimic estrogen, and thyroid-disrupting chemicals (TDCs) interfere with thyroid hormone.

EDCs cause inflammation, weight gain, and insulin resistance, and stimulate cells to grow when they shouldn't—causing problems like early puberty in girls and breast cancer in women.

Endocrine-disrupting chemicals not only interfere with our sex hormones (estrogen, progesterone, and testosterone), they also disrupt our metabolic hormones (i.e., insulin and thyroid hormones), and they have also been shown to activate the stress response, increasing cortisol. Even an exquisitely tiny amount of these signaling molecules can trigger a dramatic response in our cells.

Interestingly, dysbiosis is a downstream effect of environmental toxicity. Various toxicants, including a number of heavy metals, have the potential to alter gut flora and modify various functions of the GI tract including digestion, bioavailability and absorption, elimination, detoxification, and immune function.

How EDCs Do Their Dirty Work

- They mimic or partly mimic naturally occurring hormones in the body like estrogens (called *xenoestrogens*, *xeno* meaning "foreign"), androgens, and thyroid hormones.
- The bind to a receptor within a cell and block the endogenous hormone from binding, especially thyroid hormones, but also estrogen and androgens. The normal signal then fails to occur, and the body fails to respond properly.
- They interfere with or block the way natural hormones or their receptors are made or controlled, for example, by altering their metabolism in the liver.

Mechanisms of obesogens and diabetogens include disruption of central weight control systems, promotion of insulin resistance, and alteration in circadian rhythms. Further, through their effects on the microbiome and also independently through the nervous system, environmental toxicants have been found to alter the stress response, increasing depression, irritability, and impulsive behavior, while reducing stress resilience.

The Toxin-Hormone Connection

Given the parallel between the increased proliferation and accumulation of EDCs in our environment and lives and the increase in our hormonal and women's reproductive health problems over past several decades, with increasing intensity in the past ten years, **we can no longer simply say "we don't know" when it comes to why women are experiencing so many hormone disruptions in our lives**. The science is on our side with literally tens of thousands of research papers demonstrating the connections. Clearly, we need to start talking about

lessening our toxic load if we want to get to the root of hormone health. Here are some of the many ways endocrine disruptors are affecting our hormone balance.

Period Problems: EDCs cause higher levels of circulating estrogen, which makes the lining of your uterus get thicker between periods than it's supposed to and it's this lining that gets shed when you have your period. A thicker lining means a lot more cramping and pain for your uterus to expel it and, in many women, can lead to much heavier periods than they'd have otherwise. In one study, women's pesticide exposure was linked to a 60–99% increased risk of having longer menstrual cycles, skipped periods, and midcycle bleeding compared with women with low to no exposure.

Premature Puberty: The two biggest factors that have been identified as causes of premature puberty are childhood obesity and high levels of exposure to EDCs, which are interrelated. Phthalates; BPA; some pesticides such as DDT, PCBs, and PBBs; and cigarette smoke are just a few of the EDCs that can cause premature puberty and weight gain. High levels of the DDT metabolite DDE and high levels of phthalates have been found in the blood and urine of girls with premature breast development and early puberty. At least six studies have shown links between PCBs, lead, and other compounds and early onset of puberty in girls. These compounds also cause weight gain.

Endometriosis: Five studies have now identified a connection between phthalate exposure and endometriosis, reporting higher phthalate concentrations in women with endometriosis than those without it, and twice the likelihood of having endometriosis compared to women with lower urinary levels, while BPA exposure has also been implicated as having a role in the formation of endometriosis. It's been shown that endometriosis is not only more frequent, but more severe in women with a higher body burden of DDT, organochlorine chemicals, PCBs, and others. Two studies noted two- to fourfold increases in risk of endometriosis in relation to dioxin and PCB exposure, and women in countries with the highest rates of dioxin exposure have higher rates of endometriosis.

Fertility: A news headline a few years back reported that yoga mats may interfere with fertility. Indeed, some do contain phthalates and/or PFRs, and like so many other products do not list these ingredients on their labels, nor are they required to. Numerous studies now confirm a relationship between dozens of common environmental exposures and fertility problems in both men and women. In studies conducted in the US, women who are struggling with fertility were found to be three times more likely to have been exposed to environmental toxins. A recent study found that certain flame-retardant chemicals may make it harder for you to have a baby. A recent study done by researchers at Massachusetts General Hospital's fertility clinic found not only that do most women have traces of flame-retardant chemicals in our bodies, but that among couples undergoing fertility treatment, those with the highest levels were 40% less likely to conceive and eventually have a baby than those with the lowest levels. EDCs can affect sperm and egg quality, and a couple's chance of conception.

The impact of BPA exposure on fertility is so great that some states, including Connecticut and California, have now banned BPA not only in food packaging, but in items like shopping receipts and airline boarding passes because these are statistically more likely to be handled by women. BPA exposure has also been associated with infertility, increased risk of miscarriage, and as a result of its impact on DNA and mitochondrial (cell) function, with decreased egg quality and embryonic health. Studies done on ovarian fluid in women undergoing IVF found much higher pesticide residues, which in turn have been associated with high risk of pregnancy loss and greater difficulty achieving a pregnancy even with fertility treatment.

PCOS: EDCs can contribute to or cause PCOS by affecting ovarian health, creating imbalances in estrogen, testosterone, and progesterone, and causing weight gain and insulin resistance. The greatest risk factor for developing fibroids is chronic exposure to estrogen, and EDCs may be a contributing factor. Rates of PCOS are higher in women with exposure to fish high in DDE and PCBs. Based on animal studies, it's thought the testosterone-stimulating EDCs play a role in the development of PCOS.

Uterine Fibroids: Uterine fibroids are not considered genetic, whereas environmental exposures are a likely contributor. Estrogen "feeds" the growth of uterine fibroids, and this is likely how EDCs factor in. A number of persistent organic pollutants (POPs) and their breakdown products have been detected in the endometrium of premenopausal women undergoing hysterectomies for fibroids. Obesity also increases the risk of developing uterine fibroids, and EDCs are obesogenic. Additionally, EDCs alter the way your DNA works; in the case of uterine fibroids, this allows for unregulated overgrowth of uterine cells.

Thyroid Problems: A number of EDCs act specifically as TDCs—thyroid-disrupting chemicals—including BPA and phthalates. In 2011, University of Michigan researchers conducted the largest national study to date of both BPA and phthalates' impact on thyroid function. They found that when exposed to DEHP, a common phthalate used as a plasticizer, thyroid hormones—free T4, total T3, thyroglobulin, and especially total T4—all decreased, which is problematic for thyroid function. Those with the highest 20% of exposure had as much as a 10% decline in select thyroid hormones! TDCs can compete with iodine, preventing it from getting into the thyroid cells where it is needed for the formation of thyroid hormone, change the shape and function of the thyroid gland, block the production of thyroid hormone, inhibit the ability to turn less active T4 into active T3, prevent the transport of thyroid hormone in the body, and prevent binding of active thyroid hormone to thyroid receptors, all of which have been shown to have the same predictable harmful downstream effects of hypothyroidism.

Toxic Fat: Struggling to lose weight or improve your blood sugar when you're doing all the "right things" is frustrating. EDCs can be a hidden cause of this problem. Called *obesogens* and *diabetogens*, they trigger changes in your cells that increase fat, cortisol, insulin resistance, and diabetes and damage your mitochondria (the energy-producing compartments in cells). EDCs, including BPA, which has been shown to interfere with the production and secretion of insulin, contribute to the epidemic of metabolic syndrome, diabetes, obesity, heart disease, and Alzheimer's. When the CDC tested the blood of 2,016 adults for the presence of POPs, they found that those with the highest concentrations had a five times greater risk of developing metabolic symptoms and a thirty-eight times greater risk of developing diabetes than those with the lowest levels.

Increased Risk of Early Menopause: If you're experiencing any of the above problems, it's important to know that this also puts you at risk for primary ovarian insufficiency (POI). It's now recognized that EDC exposure can disrupt ovarian follicular formation enough to cause ovarian burnout and premature or early menopause. Women over thirty with the highest EDC exposures were six times more likely to be menopausal than women with lower exposure levels. While going into menopause a few years earlier might not seem like a big deal, risk of heart disease increases for each year earlier of menopause, and POI is associated with osteoporosis, heart disease, and increased risk of dementia, in addition to the risks of the long-term use of hormone replacement therapy to prevent these other disease risks.

Timing Matters

The effects of EDCs vary depending on when in our lives we're exposed to them. Exposure during what are called *critical periods of development*, for example, in utero, early childhood, and puberty, can set the stage for reproductive and hormonal health throughout life. **"Prepollution"** as it's called, can set the template for the child's health later in life—or disease development including obesity, diabetes, heart disease, and even hormonal and gynecologic problems in women—including endometriosis and fertility challenges—and explains many of the intergenerational impacts that could be affecting us as adult women now. The fact that these conditions can take root before we're even born is important to understand so you stop blaming yourself. The reality is that some shit just happened to us before we had any say over our bodies—and now we're paying the consequences. It's nobody's fault. Well, that's not exactly true. Doctors knew. Scientists knew. Industry knew. But our moms didn't. And not everything that happened to our cells and genes is fully reversible.

Some EDCs do their damage when we're in our teens or adult years; for example, some are known to target the ovary and cause reproductive health problems, such as infertility and POI, and most can cause abnormal hormone levels. It's important to take this in because without understanding this impact, you might assume it's you who is broken, when it's the world you were raised in before you ever had a choice of what you were exposed to. And it's why with some conditions, you can make an enormous difference in how you feel, but because cellular changes may have started before you were even born, you can't always 100% reverse, for example, every bit of endometriosis—and I always want to be both hopeful and completely realistic with you.

Where Toxins Hang Out

In Your Foods

There's a lot more to our food than just what we think we're eating. The hidden "ingredients" include a whole range of additives, coloring, preservatives, stabilizers, herbicides, pesticides, plastics, and—get this—pharmaceuticals, industrial solvents, heavy metals, and recreational drugs, to name a few of the literally thousands of contaminants that make their way from industry and agriculture into our bodies.

In 2016, researchers studying fish in Washington's Puget Sound found over eighty pharmaceuticals, plus residues of personal care products, anticoagulants, fungicides, other antibiotics, and antiseptics, in salmon that were destined for our dinner tables. Over 70% of the antibiotics prescribed in the US are unnecessary, and on top of this unnecessary insult, 50% of all antibiotics produced in the US end up in our meat as a result of being fed to cattle to make them grow fatter, faster. Heavy-metal contamination in our food is also a serious issue, occurring largely as a result of industrial use that has entered our soil and water systems. Examples include cadmium from batteries; lead from paints and gasoline, which, even though removed from such use in the 1970s, remains pervasive in soil; PCBs from manufacturing; and more. Arsenic, an element in the earth's crust that is naturally found in water, air, and soil, has also been used industrially and is a common soil contaminant. Rice, in particular, leaches arsenic in the soil and then stores it in the rice itself. Arsenic acts as an endocrine disruptor, affecting your sex hormones, as well as your blood-sugar-regulating hormones and weight, and most rice is now contaminated, as are concentrated rice products, for example, rice syrup, which is found in many "health food" granola bars and cereals. The problem was first identified when pregnant women who consumed rice-syrup-containing produce were found to have high blood levels of arsenic. The problem is serious and widespread.

In Your Water

Disturbingly, the same types of chemicals that have been found in those fish, for example in

Puget Sound or in polar bears in Antarctica, are in our drinking water and in our food supply. Perchlorate, for example, a component of rocket fuel, is an endocrine disruptor that interferes with the thyroid gland by competing with the nutrient iodine, which the thyroid gland needs to make thyroid hormones. Perchlorate contaminates the drinking water of almost seventeen million Americans (of note, the FDA also found contamination in 75% of the twenty-seven types of food sampled, with the greatest accumulation in dairy products). Atrazine has been found in water systems serving nearly thirty million Americans in twenty-seven states. And while Flint, Michigan, is an extreme example of lead contamination in water, municipal water systems in numerous major cities are contaminated with lead, arsenic, and other heavy metals that make their way into our homes and affect our hormones.

Not only do decontamination methods fail to remove most of the contaminants from the water supply, but given loose regulations and lobbying efforts—we're talking about big money here—decontamination facilities have consistently, for decades now, managed to avoid raising their standards. It is known that these environmental toxins end up in our water supply; we are all getting exposed unless we're getting well water and filtering.

What's in Cosmetics: It Isn't Pretty

You've been making big changes in your diet to eliminate toxic food triggers. You want to support that good work with clearing out your cosmetics and body products. Beauty goes more than skin deep. From the time we are teens, the average woman puts on dozens of chemicals in the morning before she leaves home for school or work, hidden in hair and body products, cosmetics, and perfumes. We absorb those chemicals into our circulation, where, like the other endocrine disruptors I've talked about, they do their dirty work of increasing our estrogen exposure. Cosmetics also contain parabens, phthalates, and heavy metals, including lead, which has been found in lipstick, cadmium, and a host of artificial dyes. Hormones, especially estrogens, are regularly added to antiaging creams because they increase collagen and help hydrate the skin, reducing wrinkling. Placental extract, which contains high concentrations of both estrogen and progesterone, is commonly added to shampoos as hair thickener. However, this adds to our overall estrogen body burden.

Unfortunately, our current formulations are a major source of endocrine disruptors in our lives, and because of our use over our lifetimes, these exposures also accumulate. Cosmetics contain a vast number of chemicals, most of which are not under the regulatory purview of the Food and Drug Administration; cosmetic manufacturers are not required to register with the FDA, and the FDA has no recall rights on cosmetics. Cosmetic manufacturers aren't even required to send consumer complaints to the FDA. Shockingly, cosmetics regulation has remained the same since the Food, Drug, and Cosmetic Act was first passed in 1938. Despite the fact that in 2014 the revenue of the cosmetic industry in the United States alone was $56.63 billion, beauty products remain an understudied source of environmental chemical exposures. The multibillion-dollar cosmetics industry bathes us in anxiety about beauty standards most of us can never achieve yet convinces us to slather up in toxic ingredients in order to try. What can you do? I'll show you in this chapter!

Why Fragrance Stinks

Have you ever gotten into an Uber and felt like you were trapped in an odorous nightmare of overpowering fake scent from car air freshener? Or sat next to someone drenched in perfume on a plane and just wanted a parachute to get out (that happened to me on a flight last year!)? You're not alone; at least 34% of people report experiencing some symptoms after being exposed to fragrance-containing products. A large study that analyzed 74 popular air fresheners found that they contain over 350 chemical and allergenic volatile organic compounds (VOCs), as well as dozens of other toxicants.

Most of the scents we are exposed to, from air fresheners to perfumes, and all the fragrances in our shampoos, skin lotions, laundry detergents, scented menstrual products, and a million other places, are the work of fragrances that are immediately absorbed via our skin and respiratory passages, and aside from causing headaches, nausea, dizziness, allergies, asthma, and cardiovascular symptoms, even in infinitesimal doses, act as hormone disruptors.

While some fragrances may include natural oils, 95% are entirely synthetic and derived from petroleum products, and even when natural oils are included, most commercial products also include VOCs, phthalates, benzene, toluene, formaldehyde, styrene, and many other endocrine-disrupting, known carcinogenic, neurotoxic, and DNA-damaging ingredients as part of the chemical cocktail that binds or disperses the scent. Independent testing done by the Natural Resources Defense Council of fourteen common air fresheners, none of which listed phthalates as an ingredient, uncovered these chemicals in 86% of the products, including those advertised as "all-natural" or "unscented." Since labeling laws don't require disclosure of any of these individual ingredients, nor that they declare containing added fragrance, most don't. So you have no idea what you're purchasing.

What's more, there's a phenomenon called *olfactory fatigue* whereby exposure to scent on a regular basis causes "scent insensitivity"—you stop smelling it so don't even realize you're being exposed to it. So while you're opening the windows in order to breathe in that car-freshener-scented Uber (been there, done that!), your driver doesn't notice the scent at all, or when you purchase a housecleaning product or body lotion and take a whiff, the fact that it is powerfully fragrant may fall on a "deaf nose."

So Many Problems with Feminine Hygiene Products

American women spend well over $2 billion per year on feminine hygiene products, and the average woman will use around 10,000 tampons or pads over the course of her lifetime. Despite this large investment and high usage, there has been limited research on the potential health risks these products may pose to women.

If you were to look at the ingredients list on your tampon or pads box, you'd find that it's very short. It doesn't tell the full story of what can be hiding in your feminine products—and causing you harm. A host of undisclosed chemicals may be found in various combinations in these products, and because tampons and pads are regulated by the FDA as medical devices, companies are not required to disclose ingredients to consumers. While the FDA recommends that tampons be free from dioxins and pesticide or herbicide residue and requests that companies provide assurances, most of the chemicals in feminine care products are unregulated by federal agencies—so neither the FDA nor the EPA has the authority to require their safety. This recommendation is not mandatory, and testing results reveal that both dioxins and pesticide residue are found in tampons. Think about that exposure to highly absorptive vaginal mucosa.

Feminine washes, wipes, and sprays—which, as we discussed in Chapter 3 ("Your Sixth Vital Sign") are completely unnecessary and can even be harmful—are regulated by the FDA as cosmetics, and therefore while they must be free of harmful ingredients, there is no preapproval process before they go to market. A key problem with all these ingredients is that they are being used in or near some of the most absorptive tissue in a woman's body. The tissue lining the vagina readily allows for transfer of chemicals into the circulatory system. This tissue is also particularly sensitive and vulnerable to the effects of potentially or known toxic ingredients and their use can affect the delicate balance of your vaginal pH, as well as causing irritation and damage to this tissue, which is your vagina's most important defense against infection. Therefore, toxic ingredients in feminine hygiene products potentially increase your risk of endometriosis, vaginal infections, allergic reactions, irritation, and rashes.

Many women also find that they experience much more painful and heavy periods when using conventionally produced pads and tampons. These and other chemicals are also found in douches, feminine wipes, and lubes, all products that do not have to be regulated the same way that foods and pharmaceuticals do, so it's basically open season on the ingredients—which increase risks of early puberty, endometriosis, and cancer, to name a few problems.

The chemicals in wipes, douches, sprays, and other similar products may actually increase itchiness, a common symptom women use them for, because they cause local irritation and allergic reactions. Additionally, feminine wipes contain a form of formaldehyde that has been associated with cancer and a chemical that was named "Allergen of the Year" in 2013 by the American Contact Dermatitis Society.

Parabens, used as preservatives in feminine care products, have been shown to have estrogenic properties and have even been detected in breast cancer tissue. Elevated paraben levels found in women's urine has also been associated with ovarian aging, a factor in reduced fertility. Advocates for healthier sanitary products and better regulations are also concerned about pesticide residues that can be found in nonorganic cotton in pads or tampons, as well as adhesive chemicals used in pads or other additives used to improve absorbency.

At Home

From laundry soap and dryer sheets, floor and tub cleaners, to mattresses, sofas, carpets, scents, solvents, softeners, flame retardants, and more, our homes and cleaning products can be less than sweet for our hormones. Cleaning product companies tell us that to keep our homes smelling fresh and looking clean we need a multitude of cleaning and air freshening products.

Women's Voices for the Earth (WVE), an independent environmental health group, commissioned an independent laboratory to test twenty popular cleaning products for *hidden* toxic chemicals—specifically looking for chemicals that were not included on the labels—from five top companies: Clorox, Procter & Gamble, Reckitt Benckiser, SC Johnson and Son, and Sunshine Makers (Simple Green). They found that twenty of the most popular products we use to keep our homes and clothes clean, including all-purpose cleaners, laundry detergents, dryer sheets, air fresheners, disinfectant sprays, and furniture polish, contain reproductive toxins.

Indoor air and dust can be exposing you to a steady stream of hormone-disrupting toxins. Indoor air is now considered more polluted than outdoor air due to the volume of toxins in home-building materials, including furnish-

Common Endocrine Disruptors in Our World

The Disruptor	Purpose	Where It's Hiding	Impact
Phthalates	Plasticizers, fragrance carriers	Most body products including shampoos, nail polishes, soaps, fragrances, air fresheners, food packaging, shower curtains, vinyl flooring, plastics, detergents, household cleaning products, and even some brands of yoga mats, to name just a few	Impairs testosterone production in animal studies, associated with POI, fertility problems, PCOS, endometriosis, weight gain, insulin resistance, and diabetes
Pesticides/ Herbicides (too many to name, so I am including the two most widely used, glyphosate, an herbicide first marketed in the 1970s under the trade name "Roundup," and atrazine, as examples)	Weed and pest killer	Glyphosate: Widely used in agricultural settings and home gardens and is a major component in producing GMO foods Atrazine: Widely used on the majority of corn crops in the US, as well as other crops, golf courses, and residential lawns. Banned in Europe in 2002, but as of 2014 in the US remained the second most widely used herbicide	Generically: associated with decreased progesterone levels and a shorter luteal phase, reduced fertility, increase in primary ovarian insufficiency (POI) Glyphosate: estrogenic activity, interferes with hormone production, affects thyroid Atrazine: ovarian disorders, altered cyclicity, PCOS, endometriosis, uterine fibroids, fetal growth restriction, pregnancy loss, breast cancer, reduced duration of lactation, and delayed puberty
Bisphenols (i.e., BPA, BPS)	A building block of polycarbonate plastic and a component of food can and packaging linings	Found in the lining of metal food and drink cans, plastic baby bottles, pacifiers and baby toys, dental sealants, computers, cell phones, hard plastic water bottles, paints, adhesives, enamels, varnishes, CDs and DVDs, plastic consumer goods, bottles, sports equipment, coating pipes, thermal paper, and certain microwavable or reusable food and drink containers	Alterations in thyroid hormone levels, estrogen levels, male and female reproductive function; disrupts immunity (associated with autoimmunity, infertility, and endometriosis); weight gain; insulin resistance (associated with PCOS); and diabetes
Brominated flame retardants (BFRs); polybrominated diphenyl ethers (PBDEs); and 2,4, 6-tribromophenol (2,4,6-TBP)	Flame retardants	Furniture, mattresses, bedding, drapery, rugs, computers and televisions; they are also in children's sleepwear, car seat covers, and nursing pillows and are applied to numerous types of furniture, sleepwear, and electronic items in order to meet state and federal flammability standards	Disrupts hormones, major impact on thyroid due to containing bromine, blocks effect of thyroid hormone on brain development and function
PFRs	A flame-retardant alternative, but can also be very harmful	Polyurethane foams used in many consumer products, including yoga mats, upholstered furniture, baby products, and nail polish	High levels have been associated with fertility problems, miscarriage, decreased success with IVF
Perfluorinated compounds (PFAs) and "Teflon chemicals" (PFCs)	Stain-resistant and nonstick, grease-resistant, and water-proofing chemicals	Cookware, waterproof clothing (i.e., Polartec, Gore-Tex), coatings on upholstered furniture and carpeting (i.e., Scotchgard, Stainmaster), and food packaging (i.e., many fast-food take-out containers, microwavable popcorn bags); drinking water is one of the most common sources of exposure to PFA chemicals	Thyroid disease, weakened immunity, developmental defects, cancer

Common Endocrine Disruptors in Our World (continued)

The Disruptor	Purpose	Where It's Hiding	Impact
Organophosphates and Organochlorides	Pesticides	Food, computers (where it leaches out as we handle them), refrigerators, flame retardants	Reduces ovarian weight, follicle growth, egg viability, fertility, and thyroid function; disrupts the immune system and the microbiome; increases autoimmune disease risk; and causes weight gain, insulin resistance, and diabetes
"Metalloestrogens": aluminum, antimony, arsenite, barium, cadmium, chromium, cobalt, copper, lead, mercury, nickel, selenite, tin, and vanadate		Cosmetics, deodorants, antiperspirants, cigarette smoke, indoor air pollution, concentrated rice products including rice syrup and granola bars that contain them	Overall interference with female reproduction function, estrogen disruption, reduced fertility, thyroid dysfunction, breast cancer

ings, electronics, and the hundreds of individual chemicals in our household cleaners, our fuel sources, insecticides, body products, perfumes, and cosmetics, all of which we're using in our home, not to mention everything that we're trafficking into our homes on the bottom of our shoes. Babies, for example, who crawl on the floor, are getting some of the highest exposures of dust, as well as contamination that we've tracked in from the environment.

One of the most shocking types of environmental chemicals, nearly ubiquitous at this point, is the flame retardants in our furnishings, computer keyboards, mattresses, and even in baby paraphernalia from nursing pillows to car seats. I mean it makes sense, right? We don't want those things to go up in smoke! But the even more shocking thing is that flame-retardant chemicals are not fixed; they can be picked up on our hands. They disperse in our environment. Every time we're typing on our computers, we're getting exposed.

For decades, Americans have been exposed to flame retardants in mattresses, upholstered furniture, foam cushions, baby car seats, insu-lation, and electronics. According to Pulitzer Prize–winning journalist Nicholas Kristof, "A generation ago, tobacco companies were facing growing pressure to produce fire-safe cigarettes, because so many house fires started with smoldering cigarettes. Tobacco companies mounted a surreptitious campaign for flame retardant furniture, rather than safe cigarettes, as the best way to reduce house fires."

Flame retardants, similar to PCBs, migrate from products to indoor air and house dust. You can inhale them, ingest them, and absorb them through your skin. These chemicals have been linked to health problems ranging from attention and IQ deficits in children to early puberty, diabetes, endometriosis, and thyroid problems, to activation of the adrenals enough to cause cardiovascular disease. Penta, a chemical that was previously packed into couches and other furniture, has turned up in the blood of babies and in breast milk around the world. The European Union banned it after researchers linked it to developmental and neurological problems in children, and manufacturers pulled it from the market. "Safer" chemicals were supposedly created as alternatives in the US, but it turns out that "Firemaster 550" and others are just as dangerous as their older cousins. The solvents in our paints, flame retardants lurking in our home furnishings—especially sofas, mattresses, and carpets, and vinyl off-gassing from our shower curtains—give you a steady, constant, accumulating dose of EDCs, and with homes that are more airtight than ever, our exposure is higher than ever, too.

Heavy Metals Are Endocrine Disruptors, Too

Medical journals from as early as the 1990s, reported on the effects of heavy metals on health. They appear to have a particular impact on women's reproductive function. They have an affinity for the pituitary, and when deposited there, which is the relay station for messages to the adrenals, thyroid, and ovaries, communication to all three is interrupted, leading to fertility and other gynecologic problems, thyroid problems, and all the downstream effects on your cholesterol, weight, heart, and brain. Heavy metals have estrogenic activity as well, so are disrupting hormones at many levels.

There are numerous examples; they are in many common products—and our foods—and are not all required to be listed as ingredients in personal care products, in foods, or on household items, baby products, or furnishings.

Let's Chat About "the Pill"

The Pill has been around since 1960, and with a 93% effectiveness for most forms (estrogen-only, progestin-only, combined estrogen-progestin) when taken correctly, there's no doubt that it was a major, hard-won breakthrough for

women. For the first time in history, we were in control of our reproduction, which helped us find safety from sometimes dangerous birth conditions, gave us more autonomy in relationships, and provided the ability to work rather than be limited by pregnancies we may not want or be ready for. Forget the maternity leave debate—back then, there was no debate. Married or not, you had to quit your job when you got pregnant or hide it until you couldn't anymore.

So on the one hand, as a dyed-in-the-wool (or "womb" may be more accurate—my mom was the first woman in her college to wear slacks to the campus!) feminist, I'm loath to criticize what has become a mainstay in women's ability to control when we do and don't get pregnant—especially during a time when our reproductive rights are being threatened.

The stigma is still there for women applying to jobs in the question that is not supposed to be asked but sometimes is, "Are you planning to have children anytime in the near future?" Further, being "on birth control" is considered a sign of responsibility in women, but women are bearing the full burden of contraceptive risk. In fact, many of my young patients in their teens have already been put on the Pill by their parents or doctor, whether to prevent pregnancy or to regulate their cycle (the latter being an illusion—it actually blocks ovulation, thus preventing a natural cycle).

A Bitter Pill to Swallow

There are things that we need to know about the Pill (and all forms of hormonal contraceptives, HCs for short) and our safety. Here's a big question I have to ask: If we're trying to avoid excess environmental hormonal exposure in our food, water, cosmetics, and household products, do we want to be taking them intentionally each day as medication when other options are available? It's at least worth asking ourselves how empowering that is, particularly when four out of five women who are sexually active have been on the Pill at some point—and many women are on it for ten years or more.

We don't have to look far to find the risks. The Pill (and this goes for most HCs, including the contraceptive ring and patch) can make women seriously unwell. Right inside the package of one popular estrogen- and progestin-containing form of the Pill, we find that it can cause:

- Blood clots

- Heart attacks and strokes, especially in smokers or women with migraines (especially migraines with aura)

- Gallbladder disease

- Breast, cervical, and liver cancers are slightly increased in Pill users.

- Lipid metabolism and inflammation of the pancreas in patients with inherited defects of lipid metabolism; there have been reports of significant elevations of plasma triglycerides during estrogen therapy. This has led to pancreatitis in some cases.

While we've been told for decades that the Pill acts in our bodies by mimicking our natural cycles, this is not accurate. The Pill overrides our natural cycles by interfering with the hypothalamic-pituitary-ovarian (HPO) axis, disrupting your body's normal hormone communication channels, and supplanting those signals with synthetically supplemented hormones. With the exception of progestin-only pills and the progestin-releasing IUD, they block ovulation—and you've learned that this is not a good thing for your hormonal well-being. But progestin-only pills aren't the answer, either. While some forms of the Pill can reduce testosterone when it is high, mak-ing them an effective acne treatment for some women, progestin-only forms of contraception can increase androgens and cause acne—and also hair growth in unwanted places (hirsutism) like your upper lip, chin, belly, and breasts. Not fun. *And there's more.*

The Pill increases risk of depression. The combined Pill increases your risk of depression by as much as 80%, and progestin-only doubles your risk. A major European study conducted by the University of Copenhagen, the largest of its kind to date, found a strong correlation between being on the Pill and developing major depression. Researchers followed over a million women, ages fifteen to thirty-four, for thirteen years and found that about 23% of the women—including many who had never struggled with depression, mood symptoms, or mental health problems prior to starting the Pill—needed to go on an antidepressant medication. This was not the first study to link OCPs (oral contraceptive pills) to depression, though it was the largest. Teens were especially vulnerable. While women on the combined pill fared the worst, progestin-only pills and the transdermal patch and vaginal ring were also associated with a higher rate of depression and antidepressant prescriptions.

The Pill can cause weight gain and metabolic syndrome. The Pill can cause weight gain (3 to 10 pounds), insulin resistance, high blood sugar, and high cholesterol, and a 2018 study showed a 35% increased risk of developing diabetes later in life if a woman had used an oral contraceptive for longer than six months at any time in her life.

The Pill can crush your sex drive. While using contraception can alleviate the fear of an unwanted pregnancy, and for women plagued by PMS, severe cramps, endometriosis, fibroids, or heavy menstrual bleeding, Pill-induced relief may well enhance sexual drive and pleasure, for 5% of Pill users there's a downside. Five percent sound like a small number? When you do the math, if ten million women are on the Pill, that's about five hundred thousand who are experiencing reduced libido. In one study, German researchers surveyed 2,612 female medical students. Among Pill users, more than a third report that it affects their sex drive.

A growing body of research shows decreased libido and impaired sexual function, and thereby a decrease in the frequency and enjoyment of sex. It's been known for decades that hormonal contraception can put a lid on sex drive for women, a result of a number of different hormonal responses including increased SHBG and progestin effects that reduce available testosterone. One in five OCP users reports negative sexual side effects, and approximately half discontinue their method as a result. Moreover, a 2006 study published in the *Journal of Sexual Medicine* revealed that not only does being on the Pill reduce sex drive, but that this symptom may persist even after discontinuing it, and that women who have taken the Pill have a greater likelihood of a *permanently suppressed sex drive* when compared to women who have never used it.

The Pill may cause vaginal pain and dryness. In addition to hormonal effects that might directly lower your libido, the Pill can make your vag dry and painful—not fun and definitely not sex-inspiring. It does this by drying up your natural vaginal lubrication (remember, ovulation gets things juicy down there and the Pill blocks ovulation), it can thin out your vaginal walls and labia making sex painful, and Pill use for more than one to two years increases risk of vulvar pain, which can make things down there uncomfortable, sex included.

The Pill may lower thyroid hormone levels. I would be remiss not to mention a less common but still worrisome potential side effect of OCPs on the thyroid. The estrogen component of the Pill, like any estrogen taken orally, raises the serum concentrations of thyroxine-binding globulin (TBG), cortisol-binding globulin (CBG), and sex-hormone-binding globulin (SHBG). As a result, the serum concentrations of total thyroxine (T4), triiodothyronine (T3), cortisol, estradiol, and testosterone increase. While levels of thyroid hormones T3 and T4 do not appear to be significantly changed, the effect of the Pill on thyroid hormone needs to be considered when evaluating thyroid tests.

The Pill may shrink your ovaries and inhibit fertility. I know that sounds crazy, but it's exactly what Danish researchers found when they compared the ovarian volume of women oral contraceptive users to nonusers. Their research, which studied 833 women ages nineteen to forty-six, showed that women who take birth control pills have 29 to 52% lower ovary volume than women who are not on the Pill, with the biggest reductions in women aged nineteen to thirty. They found that women who were taking the contraceptive pill had 19% lower AMH (anti-Müllerian hormone) than those who weren't taking the Pill. The higher the number of eggs remaining in the ovaries, the higher the level of AMH in the bloodstream. Therefore, a low level is considered to be a sign of a low ovarian reserve, that is, few remaining follicles, a risk for both reduced fertility and primary ovarian insufficiency. In another study, ovarian volume of HC users was nearly 50% lower than nonusers, and in yet another study of *former* users who'd been off HCs for at least a year, when compared with nonusers, their ovarian volume was 58% lower. In younger women taking the Pill, hormone levels associated with the ability to make mature, healthy eggs are more like those of older women than they are like the levels of younger women who don't use these contraceptives, according to the study. While further studies, including one study of over seven hundred women, show that discontinuation of the Pill should allow the ovaries to return to their normal size within about three months, and AMH levels to normalize, for women planning to get pregnant soon after coming off the Pill, this can lead to some delays—sometimes of a year or more.

Not surprisingly then, the Pill has been associated with delays in conception to the tune of sometimes up to eighteen months. Therefore, if you plan to conceive and are on the Pill, you might want to plan ahead, take delays into consideration, and keep this in mind if conception is taking longer. It doesn't mean you are infertile or need to rush to fertility treatment, even if assessment of your cycle length, ovulation, or hormones show abnormalities that suggest a fertility problem. These may just be due to temporary post-Pill dysregulation. These delays may be similar with other HCs; it can take up to eighteen months for cycles to return to normal after Depo-Provera use, and while the IUD is lauded for allowing a quick return of fertility, there are often delays with the post-progestin-based IUD as well. On all methods, however, most women trying to will conceive by twelve months after stopping the HC.

The Pill depletes nutrients. While not a symptom in itself, nutritional deficiencies can cause a host of symptoms and hormonal imbalances. They are also a problem for women who come off the Pill and hope to get pregnant right away because low nutrient status has been associated with fertility problems, and low nutrients in mom can also mean low nutrients in baby. The Pill has been associated with robbing a number of nutrients, including B vitamins and magnesium. A recent study also found that vitamin D levels drop soon after stopping the Pill. In fact, vitamin D levels were 20% lower in women who'd just come off it than in those not taking it.

The Pill causes oxidative stress and increases inflammation. The Pill has also been found to cause oxidative stress, which is known to result in significant enough cellular damage that it's a major risk factor for cardiovascular disease, cancer, and dementia, but also endometriosis, fertility problems, ovarian dysfunction, and more, which is why I cover it extensively in the next chapter. In one study of women athletes using the combined Pill (estrogen and progesterone), elevated levels of blood markers of oxidative stress were found in 92.9% of OCP users compared to only 23.5% of non-OCP users. Here's a crazy fact: use of the Pill also overrides some of the beneficial effects of the very nutrients and phytochemicals used to combat the effects of oxidative stress (and which we'll be examining more in the next chapter). This is important, because your use of the Pill may be sabotaging some of the benefits of your healthy diet (and supplements) while increasing risk of cardiovascular disease and reducing exercise effectiveness.

The Pill can increase autoimmune disease risk. Autoimmune disease is one of the top ten leading causes of death in women in the US. There is good evidence that hormonal contraceptive use (including the Pill, Norplant, the NuvaRing, and other forms) is associated with an increased risk of several serious autoimmune diseases such as Crohn's disease (which causes inflammation of the bowels), lupus (which causes inflammation in many organs), and interstitial cystitis (which causes inflammation in the bladder).

The Pill May Block Detoxification. Problematically, in the midst of everything else the Pill is doing, when an estrogen-containing version of the Pill goes through detoxification, it may get broken down into potent and hazardous reactive intermediates. And also troubling is that the Pill may interfere with the absorption of important nutrients needed for detoxification.

If you're taking the Pill, remember it can have a wide range of health effects, regardless of whether your doctor, mother, sister, or friends say that it doesn't. And keep in mind that you can't have a normal cycle on the Pill or any other hormonal birth control; it's suppressing your cycle.

What If I Need the Pill for Medical Reasons, Like PCOS or Heavy or Painful Periods?

Most women who are on the Pill are not on it for contraception; at least 50% of women are prescribed it for hormonal symptoms including painful periods, acne, migraines, PCOS, hypothalamic amenorrhea (HA), irregular cycles, and endometriosis. For the most part, it is a stopgap measure. While OCPs can be temporarily effective for reducing acne in many women, as well as symptoms associated with polycystic ovary syndrome and endometriosis, the Pill doesn't get to the root causes of these conditions—for example, nutritional insufficiencies or food triggers, high levels of exposure to environmental toxins, gut imbalances like dysbiosis, or slow-functioning detoxification. While I understand how debilitating symptoms like endometriosis pain and heavy periods or severe menstrual cramps can be, the Pill is not healing you from the inside out. In the long run, the Pill can make acne worse, and I've had many women develop rebound side effects after going off OCPs. For some conditions, like PCOS with insulin resistance, you could be making the insulin resistance worse.

Sometimes your symptoms are so severe that you might use the Pill under the supervision of a health care professional who can help you bridge a natural and hormonal approach, but keep in mind that the Pill is not an optimal long-term solution. Once you start to trace your symptoms back to their root causes, you can start to see how everything in the body is interconnected and can often start to heal your painful periods and other issues. If you do need to be on the Pill, make sure to take a multivitamin to replenish the nutrients it depletes; supplementation with vitamin B6 has been shown to relieve depression caused by birth control pills.

How to Get Off the Pill and What to Expect

Coming off the Pill is, on the one hand, straightforward: you simply stop taking it at any point in your cycle—it does not require that you wean off it. Statistically, 80% of women who went on the Pill for contraception begin cycling normally within three months of going off the Pill, especially if they were cycling normally prior to starting it. Some women, though, experience a bumpy ride coming off the Pill with a delayed return of normal cycles—and thus fertility—for some women as long as a year to eighteen months.

I first coined the term "post-OC (oral contraceptive) syndrome" in 2008 in my textbook, *Botanical Medicine for Women's Health*, as one of the possible causes of irregular periods and other hormonal symptoms in women coming off birth control. To be clear, there is no formal condition known as post-OC or post-Pill syndrome, and there is controversy over the extent to which women experience problems. Yet many experience acne, heavy periods, no periods at all, cramps, and more. This appears more likely if you were put on the Pill for reasons other than birth control, but some women experience new hormonal imbalances only after stopping the Pill.

The Most Common Post-Pill Symptoms:

- Irregular or skipped periods

- Heavy menstrual bleeding

- Ovulation pain and menstrual cramps

- Breakouts

- Bloating

- Mood swings

You can experience post-Pill symptoms whether you've been on it for a couple months or many years, though in my experience women who've been on for several or more years—and certainly those on it for close to or over a decade, which is incredibly common—are more likely to experience more pronounced hormonal imbalances when they come off the Pill.

Ideally before discontinuing the Pill, or at the same time as you discontinue it, to possibly help preempt many of the above symptoms, *replace the nutrients that the Pill depletes.* **Take a multivitamin and mineral supplement for at least three months post-Pill.** Additionally, because vitamin D levels may also drop after coming off the Pill, and most multivitamins don't have much vitamin D, take 2,000 units daily for three months as well. Continue to eat for Hormone Intelligence, emphasizing nutrient-dense foods at every meal: dark leafy greens and other phytonutrient-rich vegetables; low-glycemic fruits like berries; pastured and organic animal protein; and beans, nuts, and seeds.

If you went on the Pill to address acne or an irregular cycle, it may have simply buried your symptoms. When you come off the Pill, there's a good chance that you're still dealing with those same imbalances, which may have gotten more pronounced over time because the root causes weren't addressed. If you went

on the Pill for birth control, you may not have been suppressing a specific medical condition or symptoms, but a condition or set of symptoms might also have emerged during your time on the Pill that were masked by it. And if you're stopping the Pill to get pregnant, you may find that you still aren't cycling even up to eighteen months later.

The Pill's power to cover up a wide range of symptoms presents another danger to women. Because we don't feel outwardly uncomfortable—aren't struggling with PMS, acne, pain, or other obvious symptoms—we don't know that something under the surface is going on, and conditions like PCOS can go untreated. PCOS is a harbinger of metabolic syndrome and type 2 diabetes in some women, which themselves are harbingers of other chronic conditions, like heart disease or nonalcoholic fatty liver disease, so not getting proper treatment is a big deal.

The wonderful news is you're now including the nutrients, herbs, and lifestyle practices in my "post-Pill protocol," which includes balancing blood sugar, boosting microbiome health and improving elimination, resetting circadian rhythm, and supporting natural detoxification. These are methods I've used successfully for over thirty years. There are a few nutrients you'll want to replenish, just because the Pill typically depletes them, which you'll see below, and some targeted herbs I use to restore the HPO axis and nourish ovarian function, which you'll learn about in Chapter 11.

Women fought long and hard for access to contraception so that they—and we—could have more control over our reproductive health. The problem is that the Pill, while very liberating in many ways, can also have significant and serious unintended consequences. It creates a very specific set of hormonal imbalances that can have short- and long-run consequences. Pill-imposed hormonal changes also mean it can take some time to restore your own natural hormonal cycles or establish a new healthy hormonal equilibrium if yours wasn't in balance in the first place, which may be why you first started the Pill.

It can take time, even with a full-on natural approach—anywhere from three to twelve months—but stick with it to get back into your own "natural flow."

The Best Nonhormonal Contraception

The good news is that plenty of methods work as effectively as the Pill—and don't have the risks and side effects. These are some of the options you can consider instead of hormonal contraception.

Natural Fertility Awareness

When your hormones are in balance, your cycle is just that—a cycle that is regular, predictable, and reliable. The word *menses* comes from the Latin word for "month," as does the word for "moon"—that is the frequency of our cycle. I use the term "moon time" to describe our cycles sometimes for this reason. When you have a regular cycle and are able to pay attention to several parameters—your personal cycle calendar, your cervical mucus, and your basal body temperature—you can combine these findings in what is called *natural fertility awareness*, or fertility awareness methods. These three methods in combination can lead to up to 99% effectiveness as a method of birth control; however, in reality, for most couples practicing fertility awareness methods, the success rate is closer to 76%. For this method to be effective, you need to track your cycles and be aware of the fluctuations in your body. I recommend it be combined with condoms

for extra security. Withdrawal is not an effective method—so don't rely on this to prevent pregnancy.

Condoms

Used properly condoms are 98% effective, emphasis added because the real-life success rates are more like 88%—you have to be comfortable buying them and remember to use them. There are also problems with slippage and size, but for the most part if you use them correctly, they do work. A problem with condoms is that the lubricated ones often have ingredients that aren't optimal for your body. Several companies make eco-friendly condoms that are free from the carcinogens found in most condoms—and some use Fair Trade rubber. You can also find lubes that are body-friendly, vagina-friendly, and pH-friendly, which means they're not going to cause you to get yeast infections and pH changes that cause bacterial overgrowth, irritation, and dryness.

Condoms are great when you combine them with an understanding of your body's natural rhythms and cycles, which some people call *natural fertility awareness*. There are a lot of different names and techniques that you can use to learn when you're ovulating (this applies only if you have a generally regular cycle). During the time you're fertile—your window of ovulation—you'll use a condom if you're not trying to conceive.

Diaphragm or Cervical Cap

Diaphragms and cervical caps are 88% and between 71% and 86% effective, respectively. They work best when used in conjunction with spermicides, which I'm not a huge fan of as they're full of toxic chemicals and they are a bit inconvenient to remember to put in. It's also important to remember that if you experience substantial body weight changes, you have to be resized. When they do fail, it's because we forget to put them in, forget to take them out, or don't want to deal with the awkwardness of them. They're not my favorite, but if you can remember to use them correctly and regularly, they do work.

IUD (Intrauterine Device)

Any woman who's over thirty may have heard horrible things about the IUD because of the Dalkon shield from the 1970s, which caused massive problems for women (infection and death). Today's IUDs are a generally safe, effective, and convenient form of contraception. I know that's probably going to sound unexpected from me, but they are the most widely used form of contraception in the Western world.

These little plastic or metal T-shaped devices are inserted through the cervix into the uterus by a midwife, family doctor, or ob-gyn during an in-office procedure. It's not comfortable to have an IUD inserted—especially if you haven't had a baby—you'll want to use a heat pack and some ibuprofen for the procedure. The IUD is the most widely used form of birth control in many European countries—we're talking progressive countries with progressive health care policies. They are considered safe for women of any childbearing age, do not increase risk of uterine scarring, and do not increase future fertility risk.

There are two basic types, a nonhormonal kind made of copper and a plastic one that is impregnated with and secretes a small amount of hormone. IUDs do not cause abortions; they primarily alter the cervical mucus so that you can't conceive and cause changes in the uterine lining that prevent implantation. The IUD has many advantages—most importantly, if you tolerate it well, you get it inserted and can basically forget about it for twelve years with the copper IUD and three to seven years with the hormonal form. If you decide you want to get pregnant, you can get it taken out and resume your natural fertile cycle immediately. However, many women do find the cramping too much to tolerate and have them removed. For most women who leave it in, the cramping resolves after six to eight months. Those who do tolerate it tend to love it as a form of birth control. With the hormonal IUD, you do get a small dose of circulating hormone, but it's small compared to oral contraceptives, the NuvaRing, or Depo-Provera, the shot.

There are incidents of an IUD migrating or causing a uterine perforation during insertion, but the risks are so small that I wouldn't advise against using one for those reasons. It is possible that a Mirena intrauterine system (IUS) may play a role in hair loss, which is experienced by approximately 0.33% of women who use one.

While the Nuva Ring can be effective and simple to use, it definitely carries some of the hormonal risks of other HCs—and it's been linked to some high-profile wrongful death lawsuits. Depo-Provera packs a pretty big punch of hormones, and I don't usually recommend it. It also causes bone density changes and all the same blood sugar changes as the Pill.

These birth control methods are all alternatives to oral contraceptives. Of all the options I've mentioned, the oral contraceptive pill in my opinion is the most hormone disruptive, and the IUD is the contraceptive I recommend most often to those who want something different than fertility tracking and condoms. But if you're willing to put the time and energy into it, my preference is using fertility awareness (cervical mucus changes, calendar, and basal temperature in combination), plus condoms. It's a safe and effective method for most women but does require mindfully sticking with it for pregnancy prevention.

The Hormone Intelligence Solution: Lighten Your Body Burden

I know that's a lot of big stuff to take in. But if we don't look at it head-on, we don't see it, and ignoring it doesn't make it go away. We have to have the information to take back our health, our power—and our environment!

Now it's time to do that by lightening your toxic exposures and supporting your natural detoxification pathways. Not only will you be making an important step toward a greener planet, but you can reduce your body burden within just a few days of making healthier lifestyle choices. For example, significant drops in herbicide and pesticide levels are measurable after just a few days of "going organic" with fruits and vegetables, and likewise, drops in blood and urinary phthalate levels are found after simply switching away from using plastic drinking cups, or reducing use of EDC-containing shampoos and shower gel. It just takes some knowledge and the commitment to shift to a cleaner, greener lifestyle. But it's easily done—even on a budget and even with a family. I know because I've been doing it for almost four decades!

To make it easier for you, I've prioritized the big changes that can make the most difference, and quickly. If you're a maniac like I am, who likes to just get it all done fast, plan a weekend "makeover" and just do it. If you can't do it all at once, peel back the layers, focusing on one of each of the following three areas each week or two until you've done a complete products makeover. I've got this all in a handy checklist you can print out at aviva romm.com/hormone-intelligence-resources.

While you're working on detoxing your products, you can jump ahead to Steps 4 and 5 in this section to support your body in doing the same!

You Are Not Dirty or Toxic

Before you start reading about detoxification, I want to emphasize something important: YOU are not dirty. YOU are not toxic. The women's wellness movement, with its endless emphasis on cleansing and detoxifying, can lead us to think we are veritable toxic wastelands, always in need of cleaning and improving. Sadly, this is based on badly outdated puritanical beliefs about cleanliness being close to godliness—and women's bodies, largely because we menstruate (and, oh heavens, because we are sexual), being anything but clean. These values found their way into the medicine of the US in the early colonial days, with "purging and puking" to clean the body and the soul, then into the health movements of the early twentieth century, all the way to their modern manifestations as juice cleanses, coffee enemas, lemon and olive oil liver detoxes, and restrictive diets. That's not what I'm talking about. I'm talking about reducing your exposure to toxins that are coming from your environment, and supporting your body's natural ability to metabolize and eliminate them—in other words, lightening your body burden.

Detoxification: What It *Really* Is

Detox. You can hardly have missed hearing about it. It's everywhere from celery juice cleanses and bone broth fasts, to colonics and coffee enemas. Some methods may have kernels of truth behind them, most don't have a shred of good evidence, and some are harmful. Taken to the extreme, detoxes can quickly get out of control; I've treated many women for the results of a detox that was too strict or went on too long. So when I use the term **detoxification**, I'm talking about something *very* different—the physiologic processes your body does every second of every day to eliminate the natural wastes that accumulate as a result of just being human, and nourishing these processes into optimal functioning.

Detoxification is the work your body does to break down products, hormones, vitamins, inflammatory molecules, and signaling compounds, which your body naturally produces, as well as exposure you get from things you ingest (prescription drugs, alcohol) and toxins, and moving them out of your body. You detoxify all kinds of wastes each time you exhale, every time you urinate or move your bowels. In the context of your hormonal biochemistry and the elimination of environmental toxins, this process is properly called *metabolic detoxification.*

Can't My Body Just Take Care of It?

Have you ever seen the *I Love Lucy* episode with the chocolates? If you haven't, YouTube it, because it will show you exactly what's going on in your detoxification system as a result of a combination system overload and not enough helpers to get the job done. Lucy and Ethel have taken a job wrapping chocolates in a candy company. At first, as the chocolates pass them on a (1950s-style) conveyer belt, they're keeping up just fine. But as the conveyer belt moves faster—and then even faster—bringing them more chocolates than they can keep up with, they have to start stashing the chocolates anywhere they can—in their pockets, down their shirts, in their hats, and finally, in their mouths, so they don't get fired.

Like those chocolates, toxins may be appearing faster than our detoxification pathways can keep up with, both because the volume is too great and because we're low on wrappers—the nutrient we need to package and eliminate them—so our body stashes them in our fat cells, bones, ovaries, and anywhere we can. Like Ethel and Lucy, we're quickly overwhelmed with packets filled with chemicals we simply can't handle. Almost all of us are experiencing this chronic combo of toxin overload and detoxification underfunctioning. As with all our microecosystems, the problem reveals the cure.

We have a well-honed, sophisticated capacity to detoxify a wide range of compounds. But the unprecedented environmental toxin exposure we're now facing, along with the fact that most of us are not getting adequate daily doses of naturally detoxifying foods in our diets, is a recipe for overload of our otherwise inherently resilient detoxification systems. Further, some of us carry genetic changes (called *SNPs, single nucleotide polymorphisms*) that make us even more prone to detoxification challenges and thus potentially increase our vulnerability—one called MTHFR is the most common.

But detoxification isn't something you have to work that hard to do—it's really a matter of learning what to avoid and following the Hormone Intelligence Diet, which reduces your exposures to toxins through eating a healthy, plant-based diet, organic whenever possible, that also provides your body with the nutrients and phytochemicals needed to optimize daily detoxification, and keeps your elimination in top shape so you can get rid of what your liver breaks down. The Hormone Intelligence Diet is inherently designed to be a low-toxin, detox-supporting plan—and lifestyle. I've been living it for 40 years—and like the rest of this plan, living it every day will make it second nature to you, too. Here are 5 steps to get you there, starting today. I recommend adding in one step each day, and turning that into your new detox-supporting lifestyle!

Step 1: Pass on the Plastic

- Skip the plastic water bottles; carry a glass or stainless-steel water bottle with you instead.

- Don't take the receipt when you shop. In most states, thermal receipts (and airline boarding passes) are coated with BPA or BPS. The exposure is high enough that it can interfere with fertility, which is why a few states have banned its inclusion—because guess who handles most of those receipts on the giving and receiving ends? Women!

- Avoid plastic cling film.

- Never microwave in plastic containers.

- Use only glass or stainless-steel food storage containers. Containers with plastic lids are fine as long as the lids don't touch the food.

- Avoid all nonstick pots, pans, and bakeware; instead use stainless steel, cast iron, glass, or enamel.

- Avoid packaged foods as much as possible; the insides of packages may be treated to prevent food from sticking and to make things like frozen pizzas slide out more easily. Ditto that for fast-food containers and microwave popcorn bags.

- Choose fresh or frozen food over canned whenever possible; if it has to be canned, make sure it is BPA free—though you might be getting its younger cousin, BPS, which isn't necessarily a whole lot better. Check whether a food's or beverage's package contains BPA using EWG's BPA product list. If it does, look for alternatives in EWG's Food Scores.

- Drink filtered or spring water.

- Consider a charcoal countertop water filter or an under-the-sink reverse osmosis filter (you or a plumber can install this and over time, it's a cost savings over purchasing bottled water).

- Get home delivery of five-gallon glass containers (plastic may contain BPS, but it's still better than what's coming out of most taps if that's all you can get).

Step 2: Do a Body Products Makeover

I prefer the Frenchwoman approach of less is more when it comes to cosmetics—it's easy, affordable, and clean. But we still have to brush our teeth, it's lovely to have a skin care routine, and if you do wear cosmetics, you need to know which ones are safe for your hormones!

To create a 100% clean beauty routine, Tara Foley, founder of Follain, shares her tips:

- Soap and lotion are the first two products I recommend you switch when starting your clean beauty journey. They're not technically "beauty" products, but they're the products we use most often (soap) and on the most body surface area (lotion).

- For your soap, make sure to avoid fragrance (a.k.a. parfum), SLS (sodium laureth sulfate), triclosan, parabens, methylisothiazolinone, and methylchloroisothiazolinone.

- In lotion, make sure to avoid fragrance (a.k.a. parfum), PEGs, parabens, petrolatum, and mineral oil.

- Go fragrance free or use only pure essential oil fragrance for soaps, shampoo, conditioner, shower gel, etc. How to identify safe-fragrance body products:

- Whenever you see "fragrance" or "parfum" on a product, make sure the company discloses what the fragrance is composed of (some companies will have a little asterisk and go into further detail on the fragrance ingredients on their website or the bottom of the product ingredient label). If they don't or won't disclose fragrance ingredients, avoid it! Or even simpler—just stick with products that do not include fragrance at all.

- Cosmetic products can be some of the worst offenders when it comes to using ingredients that are harmful to people and planet. This includes ingredients like coal tar in most conventional mascaras, cyclic silicones in most foundations, and PEGs and parabens in almost all conventional makeup. Tara's own makeup bag (and mine, too!) contains products made mainly of real ingredients that take care of my skin just as well as my skin care products would. Her concealer and even blush are based in coconut oil. Her mascara and brow gel are mainly based in beeswax. And so on and so forth. The best part: clean makeup has come so far over the years, and these products work so well!

The easiest way to make the transition is to find a few brands that you love and feel are most affordable to you, from a source like Follain, Credo, or the Detox Store, all of which have online and brick-and-mortar shopping options, and purchase anything that gets broad coverage (foundation, lotion, moisturizer, sunscreen) and anything for your lips (balm, gloss, lip color) 100% clean and organic. Then, over time, gradually scale up so that all your cosmetics are 100% clean beauty.

A few more important tips are to:

- Use less nail polish, and when you do get your nails done, go for a "10-free" brand—one free of at least the worst of the chemicals that get breathed in and absorbed.

- Choose a natural, fluoride-free toothpaste.

- Avoid aluminum-based deodorants and don't use antiperspirants that block sweating and add to your toxic load. Instead, use a natural deodorant—there are brands that work well, don't stain clothes, and still leave you feeling fresh and confident.

Step 3: Home Sweet Home

Optimally, we'd all paint with only non-VOC paints, have nontoxic oil-treated wood floors, natural fiber rugs (wool, cotton), untreated natural fiber sofas, and organic cotton or coconut husk mattresses (and no, I'm not kidding about all this). While that might be 100% practical for most folks, here are steps you can take that are easily affordable and within reach.

Greener Cleaners

Clean and green housekeeping is easy; it's amazing what vinegar, baking soda, a little lemon, and some "Bon Ami" (made only from feldspar, a naturally occurring mineral) can do, but if that's too "crunchy" for you, there's no shortage of natural cleaning products on the market to replace the outdated toxic ones. Here are some steps to take:

- Green up all your household cleaning products with simple products that have only a few natural ingredients in them. Use the EWG's Guide to Healthy Cleaning. You can have a sparkling clean home without any toxic products.

- Don't use air fresheners in your home, car, or anywhere—ever. They contain phthalates, benzenes, and other endocrine disruptors.

- Have a no-shoe policy inside your house, which can massively reduce the number of contaminants you're tracking in from outdoors—doubly important if you have little ones who crawl or spend a lot of time playing on the floor.

- Use a vacuum with a HEPA filter and dust with a wet rag frequently to prevent chemically laden dust from accumulating.

Home Makeover

Admittedly, this is a 2.0 level of greening up your life but it's something to keep in mind if you are repainting, redecorating, doing a baby's room, or setting up a new apartment or house. IKEA, West Elm, and even Target have greener home furnishing options now that make having an eco-friendly home a more affordable possibility.

- If you do have a foam-filled mattress or sofa cushions, keep them covered.

- Avoid dirt- and spill-resistant fabrics as these have usually been treated with endocrine-disrupting chemicals like Scotchguard and Stainmaster. Having raised four kids and having two grandkids—with gray untreated wool sofas—I promise, there are lots of natural stain-removing tricks online!

The Great Outdoors

Lawns, gardens, and decks can be hidden sources of herbicide, pesticide, and arsenic exposures. Switching to these more ecological options can reduce your risks:

- Skip toxic herbicides and pesticides in favor of natural landscaping, garden, and insect management. You may have a few more weeds, but you'll have far fewer worries!

- If you have a home built before the 1980s, or your home is newer but built on an old homesite, get your garden soil tested for lead before eating produce grown in that soil.

- Wooden playsets, garden beds, and decks made before 2005 are likely to contain arsenic; you can have yours tested. If positive, replace them with new ones if you can; if not, at least replace high-traffic areas, seal the rest, and always wash hands after contact.

- Use only natural bug spray and suntan lotion.

Step 4: Turn Up the Volume: Support Natural Detoxification

To turn down the noise in your endocrine system, you're already doing the work of dialing down your toxin exposures. Now you're also going to gently turn up the volume on your natural detox systems by showing your liver some love and making sure your elimination is in tip-top shape. This is such a gentle approach that it's safe if you're trying to conceive or breastfeeding. It's easy from here, because you're already doing 99% of this by eating for Hormone Intelligence, getting the nutrients you need to support detoxification, and the gut care you need to ensure that you're eliminating toxins.

Your diet can provide all the micronutrients, minerals, and powerful phytochemicals you need for optimal liver health, which is why I include the food sources for the nutrient supplements that optimize detoxification, and emphasize these in the meal plan for this week, and going forward. Sometimes, though, when you're actively treating a condition or you've been in "body burden overload," a little boost can get your nutrient "tank" from "below the empty line" to full. The nutrients and herbs below give your detoxification systems that extra support.

Love Your Liver

Your liver plays a major role in blood sugar balance, cholesterol formation, conversion of thyroid hormone into the active form, and the production of sex-hormone-binding globulin, which helps to regulate your hormone levels. It's also the clearinghouse where metabolic detoxification occurs.

Metabolic detoxification is a series of highly coordinated phases that take place in your liver that filter non-water-soluble products, which includes your hormones, most pharmaceuticals, fat-soluble vitamins, most environmental toxins, and even everyday exposures like alcohol, out of your bloodstream; break them down into water-soluble by-products; and package these into nontoxic compounds that can be eliminated out of one of your natural garbage shoots (urine, stool). When your liver isn't breaking down and binding estrogens effectively, or your microbiome isn't doing its part in eliminating them, you can end up with too much of the wrong kind. Loss of detoxification resilience is one of the downstream effects of exposure to environmental toxins. Additionally, the immune system is put into a chronic state of overload due to the constant low-level inflammation being triggered by toxins in our body.

Power Foods for Detoxification

Overall, low phytonutrient and phytochemical intakes have been associated with impaired ability to detoxify environmental toxins. Detoxification is a highly nutrient- and phytochemical-dependent process. All that heavy lifting gobbles up vitamins, minerals, and phytochemicals, so we have

5 Steps You Can Take to Protect Yourself from Flame-Retardant Chemicals

- Wash your hands before you eat, especially if you've been typing on your keyboard.
- If you have wood floors, damp mop regularly to remove as much chemical dust as possible; if you don't have wood floors and can afford to, switch to wood flooring.
- Foam furniture and mats made without chemical flame retardants should say so on the label. If you purchased your furniture before 2015, there's a good chance the manufacturer treated the cushion foam with toxic flame-retardant chemicals. If you are just furnishing your home, decorate with wood and consider futons made of organic cotton materials rather than foam for your chairs, sofas, and bedding.
- Avoid upholstered furniture and carpet padding made with polyurethane foam.
- If you have babies or toddlers, purchase flame-retardant-free nursing pillows, car-seat covers, and baby clothes.

to keep them replenished to meet the demand. These include B-complex (especially B1, B3, B6, and B12), choline, magnesium, selenium, zinc, folate (which I recommend in the form of methylfolate), iron, calcium, copper, glutathione, sulfur, amino acids, and others. Insufficient amounts of any of these can inhibit or prevent the detoxification of numerous medications, alcohol, caffeine, hormones, and environmental toxins.

Hundreds of studies show the power of phytonutrients, vitamins, and minerals for boosting your body's natural detoxification mechanisms. You're already well on your way with the Hormone Intelligence Diet. These are just some of my favorite detoxification "power foods" as examples of the marvelous way eating for Hormone Intelligence naturally nourishes detoxification.

Yup, Those Greens! I know, I know. I keep saying it. But there's a reason—kale, collards, broccoli, Brussels sprouts, broccoli sprouts ("microgreens"), bok choy, and napa cabbage are the queens of detoxification. When you digest them, they release chemical compounds called *glucosinolates*, *indoles*, and *sulforaphanes* that ramp up detoxification. Plus, the fiber from these greens helps you directly clear out estrogen from your intestines before it can be reabsorbed into circulation, and it feeds

Be Kind to Your Vagina

Given that we menstruate for, give or take, 4,000 days of our lives, what you use for period products deserves a second thought and makes a lot of good sense. When it comes to traditional feminine hygiene products, other than soap and water in the shower, or a bidet if you have one, you just don't need them! I quit using conventional sanitary pads and tampons in 1982 when reports first started coming out about their high content of dioxin, pesticides, and other toxins that act as carcinogens and endocrine disruptors and switched to organic products and have never gone back to the "regular" brands. Here are the top options for both conventional period products and those not so widely known:

- Purchase only unscented pads, tampons, toilet paper, and other products intended for down there; scents are endocrine disruptors and are absorbed into your bloodstream from your vag, too.

- Choose disposable menstrual pads and tampons made from organic cotton and other organic fibers that are manufactured with non-chlorine bleach. These offer the convenience of disposability and are more environmentally friendly than many of the larger commercial brands.

- The menstrual cup has been around since 1937 and was invented by a woman (Leona Chalmers). Pros: Earth friendly, reusable, lasts years, inexpensive, and many women find them easy to use, reliable, and effective. They are considered safe to use while exercising, traveling, and sleeping for up to six hours. Cons: Women with heavier flow find that overflow can lead to leakage, so they have to also use a pad on heavier days; many women report it being less than convenient and hygienic to have to rinse their cup, when changing it in a public bathroom, for example.

that fabulous microbiome of yours, amplifying hormone and toxin neutralization and elimination.

Garlic, Onions, Leeks: These foods are such a normal part of our diets that you may forget they are medicinal herbs. Their rich sulfur content, as well as other compounds, powerfully increases detoxification. They also increase glutathione and another compound called superoxide dismutase (SOD), both of which the Pill burns through or blocks, which is part of why the Pill interferes with natural detoxification.

Avocado: Perhaps one of the richest glutathione-containing foods in town, avocados support detoxification. They're also high in potassium, which is calming, have 20% of the daily recommended amount of folate, are rich in PMS-preventing vitamin B6, as well as a host of other B vitamins, give you a nice dose of magnesium and important trace minerals, and help your body to absorb fat-soluble vitamins. They balance blood sugar and reduce metabolic syndrome, too. One study showed that adding avocado or avocado oil to either salad or salsa can increase antioxidant absorption up to fifteen times, and another found that people who eat avocados regularly enjoy overall better health than those who don't! Now just think about guacamole (see Guacamole

---

- Washable "period panties," which absorb about two to four tampons' worth of menstrual blood, are the most recent innovation in period products and allow you to change your undies a couple of times per day rather than ever having to use a pad or tampon again. Pros: Earth friendly, no more pads or tampons, 100% reusable, can last a few years. Cons: Expensive; when you do have to change it, it could mean stripping off clothes rather than just the pad, and so on. Then you also have to stash and carry the used one until you get home; inconvenient while traveling.

- Although less convenient, cotton reusable pads that you wash at home are an environmentally and body-friendly choice. For nearly three decades I used reusable cloth pads that I washed at home, supplementing with organic cotton pads and tampons when I was at work, or out and about. Pros: Earth friendly, reusable, last five years or more, organic, zero waste other than wash water, comfier than you might think, you never run out, cost nothing but a modest initial investment. Cons: Washing; what to do with dirties when you're out, no plastic so bleeding through is possible, inconvenient while traveling because they need washing.

With reusables, careful cleaning of products after use is essential. In one study of colonization of microorganisms during menstruation among women using various menstrual products, cultures from users of sea sponges were found to have significantly higher colonization rates with *S. aureus*, *Escherichia coli*, and other *Enterobacteriaceae*. The association of sea sponges with a high rate of *S. aureus* colonization suggests that they are not an alternative to tampons for women seeking to decrease the risk of toxic shock syndrome, and I don't recommend that choice.

Mash, page 345)—the perfect duo of avocados and garlic—for your health.

Eggs: Eggs provide important amino acids needed for detoxification and are rich in choline.

Legumes: Make sure to include legumes in your diet, they're rich in detox-boosting proteins and phytochemicals.

Berries: Talk about awesome medicine for the body and deliciousness, too! Blueberries, red raspberries, strawberries, and blackberries are especially packed with flavonoids that support detoxification. That's why they're an important part of this plan.

Seeds: While flaxseeds certainly pack a powerful punch for your hormones, increasing the length of the luteal phase and reducing cycle-related symptoms including PMS, other seeds that you can easily enjoy daily that boost detox include sesame seeds, a rich source of copper, and pumpkin seeds, rich in zinc.

Dark Chocolate: YES! More benefits to dark chocolate. Rich in phytochemicals, dark chocolate makes the list of foods that support detoxification!

Turmeric: Used in Indian cooking for thousands of years, this bright yellow herb has become famous for its ability to support our natural detoxification processes. Curcumin, an active compound, helps the body slow its roll on breaking down toxic chemicals long enough for the body to be able to do it effectively and efficiently without causing you to build up what are called toxic intermediates when the two phases of liver detoxification are out of sync. It also boosts up your body's natural anti-inflammatory production. You can also use it in cooking or in your favorite smoothie.

Green Tea / Green Tea Extract: This "food" boosts liver detoxification, helping you to break down and get rid of toxins, while acting as an antioxidant, putting out the fires of inflammation around your body. It can be taken

---

Love Your Liver Bitters

Combine ¼ ounce of each of the following tinctures in a 2-ounce glass bottle with a dropper: dandelion root, burdock root, artichoke leaf, yellow dock root, angelica root, fennel seed, and ginger. Use in the Love Your Liver Bitters and Tonic recipe on page 371, or simply squirt a dropperful into a ¼ cup of water and take daily after dinner (not for use during pregnancy). While you can eat leafy greens freely, do not use bitter herbs if you have any of the following conditions: kidney stones, gallbladder disease, hiatal hernia, gastritis, or peptic ulcer.

Another way to introduce bitters—that is my favorite—is with herbal bitter elixirs.

---

as a tea, but in extract form it is a potent supplement for weight loss, hormonal balance, and detox. If you are very sensitive to caffeine, use a decaffeinated extract.

Bitters: The bitter taste was an important part of our ancestral diet but has been replaced by a general distaste for it in favor of sweet and salty. Bitters are powerful digestive stimulators, aid in detoxification and bile flow, improve peristalsis and elimination, stimulate the pancreas and help regulate blood sugar, insulin, and glucagon, and help the gut wall repair damage. Because of the gut-brain connection, they can reduce depression and improve mood. Had your gallbladder removed and thinking, well, now what? Bitters can help keep things moving. The simplest way to introduce bitters into your daily life is to eat dandelion greens, endive, radicchio, and arugula, all of which can be incredibly delicious when you know how to prepare them. The trick is to use some "acid" (i.e., citrus or vinegar) and a pinch of salt to mellow the taste.

Healthy Gut, Better Detoxification

A healthy microbiome and daily evacuation help your body effectively eliminate waste products from the breakdown of both environmental and naturally occurring hormone metabolites and other products.

Once your liver has packaged spent hormones and other toxins, you've got to get them out of the body. That means having a complete bowel movement at least once a day. Estrogen metabolites are excreted into the small intestine through bile; they are "soaked up" by fiber in the small intestines and eliminated when you poop. If the diet lacks fiber, bile along with the estrogen metabolites are reabsorbed, adding an unnecessary estrogen burden to the body.

Focus on getting plenty of fiber in your diet (the Hormone Intelligence Diet provides this), get plenty of exercise, and stay hydrated. Improving the health of your microbiome will help with regularity, too. So continue to pay attention to getting your daily dose of probiotic foods and don't skimp on any of the veggie dishes in the meal plans. Still not pooping daily or at least most days? Revisit page 200 for tips on getting things moving.

Make Sure to Rest

Chronic lack of sleep can reduce detoxification. Studies show that glutathione levels are lower in those suffering from insomnia and sleep deprivation. So if you glossed over the

Girl, Go Wild!

Wild foods bring us a plethora of trace nutrients and powerful phytochemicals that are tremendously hormone healthy and also, according to studies on the relationship between humans and plants, important for DNA functioning and cellular repair. Do you have to become a food forager? No! You can find wild foods at your local natural food store or farmer's market.

Here are the wild foods to look for. You can substitute a wild source any time you see one of these items in the meal plans:

- Wild berries

- Wild-caught fish

- Wild-harvested leafy greens (i.e., dandelion greens, lamb's quarters, violet leaves)

- Wild-harvested roots (i.e., dandelion or burdock root)

- Seaweeds (e.g., alaria, wakame, dulse, kombu)

- Wildflower honey

Note: Wild mushrooms or herbs can be mistaken for or accidentally mixed with toxic ones, so only use those from credible sources!

importance of sleep and healthy circadian rhythm, start making that a priority on your hormone-health list! Ample, restorative sleep each night may help boost your detox game.

Step 5: Boost with Botanicals and Nutrients

Love Your Liver Foods and Nutritional Supplements

For doses, see the Botanical and Supplement Quick Reference Guide on pages 372–81.

B Vitamins: Found in numerous foods, and also in most complete multivitamin and mineral supplements, B vitamins are essential not only for a healthy nervous system, but for hepatic detoxification. Particularly important is methylated folate, critical for the methylation process of detoxification. Folate helps to mitigate the risk of environmental exposure to endocrine disruptors. Dutch investigators measured the urinary levels of BPA and phthalate of nine hundred pregnant women and compared the results with how long it took them to conceive. They found that in those with ample folic acid intake, it did not take longer to get pregnant, even with detectable levels of bisphenol or phthalate exposure, whereas those not taking adequate folic acid were more likely to experience fertility challenges and adverse effects from these chemicals. Also important are vitamin B6, needed for glutathione production and beneficial in preventing PMS and other period problems and for boosting ovulation (think better progesterone levels) and fertility, and vitamin B12, which is part of the methylation process.

Broccoli Extracts (DIM, Sulforaphane, Indole-3-Carbinol [I3C]): I3C is converted to DIM upon digestion. It potently increases detoxification and helps to metabolize estrogen. It's used for symptoms of excess estrogen, endometriosis, cyclic breast pain, PMS, cervical dysplasia, and uterine fibroids. Food sources include broccoli, broccoli sprouts, and to some extent other Brassicaceae vegetables, and you can also supplement with DIM or I3C.

Glycine: This amino acid and neurotransmitter is essential in the detoxification pathway. It upregulates glutathione production and can help protect and heal intestinal cells. It also improves sleep, alleviates fatigue, reduces depression, and improves blood sugar balance; it's also a main component in collagen production. Food sources include fish, meat (especially in tough cuts like the chuck, round, and brisket), and legumes; it's also in dairy products, which partly explains the warm milk before bed. You can also supplement with the powder form, which is sweet tasting, so can even be added to tea, coconut yogurt, oatmeal, smoothies, Chocolate Avocado Mousse (page 365), and other foods just before serving.

Let Go of Toxic Stress

Did you know that stress is considered a toxin? There's even a term for it: toxic stress! It's any situation that results in prolonged activation of the stress response, making it hard for the body to recover and leading to health dysfunction. As women, toxic stress is all too common. Reflect on toxic situations you might currently be facing in your life: your job, living situation, or relationship, and consider what you might be able to do to shift the energy—or situation—for yourself. It may be a small step or it may be a grand gesture that you've been too afraid to make for a long time.

Vitamin C (Ascorbic Acid): Raises red blood cell glutathione by nearly 50% after just 500 mg/day. Top food sources include cantaloupe, citrus fruits and juices (such as orange and grapefruit), kiwifruit, mango, papaya, pineapple, strawberries, raspberries, blueberries, and cranberries.

N-Acetyl-Cysteine (NAC): This supplement is one of the most important for detoxification because it increases glutathione. Glutathione helps to clean up heavy metals, as well as other environmental toxins, without binding to your own nutrients. As you'll learn in the next chapter, glutathione is also one of the most important antioxidants for preventing and repairing cellular damage—including to our ovaries, thyroid, and endometrial tissue. It's most specifically used for endometriosis and fertility support. NAC is not found naturally in food sources; the body converts NAC to cysteine. Cysteine is found in most high-protein foods, such as chicken, turkey, eggs, sunflower seeds, and legumes. Vegetables like broccoli, garlic, red pepper, and onion are also significant sources of cysteine. A number of herbs increase the body's natural production of glutathione; see herbal supplements below.

Detoxification-Supporting Herbs

For doses, see the Botanical and Supplement Quick Reference Guide on pages 372–81.

Curcumin: This key active ingredient in turmeric boosts one of your body's most important detox chemicals, glutathione, and also enhances detoxification enzymes in general. It is specific for leaky gut, acts as an anti-inflammatory, and has adaptogenic activity useful for anxiety. Turmeric as a cooking spice—and if you have access, the fresh root—can be used in cooking or smoothies. It's also taken as a powder in capsules for its anti-inflammatory effects. At about 2 grams daily, the powder is also healing for your gut lining.

But to get the liver detoxification and antioxidant benefits, you have to use it as the extract, curcumin, which is taken as a supplement.

Milk Thistle: Protects and heals hepatic cells, supports both Phase 1 and 2 detoxification, and increases glutathione. While they're not usually thought of as a food, milk thistle seeds are edible and tasty. You can grind them like you would flaxseeds and add 1 to 2 tablespoons to your parfaits, puddings, smoothies, salads, and so on, or supplement with capsules or tincture.

Artichoke Leaf Extract: This extract supports liver detoxification and acts as an antioxidant, while increasing the amount and availability of natural detoxification chemicals produced in your body, especially in your liver. Take it as a tincture or in capsules.

Green Tea Extract (Decaffeinated): Green tea boosts liver detoxification, enhances glutathione production, and supports healthy gut flora. The active ingredient, EGCG, is also an antioxidant, supporting cellular health and reducing inflammation. In extract form it is a potent supplement for symptoms associated with estrogen excess, including PCOS, female pattern hair loss, and uterine fibroids. Drinking one to two cups of green tea daily is certainly healthy, but to get the hormonal benefits, supplementation with the extract is recommended over the eight cups you'd need for benefits of the tea.

St. John's Wort (SJW): This herb often comes with warnings about not taking it with medications. The reason for this is that SJW increases the rate of clearance of medications from the body. How's it doing this? By increasing hepatic detoxification. When it comes to a small group of medications that SJW does this to, it's a problem because it can lower the amount you're getting below the intended dose. But when it comes to estrogen, it can be a good thing. In fact, one of the cautions with SJW is not to take it with an estrogen-containing form of the Pill because it could interfere with effectiveness. While no pregnancies have ever been reported as a result, lower blood estrogen levels have, because it's enhancing detoxification. Keep in mind that excess estrogen can cause depression and contribute to numerous hormonal symptoms, and SJW is known for its effectiveness as an antidepressant. Specific indications include symptoms of estrogen excess, depression, and anxiety.

Pycnogenol: An extract of maritime pine bark, pycnogenol reduces inflammation, oxidative stress, cellular membrane and DNA damage, and damage due to the impact of chronically elevated blood sugar on the cells. It contains the same compounds, procyanidins, that make cacao, green tea extract, grape seed extract, and berries so health promoting and protective. Specific indications include improved cognition and focus, increased sense of well-being, reduction in inflammatory cytokines (after just five days of use), lasting reduction of symptoms with endometriosis, reduced menopausal symptoms, reduction in wrinkles, and improved osteoarthritis pain. It may also reduce fat accumulation that happens as a result of inflammation and improve insulin sensitivity. Food sources include grapes, apples, cocoa, tea, nuts, and berries, and it can be taken as a supplement.

For How Long Do I Support Detoxification?

Reducing body burden of some toxins, like herbicides and pesticides, can happen quickly; reducing heavy metal burden may only happen over a matter of years. And remember, no matter how much we clear up our own act, we're still getting some level of constant toxicant exposure that is beyond our control. Therefore, detoxification is a lifelong relationship with your environment and detox pathways. Does that mean lifelong supplements? Not at all. It means making Hormone Intelligence a way of life, not just a short-term fling.

revitalize cellular repair

REJUVENATE YOUR OVARIES

She sings from the knowing of *los ovarios*, a knowing deep within the body, deep within the mind, deep within the soul.

—**Clarissa Pinkola Estés,** *Women Who Run with the Wolves*

I can't believe it: You're in the last week of the Hormone Intelligence Plan! Congrats. That's huge! Let's now give *los ovarios* the direct attention they deserve given all the hard work they do!

I've generally been referring to inflammation as the "Mother of Root Causes." In this chapter, we're going to take healing inflammation one step further with specific support to repair any damage that may be affecting your powerhouse organs that often take a big hit and send your cycles and systems into chaos: your ovaries. You'll learn how to take the steps that can rejuvenate your ovaries back to optimal health. Not only will your ovaries benefit, but so will your thyroid and endometrial tissue, your endocrine, immune, and nervous systems, your hair and skin—and your vitality.

Let's wrap this beautiful gift to yourself with a bow by giving your ovaries, and with this, all your cells, the extra spark they deserve as you continue what you've learned in the preceding chapters.

Out of the Frying Pan and into the Fire: Oxidative Stress

What is it about inflammation that makes it so problematic when it gets out of control? Largely, it's a phenomenon called *oxidative stress* and it's terribly damaging to cellular structures and functions, taking a particular toll on your ovaries, because along with aging our hair, skin, and other organs, it accelerates aging of our ovaries.

Hormone Intelligence:
Revitalize Your Cells, Rejuvenate Your Ovaries

- Learn which foods specifically nourish and can even revitalize your ovaries.
- Discover the nutrients and herbs that give your ovaries the first aid they need for regular cycles and ovulation, fertility, and more.
- Start a movement practice to mobilize your mitochondria (you'll also learn what these are and why they're so important) to restore and optimize ovarian function—as well as boost your energy and vitality.

Oxidation is a natural process occurring constantly within our cells as a by-product of chemical reactions that require a great deal of energy, and among those cells, the ones in your ovaries require a tremendous amount. When oxidation occurs, which is constantly, free radicals are generated. A **free radical** is a molecule that is missing an electron. This makes it highly unstable, so it seeks another molecule to feel whole again. The only problem is that along the way, it can cause some damage to your cell membranes, other parts of your cell, and your DNA. It's a big deal. Most free radicals are rogue forms of oxygen, and thus are called *reactive oxygen species* (ROS). Too much oxidation and you end up with oxidative stress. As you can imagine, free radicals aren't just happy hippies. Like hormones, they are signaling messengers, and as such, can affect the cross talk between your brain, cells, and hormones.

What's the problem? You might be able to guess! We're back to the story you're now familiar with: the mismatch between the amount of oxidative stress we're facing and our ability to keep up with it in real time, before it causes damage. What causes oxidative stress? All the other issues you're resolving with this plan: not

getting enough fruits, vegetables, nuts, seeds, fish, and high-quality oils, and thus their important antioxidant phytochemicals and nutrients; getting too many of the foods that cause inflammation; cell-damaging environmental toxin exposures; poor detoxification leading to increased reactive toxins in our system; insulin resistance and hyperglycemia; low microbiome diversity and quality, which prevents us from making use of our dietary antioxidants, stress, and not getting enough sleep and R&R to allow for healing.

Mitochondria: The Hidden Powerhouses of Ovarian Health

Perhaps you remember from high school or college biology that **mitochondria** are organelles, subcomponents of your cells, whose job it is to provide about 90% of your body's energy in the form of ATP. It's like the solar energy for our cells! That's how they earned their nickname: the powerhouses of our cells. Your cells rely on mitochondria not only to provide fuel for cellular survival, but also to act as the critical self-destruct button on old or damaged

Oxidative Stress and Your Mitochondria

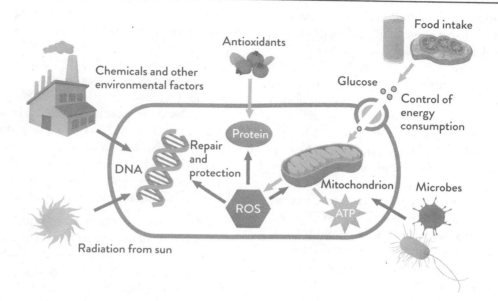

cells. Most ROS and oxidative damage originate intracellularly in the mitochondria, where these ROS can also damage mitochondrial DNA. Repeated injury results in a cumulative loss of function. And guess what? Those lovely ladies called your ovaries are the home of your oocytes, which have more mitochondria than any other cells in the body.

Oxidative Stress and Mitochondrial Roots of Hormone Imbalance

Both oxidative stress and mitochondrial function have a tremendous influence over ovarian health. Impairment of mitochondrial function can exert a significant negative effect on hormone production and regulation, as well as gynecologic conditions. Oxidative stress influences our entire hormonal and gynecologic

life span and health span. Here are just a few of the ways oxidative and mitochondrial stress show up in our health as women:

- **Sex Hormone Production:** Ovarian mitochondria are responsible for blood flow to the corpus luteum, as well as for synthesizing your sex hormones, particularly progesterone, by shuttling cholesterol needed for its production into the ovary. Slow mitochondrial function means low sex hormone production. Adding another layer of complexity, mitochondria also control steroid production in the adrenal glands. Any impairment of mitochondrial functioning can adversely influence hormone production and regulation.

- **Anovulation and Luteal Phase Dysfunction (also called *luteal phase defect*, a term I don't prefer, as it's not a defect, but a correctable problem):** Ovarian mitochondria produce the energy needed for ovulation. Without ovulation, you have low progesterone, leading to a phenomenon called *luteal phase dysfunction*. Symptoms include irregular menstrual cycles, moods, and fertility challenges, and all the other symptoms of low progesterone (see page 34). Luteal phase dysfunction is found in up to 10% of women with fertility challenges, and up to 35% with recurrent miscarriage, thought to be due to underdevelopment of the uterine lining because of the low progesterone levels. Recurrent miscarriage and fertility problems have been linked to low levels of antioxidants, including vitamins C and E, and glutathione in the blood and cells, which makes sense as this also contributes to mitochondrial damage and free radicals.

- **Thyroid Problems:** In yet another bidirectional hormone relationship, your mitochondria drive the energy for your thyroid, and your thyroid provides energy for your mitochondria; mitochondrial dysfunction can drive thyroid function down, and oxidative stress can damage and cause inflammation in thyroid tissue, which can lead to Hashimoto's, hypothyroidism, fatigue, and hair loss.

- **PCOS:** Women with PCOS have markedly elevated blood levels of oxidative stress and inflammatory markers (due to variability among women for a variety of reasons, these are not reliable diagnostic indicators of PCOS). Oxidative stress, in turn, increases androgen production. However, androgen-reducing conventional medications do not reduce inflammation or oxidative stress. Mitochondrial dysfunction also increases insulin resistance, and like

so many interconnected relationships, insulin resistance creates inflammation and oxidative stress, increases androgen production, and leads to many of the symptoms of PCOS. Insulin resistance also negatively impacts mitochondrial dysfunction. It's not clear which comes first, insulin resistance causing mitochondrial dysfunction, or the other way around, but we do know that reducing insulin resistance improves mitochondrial function and improving mitochondrial function decreases insulin resistance. The Hormone Intelligence Plan does both.

- **Endometriosis:** Endometriosis is an inflammatory disease with high levels of oxidative stress (though as with PCOS, blood markers of it are not reliable diagnostic indicators) particularly in the peritoneal cavity, where endometrial lesions are most common. Oxidative stress in the peritoneal cavity of women with endometriosis is one of the main causes of infertility. Researchers are now looking at targeting oxidative stress as a line of treatment for endometriosis. But you don't have to wait; you can do it yourself with Hormone Intelligence.

- **Fertility, Miscarriage, and Pregnancy Problems:** Mitochondrial health influences egg quality. Oxidative stress has a major impact on fertility, decreases success with assisted fertility techniques, and leads to less healthy oocytes at all levels of development. Lack of ovulation due to mitochondrial dysfunction also makes it impossible to conceive. And if you do ovulate, poor corpus luteum formation due to mitochondrial problems could lead to decreased β-hCG, the hormone needed to maintain a healthy pregnancy for the first trimester, so there's an increased risk of miscarriage. Healthy ovarian mitochondrial function is associated with the health of the early embryo when we do get pregnant, and oxidative stress has been linked to pregnancy problems including low birth weight babies and preeclampsia.

- **Skin and Hair Health:** One more important bit about oxidative stress: it ages you faster on the inside—and the outside. This process has a technical name: **inflammaging**. Yes, that's a real thing. And not to appeal to vanity here, but our skin and hair may reflect our inner ecosystem. Skin and hair follicles are dense with mitochondria and highly regulated by thyroid hormones. Considering that hair generation and growth is an energy-intensive process, meaning it relies on your mitochondria, hair loss can be a sign of decreased thyroid and/or mitochondrial function, and premature aging (i.e., early or excessive wrinkling) can be another.

- **Loss of Ovarian Reserve:** We're born with between one and two million follicles. As we age, this number declines gradually, and by the time we reach menopause (international average age for this is 52 years old), those follicles are depleted. The number of follicles we have remaining at any given time is our "ovarian reserve" or egg quantity. When your ovaries are not getting the nourishment they need from your diet, or the attack they're under from oxidative stress exceeds their ability for self-repair, you can experience premature ovarian aging. Almost 20% of women consulting for infertility show signs of premature ovarian aging. When the damage becomes extensive, this can lead to ovarian burnout or primary ovarian insufficiency (POI), which affects 1 in 1,000 women by age thirty, and 1 in 100 by age

forty. Premature loss of ovarian function can not only affect your plans for having kids, but can also affect the heart, bones, and brain, dramatically impacting your health span.

Mitochondria Need a Healthy Ecosystem, Too

Mitochondria are fascinating in that initially, as in way back when we were first on the planet, they were bacteria that lived symbiotically in our cells. We became so interdependent that they stopped being independent organisms and became organelles—a part of our own cells. Another interesting thing about mitochondria is that their DNA is the only DNA in our bodies, male or female, that comes only from our moms (remember, all other DNA is 50/50 from mom and dad). Given that they're so remarkable and have been around awhile, it would seem they're pretty resilient, and they are, under the right circumstances.

- They require proper nutrients and cofactors, without which their function quickly tanks and ROS activity increases.

- Not only do they help to regulate hormone function, but they are also regulated by it, especially by T3. If you have hypothyroidism, there's a good chance your mitochondria have slowed down, too.

- They can be damaged by many medications and environmental toxins.

- Anything that messes with your epigenetics can mess with the mitochondrial DNA, altering its function.

Fortunately, you're already addressing all these roots of oxidative stress with the Hormone Intelligence Plan (isn't it amazing to know that you're already healing?). It's also why I saved adding in this extra bit of ovarian support for last. But there are some additional steps you can take to nourish your ovaries even more and that are nourishing for your thyroid, endometrial tissue, and your longevity.

Two Common Meds That Can Put a Damper on Your Ovaries

A Little-Known Pill Side Effect: In addition to the general nutrient depletion that I describe from taking the Pill (page 221), estrogen-containing birth control pills interfere with cellular repair by using up the nutrients these processes require, including vitamin C (ascorbic acid), vitamin E, β-carotene, magnesium, selenium, zinc, and coenzyme Q. Additionally, the Pill depletes glutathione and other naturally produced antioxidants by creating more oxidative stress. One study found that compared to women not taking the Pill, nonsmokers taking the Pill had 37% lower coenzyme Q10 levels and 23% lower vitamin E levels. Another study, this time among women athletes taking the Pill, found that taking the Pill negated even the positive antioxidant benefits of a diet high in antioxidant foods like fatty fish and dark chocolate, which makes it harder to repair exercise-induced cellular and muscle damage. Because contraceptives are taken over an extended period of time, even subtle effects can add up. If you do need or choose to stay on the Pill, for health or contraceptive reasons, a progestin-only option can help you avoid some of the common Pill-related side effects, including nutrient depletion. Whatever form you take, staying on a multivitamin or a prenatal vitamin that contains the commonly depleted nutrients can offset some of the nutrient losses and protect your mitochondria.

Nonsteroidal Anti-inflammatory Drugs: In 2015, a study demonstrated a decrease in ovulation in women taking NSAIDs. In this study, thirty-nine women of childbearing age used prescription doses of diclofenac, naproxen, or etoricoxib for ten days. After this time, medical assessment showed that their ovulation was suppressed. When the NSAIDs were discontinued, ovulation resumed, usually in the following month. Another recent study focusing on fertility and NSAID users found that women with rheumatoid arthritis taking NSAIDs were more likely to have unexplained delays getting pregnant in comparison to people with RA who were not using NSAIDs. If you do have chronic pain, keep NSAIDs to a minimum, avoiding prescription-level doses; use just the occasional OTC ibuprofen in the form of Motrin or Advil, for example, no more than a couple of doses in any cycle. I also share alternatives for mild-to-moderate pain relief in Part Three.

Should I Get Tested for Oxidative Stress? What about for Ovarian Reserve?

While there is testing available for oxidative stress, it is typically costly and not something your primary care provider likely offers. Also, the reality is that most of us are experiencing some amount of it. Dietary and lifestyle changes to reduce it are important for your health now, and for graceful aging in the long run, regardless. So I don't recommend pursuing testing for this.

There are numerous limitations to the value of ovarian reserve testing, so in my practice I only recommend it when I suspect primary ovarian insufficiency (POI) and am assessing a woman for fertility testing and treatment, or for egg retrieval for freezing.

The simple tests that are usually used to assess ovarian reserve are:

- AMH level: Oddly, there are no agreed upon standards for AMH, so you have to go with the reference range given on the report by the lab you use. In general, a level well above the laboratory's lower threshold for normal suggests adequate ovarian reserve. As the level falls below the lower limit of normal, the odds of reduced ovarian reserve increases, with very low levels suggesting very low ovarian reserve.

- Day 3 follicle-stimulating hormone (FSH): Should be less than 10 mIU/mL.

- Estradiol: This is a bit more controversial but is often included in an ovarian reserve test panel.

The premise of these tests is that women with good ovarian reserve have adequate AMH levels and sufficient production of ovarian hormones early in the menstrual cycle, which keep FSH at a low level. These tests do not give us the whole picture. The most current research shows that even low AMH doesn't tell us who can—or can't—get pregnant, yet the information can cause serious worry for women already worried about their fertility. They can't tell us anything about egg quality, either. PCOS is associated with high AMH, so sometimes this is tested as part of a PCOS workup, though again I don't usually do this in my practice unless a woman doesn't meet the clinical criteria for PCOS (see page 76) but seems to have the condition based on irregular cycles or fertility challenges.

When and why would they ever be helpful? AMH and FSH may help us to measure ovarian reserve, which can be important to know if you are trying to get pregnant and are having trouble. If you know you have fewer eggs than average for your age, then you can take steps to address this both with the Hormone Intelligence Plan and targeted supplements below for improving ovarian health, oocyte formation, and quality.

The Hormone Intelligence Solution: Revitalize Your Mitochondria, Rejuvenate Your Ovaries

Nourishing your ovaries is probably not something you considered doing before picking up this book! Yet whether you're trying to regulate your cycles, improve ovulation or increase your progesterone levels, reverse PCOS and reduce androgen levels, conceive (and have a healthy pregnancy), or prevent or reverse the early onset of primary ovarian insufficiency (POI), your ovaries have a say. And who doesn't want to slow down the impact of the aging process—ovarian and otherwise!

While the entire Hormone Intelligence program has been geared toward restoring healthy brain-ovary communication, removing the obstacles to healthy ovarian function, and providing the nutrients your "ladies" need for health, giving them some directed extra tender loving care can more quickly help you reach your goals. Because healthy ovaries are central to so many of the hormonal imbalances most women are facing, rather than repeat them in numerous Advanced Protocols, I share them here.

One of the most promising areas of research in improving ovarian function and egg quality has to do with improving mitochondrial function and reducing oxidative stress. It can get your cycles back on track, improve your hormone balance, and enhance your fertility if you're trying now and preserve it if you want to try later. And anything that improves mitochondrial function can also improve insulin resistance and thyroid function, hair and skin, energy, strength, and vitality. Sound like a plan? It does to me! If you're moisturizing your skin to prevent wrinkles, think of this as skin care for your ovaries!

Step 1: Eat for Ovarian Health

The most effective and healthful approach to reducing oxidative stress, increasing cellular repair, and supporting mitochondrial function is through the quality of our diet. But not just any diet. The traditional Mediterranean diet has been shown to create the optimal environment for doing all these. And it's the very foundation of the Hormone Intelligence Diet. So you're already on your way!

Phytonutrient Power

If you're following along with the Hormone Intelligence Diet, you're now getting the abundant fruits, vegetables, nuts, seeds, and herbs rich in phytochemicals like polyphenols, bioflavonoids, and numerous others, that are present in our diet when we eat a rainbow, consume a variety of seeds, nuts, oils, and so on—all of which prevent and reverse oxidative damage daily, while also supporting detoxification, gut health, our nervous system, and so

much more. Unlike with specific antioxidant supplements, we absorb more of these nutrients when we get them from our diet, but the key is microbiome health—we can't make use of these nutrients, even from dietary sources, without gut flora that process them into available forms we can then use.

Can't I Just Take Antioxidants?

Antioxidants are the body's natural antidote to oxidation. Your body uses nutrients from your diet, notably from fruits, veggies, seeds, nuts, and healthy fats (getting the picture here?), and also naturally generated internal chemicals like glutathione, which you learned about in the last chapter, to neutralize those ROS (and other types of free radicals). Antioxidants "lend" that missing electron. When we are well nourished, or when oxidative stress isn't out of control, we have the materials on hand that we need to supply those missing electrons.

While it might seem logical to just take antioxidant vitamins to reverse oxidative damage and call it a day, unfortunately a current review of the science suggests that antioxidant supplements bomb out as general treatments for oxidative stress. Most studies show that we only absorb the smallest fraction of the allegedly helpful antioxidants that we ingest when we take them as supplements. However, this doesn't negate the very important science that shows us that eating a diet rich in the foods that have been considered the highest in antioxidants does improve overall health and reduce chronic disease, and that it's best to use antioxidants targeted for specific conditions that have been proven to work. For example, in one study, fifty women, 19 to 41 years old, with pelvic pain and history of endometriosis and infertility, all scheduled for surgery, were randomly assigned to two groups. One group was given a vitamin E (1,200 IU) and vitamin C (1,000 mg) combination daily for eight weeks; the other group, a placebo. Forty-three percent of the women who received these "antioxidants" had improvement in "everyday pain," and 37% experienced reduction in period pain and 27% in painful sex. In the placebo group, there was minimal to no change in these symptoms. Further, the antioxidant group had a significant decrease in peritoneal fluid inflammatory markers, compared with women not taking the antioxidants. So how do you increase antioxidants and mitochondrial function and reduce oxidative stress?

Eat More Seeds

If you've been exploring women's wellness online, you may have come across articles touting the miracles of seed cycling for regulating the menstrual cycle. In case you missed it, the logic of seed cycling is that by eating certain seeds at different phases of the cycle, the varying lignan (phytoestrogen), fatty acid, and micronutrient properties of the seeds will provide the optimal nutritional support at the right time. Unfortunately, while intriguing, it is not substantiated.

Yet, like so many wellness trends, there is, excuse the pun, a seed of truth. In this case, seeds are indeed healthful for hormone balance. For example, studies show that vitamin E and omega-3 and omega-6 fatty acids in flaxseeds, sesame, pumpkin, and sunflower seeds are essential for hormone production and ovarian follicular function. We also know that zinc, present in meaningful concentrations in pumpkin and sesame seeds, helps to improve progesterone levels and the formation of the corpus luteum, and gets the endometrium prepped for implantation. Seeds are rich in selenium, which supports ovulation and fertility, as well as liver detoxification phases, as we talked about in the last chapter. Lignans,

which flax and sesame seeds are especially rich in, are converted to enterolactones in the presence of healthy gut flora, which help keep your estrogen levels healthy.

So, while seed cycling does not have any scientific merit, eating more seeds as part of your overall daily diet does. If you find the structure of seed cycling useful, feel free to continue with it. There's no harm to it. The most important thing is to get a diversity of seeds into your diet, in ample amounts. Mix it up, and make sure to consume some combination of seeds every day.

Flaxseeds: Studies have shown that eating flaxseeds increases luteal phase length and reduces the number of anovulatory cycles, as well as improves the progesterone-to-estrogen ratio in the luteal phase, so if you're skipping periods or have low progesterone, adding flax to your diet is a great choice. Flax has additionally been found to decrease stress hormones and stress perception, which could have positive effects on your cycle as stress is one of the overarching signals that most influences sex hormone levels. After menopause, they also have protective effects against breast cancer. Flax is also a superstar for your overall health. In addition to its sex hormone effects, it has also been shown to reduce cardiovascular risk profile and decrease Hemoglobin A1C levels in type 2 diabetes, making them a great addition to your diet if you have PCOS with insulin resistance or elevated blood sugar. Most of these studies tested 10 grams of flax a day; I recommend women consume 2 tablespoons of ground flax daily, which is a bit above this amount, and also gives you a healthy fiber dose. Sprinkle on your cereal, add to your smoothie, or use as a salad topping.

Sesame Seeds: Sesame seeds have been shown to influence female hormones and may be particularly useful for women with PCOS.

One of the simplest and most delicious ways to incorporate sesame seeds into your diet is by using organic tahini (sesame seed butter). All you need is 1 to 2 tablespoons at a time; you'll find recipes that include tahini in Part Four.

Pumpkin and Sunflower Seeds: These seeds contain important micronutrients and fatty acids that are beneficial for menstrual health. For example, zinc, which is highest in pumpkin and sesame seeds, may increase the formation of the corpus luteum and support healthy progesterone levels in the second half of the cycle.

See the recipes in Part Four, like Not for the Birds Seed Crackers, Seed Power Bites, Toasty Savory Nuts and Seeds, and Women's Bliss Bites, as well as others, for delicious ways to get more seeds into your diet.

Step 2: First Aid for Your Ovaries

A number of nutrients are critically important for effective mitochondrial functioning, including vitamin C (ascorbic acid), coenzyme Q10, L-arginine, L-carnitine, riboflavin, and alpha-lipoic acid. In my practice, I include these to protect and restore ovarian reserve, improve ovulation and fertility, reverse insulin resistance, and as part of my PCOS care plans. The most compelling studies suggest that a combination of these various supplements might be most effective for optimizing mitochondrial function. Combination products are available on the market. However, those studies have not looked specifically at ovarian function. This group of supplements is considered safe at recommended doses per the National Institutes of Health Office of Dietary Supplements.

Supplementation support is optimal for any woman who is not ovulating, is trying to conceive, is having fertility challenges, or who has PCOS or signs of primary ovarian insufficiency (POI). These are discussed further in specific Advanced Protocols, but again, the nutrients below, whether through the diet, or diet plus supplements, are universally supportive of ovarian health. For doses, see the Botanical and Supplement Quick Reference Guide on pages 372–81.

B Vitamins: You can't make ATP without B vitamins. Riboflavin (B2) is one of the essential nutrients fueling the shuttles that bring energy from your diet (amino acids, glucose, lipids) into your mitochondria, fueling ATP production. **Folic acid / folate** is very important for ovarian health and mitochondrial function. Make sure you're taking a multi with B-complex vitamins, with the methylfolate form so you're able to use it if you have the MTHFR SNP.

Vitamin C (Ascorbic Acid): Your ovaries depend on vitamin C to quell the fires of oxidative stress that are generated in the highly energy-intensive process of maturing your eggs for ovulation and creating the corpus luteum. This is why our ovaries are one of the highest vitamin C concentrated areas in the body. The concentration of ascorbic acid is higher in our ovarian follicular fluid than in our blood. Vitamin C has been associated with reduced ovarian function and infertility and has been shown to improve ovarian function, reduce oxidative stress, and increase progesterone levels.

If you're including the recommended 8 to 10 daily servings of fruits and veggies, you're already increasing vitamin C intake, which has been shown to improve fertility because it's restoring ovarian function and ovulation. However, if you're having low progesterone symptoms (page 34 for a refresher), aren't ovulating, or are having trouble getting pregnant, supplementing is a smart idea. Specifically, 750 mg/day of vitamin C has been shown to increase progesterone in women with both low progesterone and luteal phase dysfunction. In one randomized trial, women were randomly assigned to receive either vitamin C or a placebo. Within three menstrual cycles, the women taking vitamin C had an average increase in progesterone on average from 8 to 13 ng/mL.

Coenzyme Q10 (Ubiquinone): Coenzyme Q10 (also referred to as CoQ10) is a powerful antioxidant that is made by your body and stored in your mitochondria. It plays an essential role in ovarian health and fertility. CoQ10 supplementation has been shown to improve ovarian mitochondrial function, ovarian health, and egg quality. As a result, it's also been shown to improve fertility, IVF, and the health of the embryo and placenta and may prevent preterm labor and preeclampsia. Your body produces CoQ10 naturally, but its production tends to decrease with age and can also be affected by environmental toxins, oxidative stress, and nutritional deficiencies, especially vitamin B6 deficiency. As you age, CoQ10 production slows, making the body less effective at protecting the eggs from oxidative damage. Supplementing with CoQ10 seems to help and may even reverse this age-related decline in egg quality. Low CoQ10 has also been associated with migraines; supplementing has been shown to reduce migraine frequency. Fortunately, you can replenish CoQ10 by getting it from your diet and supplements. Food sources: fish, meats, and whole grains.

L-Arginine: Arginine is an amino acid involved in many metabolic processes. After ovulation, the corpus luteum requires abundant blood flow for luteal function, particularly for importing the large amount of cholesterol needed for progesterone production, and then distributing it through your body. This flow can get blocked, preventing progesterone production and delivery. Additionally, decreased blood flow causes oxidative stress. L-arginine treatment improves luteal function by improving blood flow.

NAC: NAC is the precursor our body uses to make the powerful antioxidant glutathione. It is rapidly depleted when we're exposed to more toxins and oxidative stress than we can keep up with. All the foods, nutrients, and herbs I taught you about in Chapter 9, including NAC and curcumin, that help you to replenish GSH are beneficial for protecting your ovaries from oxidative stress and premature aging and should be a part of your Hormone Intelligence lifestyle.

Melatonin: In addition to its benefits for sleep and circadian rhythm, melatonin is a powerful antioxidant. A certain level of ROS is required for normal ovulation (follicular rupture) and corpus luteal function; it's thought that the purpose of the high volume of melatonin found in the healthy ovaries of women in peak fertility years is to counterbalance this oxidative stress, protecting the corpus luteum—and ovum—from damage. An imbalance of ROS results in oxidative stress and this has been identified as a potential cause of luteal phase defect.

Selenium: Selenium acts as an antioxidant in the ovaries as well as the thyroid, promotes healthy follicles in the ovaries, and because it protects again DNA damage in the oocyte, can help protect against miscarriage and birth defects caused by oxidative stress–related DNA damage.

Step 3: Try Vitex: The Classic Herb for Women

While there are dozens of herbs for women's health, so many that I wrote a textbook on the subject (*Botanical Medicine for Women's Health*), there's one that stands out among them for ovarian support: vitex.

Also known as chasteberry or chaste tree, the use of this herb for "women's conditions" dates back thousands of years. Science has shown us why. It works by restoring signaling between the pituitary and ovaries, by increasing luteinizing hormone (LH) and reducing prolactin. As such, it encourages ovulation, which in turn increases your progesterone levels. It also increases estrogen slightly. It has proven beneficial in reducing PMS symptoms, including mood swings and breast pain, restoring period cyclicity and ovulation, improving fertility, and easing symptoms in perimenopause. Its efficacy in treating many of these symptoms make it one of the most widely used treatments in Germany, where herbal medicine is a standard part of regular medical care.

While symptoms may shift within a matter of weeks, it's typically best to take vitex for a minimum of three months. For dosing, see the Botanical and Supplement Quick Reference Guide on pages 372–81.

In a very small subset of women vitex may cause depressive symptoms. In some women, these clear up after just a few days on the herb; if you feel just mildly blue after starting it, you can push through for a few days and see if symptoms clear; if not or if you experience major depression, this herb is not for you. No fear; just discontinue it. Your mood should clear within a day or so. While cautions about use with fertility treatment due to ovarian

Ovarian Cysts 101

Your ovaries are normally the size of olives, or about 2 to 3 centimeters across. When an ovary gets enlarged, due to an ovarian cyst or cysts, it can be very painful and worrisome to you. An ovarian cyst happens when fluid accumulates within a thin membrane inside the ovary. Most ovarian cysts are small and harmless and usually occur without any symptoms. The size can range from as small as a pea to larger than an orange. Ouch.

The term *cyst* itself may sound alarming, but remember, your ovaries are busily creating cysts every cycle—follicles that then either produce and release an egg (ovulation) or shrink and disappear. Most ovarian cysts that become painful are a result of this process going wonky. These are considered **functional cysts**, and if it just happens once or extremely rarely, they are not a cause for concern or treatment. But if you're getting them regularly, you'll want to consider underlying causes, which can include hypothyroidism (including the subclinical form), PCOS, and endometriosis.

Other types of cysts occur that are also harmless, unless they become so large that they cause severe pain, rupture, or twist (ovarian torsion)—any of which may be an exceptionally painful situation and the latter requires prompt surgical intervention.

Symptoms of an ovarian cyst can include:

- Irregular and possibly painful menstruation
- Pelvic or abdominal pain that can be persistent or intermittent, dull and aching or sharp, and may radiate down the backs of your thighs or into your lower back
- Pain or discomfort during sex or with other pelvic movements (i.e., exercise, yoga)

hyperstimulation can be found on the internet, there is only one case of this reported in 1994 in the medical literature; a woman was undergoing in vitro fertilization (IVF) treatment who showed signs of mild ovarian hyperstimulation.

FertilityBlend: While I don't usually recommend proprietary products in my books, a study looked at a product containing a combination of the herbs and supplements I've mentioned to you, bringing home the potential value of making a few targeted herbs and supplements with good science behind them a part of your personalized Hormone Intelligence Plan, so I wanted to share this with you.

A product called FertilityBlend contains a combination of vitex, green tea, L-arginine, vitamins (including folate), and several minerals. Researchers look at its effects on progesterone level, basal body temperature, menstrual cycle length, pregnancy rate, and side effects. Ninety-three women aged 24 to 42 years, who had tried unsuccessfully to conceive for 6 to 36 months, were divided into two groups. After 3 months, the 53 women in the Fertility-Blend group had increased midluteal phase progesterone levels, increased evidence of an ovulatory rise in BBT, and 14 of the 53 women (26%) were pregnant. Three additional women conceived after 6 months on FB (32%). Little

---

- Abdominal bloating or distention
- Frequent need to urinate
- Pain with bowel movements, new onset of constipation, or a feeling of bowel pressure, especially in conjunction with any of these other symptoms

How are ovarian cysts confirmed/diagnosed? Vaginal ultrasound is the diagnostic technique of choice. It's very safe, doesn't require radiation or surgery, and can be done in the office with your participation by an ob-gyn, family doctor, certified nurse midwife, or nurse practitioner. Sometimes cysts come on suddenly and are so painful women go to the emergency department and get the diagnosis there.

How can ovarian cysts be prevented? Keeping ovulation regular is the best prevention of functional cysts. Mitochondrial support is an important part of this. The plan in this book should prevent and help reverse common ovarian cysts.

How are functional ovarian cysts treated? Watchful waiting, especially with small cysts just a few centimeters in size, is the primary treatment. Surgery is usually only needed if the cyst is large, persistent for three or more months, or growing; if the cyst is persistent, sometimes the Pill can help short term as a way to avoid surgery. Treatment of other types of cysts should be discussed with your care provider.

Could it be cancer? Rarely, a cyst is a symptom of ovarian cancer, though truth be told, and sadly, ovarian cancer symptoms often come in late stages, and currently there is no preventative screening. Therefore, even though most symptomatic ovarian cysts are harmless, if you have persistent symptoms, it's important to get an ultrasound and appropriate follow-up if there is any concern.

change was seen in these parameters in the 40 women in the placebo group, and only 4 of those women conceived.

Step 4: Move for Cellular Health

Overexercising can put a damper on ovarian function, but **high-intensity interval training (HIIT)**, while giving you a great workout, is a win for your ovaries and general health, even keeping your cells younger for longer. A 2017 study published in the journal *Cell Metabolism* found increased mitochondrial function, improved insulin sensitivity, increased muscle tone, and a marked reduction in cellular aging. It's easy to learn and can be done almost anywhere, as long as you are able to support your own weight. If you are wheelchair or bed bound, a personal trainer can show you how to adapt this to your abilities in just one or two sessions, or you can find helpful videos online.

The HIIT Mini Workout, also called the 7-minute Workout, is a series of simple exercises done for 30 seconds each, with a 10-second rest between exercises, with the whole series repeated twice. Ideally, do it daily, or at least four times each week. If you don't have a stool for step-ups, skip that one and double up on a different one. Here are the moves—each done for 30 seconds. You can find the workout online, too.

- Squats
- Lunges
- Plank
- Side plank
- Pushups (you can do a modified version)
- Triceps dip
- Jumping jacks
- Crunches
- Wall sit
- High-knees running
- Chair step-up

And nothing beats walking. Do you need 10,000 steps a day to make a difference? A recent study found that 7,000 is optimal, but even 4,000 steps a day is fantastic for promoting health and preventing chronic disease. Don't have a Fitbit? I don't, either, so I'll translate: if you have an average length stride, you'd cover 4,000 steps on a slow 1.8-mile walk.

Step 5: Phone a Friend

If you recall from Chapter 3 when we talked about cycle sense, progesterone increases your desire to hang out and connect with others, but social closeness also boosts your oxytocin, which in turn ramps up progesterone levels and is good for your ovaries!

get personal

THE HORMONE INTELLIGENCE
ADVANCED NATURAL PROTOCOLS

The Advanced Natural Protocols offer you an "at a glance" selection of the top targeted adjunct therapies you can use to quick start your healing or use as next-level support along with the important, foundational changes presented in the core Hormone Intelligence Plan in Part Two.

These protocols presuppose that you're following those core recommendations, which are therefore not repeated here, with the exception of an occasional key point or added nuance specific to a symptom or condition.

As a quick reminder, refer to these chapters/pages when I mention the following topics:

The Hormone Intelligence Diet (food, diet, nutrients)	Chapter 6 (pages 99–135)
Mind-body, self-care, lifestyle, HPA axis, reducing stress, etc.	Chapter 7 (pages 137–58)
Sleep, circadian rhythm	Chapter 8 (pages 159–82)
Gut health, vaginal microbiome	Chapter 9 (pages 183–204)
Environmental exposures, toxins, detoxification, elimination	Chapter 10 (pages 205–38)
Reducing inflammation, oxidative stress, mitochondrial function, and repairing ovarian function	Chapter 11 (pages 239–52)

As an author, I pour my heart and soul into my books, trying to pass along everything I possibly can, but, alas, one is only allowed to write a book with so many pages! If you're hungry for an even deeper dive into Hormone Intelligence, join me online at avivaromm.com. You'll find additional resources, courses, a membership, and group programs that include community connection with support from me and my wonderful women's health team.

Herb and Supplements Doses

For your convenience, all herb and supplement doses in Part Three are listed in the Botanical and Supplements Quick Reference Guide, starting on page 372.

period and pms
ADVANCED PROTOCOL

If your periods have your panties—and your uterus—in a twist each month, if you struggle with heavy or irregular periods, you're not ovulating, or you have cyclic breast pain, acne, or headaches, and you want to get a head start on treating these while you're just starting the Hormone Intelligence Plan, or if you're well into the plan but period symptoms are still raining on your parade now and then, you'll find extra help in this section.

While the Hormone Intelligence Plan will address the core imbalances leading to these symptoms, the Advanced Protocol gives you additional supportive tools, nutrients, and herbs you can use for symptom relief and to augment healing the root causes, while the core plan has a chance to do its work. Remember, period pain can also be due to an underlying gynecologic condition, most commonly endometriosis or adenomyosis, so these conditions need to be taken care of directly as well. See those relevant sections of the book too, but these remedies can still help for symptoms that show up around your period.

All herb and supplement doses are listed in the
Botanical and Supplements Quick Reference Guide, starting on page 372.

Menstrual Cramps and Period Pain

If you're just starting the core plan and period cramps are raining on your parade, or you need to ease the occasional crampy period, these recommendations can make your cycles much more comfortable. If you struggle with severe menstrual cramps follow this protocol along with the Hormone Intelligence Plan in Part 2 to amplify your success.

Lifestyle

- Low-level **heat** from a heating pad or hot water bottle applied to your lower belly or lower back is as effective as ibuprofen for menstrual cramps.

- Scent up your room, a hot shower, or warm bath with diffused lavender, clary sage, and rose **aromatherapy oils** to improve period pain and promote relaxation.

- **Aromatherapy abdominal massage** or Arvigo massage can also ease period pain.

- **Switching from tampons to pads** brings huge relief from menstrual cramps for many women.

- **Exercise** can prevent and reverse period pain and depression and boost your mood.

- **Yoga** can relieve menstrual discomfort severity and duration, balance hormones, and reduce stress, depression, and anxiety. See Yoga for an Easier Period (below).

- **Go for the Big O** (orgasms, alone or with a partner) to relieve pelvic discomfort and period pain.

Food

As part of the Hormone Intelligence Diet:

- **Emphasize plant-based** meals.

- **Eliminate red meat** or eat only sparingly if needed for iron during or after your period.

- **Eat omega-3-rich fish** up to three times per week.

- **Try going vegan** even for just two cycles to dramatically reduce menstrual cramps.

Mind-Body

- Better **sleep** can reduce period pain—and your ability to cope with it.

- Hit **pause more often,** building in time for period self-care and honoring your **cycle sense** (page 51).

Nutrients

- **Fish oil** taken daily reduces the need for ibuprofen in as short as three months.

- Lower **calcium levels** are linked to period pain; take calcium daily to reduce pain in 3 menstrual cycles.

- **Magnesium** taken for 5 days before and the first 3 days of your period may reduce menstrual cramps and low back and leg aches.

- Include **vitamin D3** daily.

- **Thiamine (vitamin B1)**, taken daily over 3 months, may improve even severe menstrual pain.

Herbs

- **Gingerroot** can reduce period pain, nausea, bloating, and headaches. Try tincture or capsules. Enjoy **WomanWise (Better Than Ibuprofen) Carrot-Apple-Ginger Juice** throughout the month (page 370).

- **Motherwort and cramp bark** reduce cramps and pain. Take just before and during your flow.

- **Peppermint oil** relieves cramps and pain. Try 3 peppermint oil capsules daily (187 mg each) on your first few flow days.

- **Cannabis tincture or CBD oil** may reduce period pain and anxiety. Take daily for 5 days before and through the first 3 days of your flow.

Conventional Approach

- **NSAIDs** (page 203) are generally safe and effective when used for a couple of days a month. For best effects start at the first hint of cramps.

- **The Pill** and other hormonal contraception (the NuvaRing, IUD with hormones) are commonly prescribed but are less effective for period pain than NSAIDs and have more side effects (page 244).

Yoga for an Easier Period

- **Cat and Cow**
  Get down onto all fours. With a deep, slow exhale, drop your belly toward the ground, gently stretching your lower back and lower abdomen. Next, with a deep, slow inhale, arch your back, tucking your tailbone under, elongating your lower spine. Repeat eight times, rhythmically inhaling and exhaling with each movement.

- **Expanded Child's Pose**
  Walk your hands forward toward the front of your yoga mat, bringing your chest and belly toward the ground, widening your knees, and dropping your hips toward the floor. Feel a delicious stretch in your hips and lower back.

- **Open-Hearted Pose**
  Place a pillow toward the upper third of your mat and lie on your back so that the lower part of the pillow lands just below your shoulder blades, and your head and neck are extended, draping off the top. Place the heels of your feet together, letting your knees drop to each side. A rolled towel or bolster can be placed under your knees for extra support. Lie in this position as you transition into the next optional practice.

- **Resting Goddess**
  Remove the pillow from under your back, but keep your legs in the same position. Lie here for 3 to 10 minutes, breathing deeply and slowly.

The Luna Yoga Flow

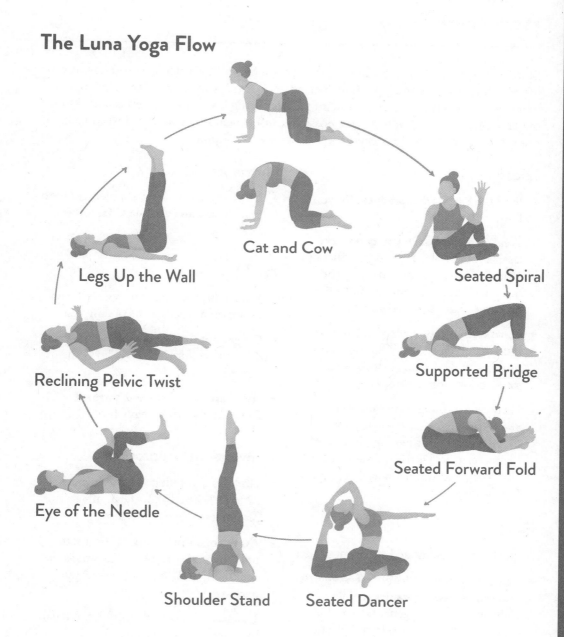

Cat and Cow

Seated Spiral

Supported Bridge

Seated Forward Fold

Seated Dancer

Shoulder Stand

Eye of the Needle

Reclining Pelvic Twist

Legs Up the Wall

Heavy Periods

Blowing through a box of tampons each cycle, a heavy flow getting in the way of your life each month, or stressing about "period accidents" is miserable. The Hormone Intelligence Plan can turn this around for you, reducing high estrogen levels and skipped ovulation, and helping you reverse possible causes including endometriosis, PCOS, or even slow thyroid function. These steps provide extra support.

Lifestyle

- Find the **best period products** for your flow.

- Wear **dark clothes** so you can worry less; if you do bleed through, a fuck-it attitude is the best one to have. The more we claim bleeding as natural, the more we change period stigma.

- Have **sex**. I know that sounds messy but it can reduce heavy flow amount, number of days, and cramps. Solo satisfaction works, too.

- Heavy periods can cause **low iron and anemia**. If you have symptoms (page 53), get your hemoglobin, hematocrit, and ferritin tested, enrich your diet, and supplement if necessary (see below).

Food

As part of the Hormone Intelligence Diet:

- Get plenty of **fiber, leafy green veggies, and fermented vegetables** to help reduce excess estrogen, and avoid exposures through dairy and plastic food packaging.

- Add **iron-rich foods**, including red meat, dark meat poultry, or vegetarian options such as dried apricots, leafy greens, lentils, and raisins.

Nutrients

- If you are low in iron, supplement with **iron chelate and vitamin C (ascorbic acid)**.

Herbs

- **Vitex (chasteberry):** can reduce heavy flow over a few months of daily use.

- **Gingerroot** or **Cinnamon Bark Powder:** 3 times/day for the first 3 days of your period.

- **Red Raspberry Leaf and Yarrow Tea:** 2 cups/day during heavy flow.

Conventional Approach

- **NSAIDs** can reduce heavy flow by 22 to 50%; used short term, it's a reasonable stopgap measure.

- An estrogen-progestin, or progestin-only form of **the Pill**, or the **progestin-containing IUD** may reduce heavy periods.

- **Tranexamic acid** can be used, but it can have serious side effects.

- **Endometrial ablation** and **hysterectomy** are options but carry risks.

Missed Periods and Skipped Ovulation

Most women skip a period once in a while due to travel, stress, or illness. But skipping three or more periods in a row or menstruating fewer than eight times a year suggests that you're not ovulating (page 69). In this section we'll focus on one of the most common causes: **hypothalamic amenorrhea.**

For skipped periods due to **primary ovarian insufficiency (POI)** (page 83), see Chapter 11. If you have **PCOS**, the PCOS Advanced Protocol should get ovulation and your period on track. If you suspect **a thyroid problem**, seek appropriate testing and treatment (page 145).

Lifestyle

- **Lighten up on exercise** by 5 to 15% or increase your nutritional intake to meet your body's caloric needs. It may take up to 6 months, but this can bring back a regular period.

Food

As part of the Hormone Intelligence Diet:

- Make sure to **eat enough**, especially healthy carbohydrates (page 119) and ample healthy fats (page 118).

Mind-Body

- **Unwind stress** and nourish your nervous system using self-care tools from Chapter 7.

- **Cognitive behavioral therapy (CBT)** may help to restore ovulatory cycles.

Nutrients

- **Vitamin B6** supports ovulation, progesterone production, luteal phase length, cycle regularity, and fertility.

- **Ascorbic acid (vitamin C)** promotes ovulation; used in skipped periods and low progesterone due to anovulation.

Herbs

- **Vitex (chasteberry)** can restore ovulation and improve progesterone and estrogen levels and cycling in as short as 3 months of daily use.

- **Flaxseeds** support regular ovulation, lengthen the luteal phase, and increase progesterone production.

Conventional Approach

- **Use a dietary approach** to achieve a healthy weight.

- **Identify and treat underlying medical causes.**

- **Implement a progesterone challenge** to bring on your period if needed; the Pill is also commonly recommended.

Premenstrual Syndrome (PMS)

PMS and PMDD (premenstrual dysphoric disorder) symptoms may resolve in one to four cycles when you hit on the right combination of dietary, mind-body, and supplement therapies for your needs. If you experience severe depression or anxiety, or any thoughts of self-harm, it's critical to seek appropriate medical support.

Lifestyle

- Preempt PMS with **extra self-care** the week before symptoms start (page 51).

- **Aerobic exercise**, 60 minutes, 3 times weekly, for 8 weeks can prevent PMS. Brisk walking counts.

- **Light therapy** is easy to do at home in a sunny window or with a light box, once or twice daily for even severe PMS and PMDD.

- **Get your thyroid checked** as hypothyroidism (page 145) may affect a large proportion of women with PMS; proper treatment can completely relieve symptoms.

- **Quit the cigs.** Smoking can cause PMS.

Food

As part of the Hormone Intelligence Diet:

- Increase intake of **omega-3-rich fish** (page 116) to 3 times weekly.

- Take 2 tbsp. of fresh ground **flaxseeds** daily.

- Low iron can cause PMS; bump up your diet with **iron-rich foods**, including red meat, dark meat poultry, or vegetarian options like dried apricots, leafy greens, lentils, and raisins.

- Eat more **complex carbs** during your luteal phase.

- **Dark chocolate** can improve mood and prevent depression.

- **Sugar, fast carbs, dairy, excess salt, and alcohol** all worsen PMS.

Mind-Body

- **Yoga and meditation** can prevent and reduce even severe PMS.

- **Reset your HPA axis** to reduce premenstrual distress and burnout and improve mood and coping.

- **Cognitive behavioral therapy (CBT)** has been shown to help reduce PMS.

Nutrients

- **Calcium** can reduce PMS headaches, pain, moodiness, and food cravings by as much as 50%.

- **Vitamin B6** alone or combined with calcium is a must for PMS.

- **Myoinositol** can be effective in preventing PMS mood symptoms.

- Try **krill oil** supplementation for 3 months.

- **Zinc, magnesium, and vitamin D3** can help prevent physical and emotional PMS symptoms.

Herbs

- **Vitex (chasteberry)** may be even more effective than fluoxetine (an SSRI medication) for the physical symptoms of PMS.

- In one study, 76% of subjects taking **saffron** experienced more than a 50% reduction in PMS symptoms.

- Take **curcumin** for a week before and into the first 3 days of your period, for relief of mood and physical symptoms in just 3 months.

- **Adaptogens** (page 156) can play an important role in healing PMS.

Conventional Approach

- **SSRIs** can help, used daily or on an intermittent schedule for as little as 10 days monthly during your luteal phase. They do have potential side effects to discuss with your provider.

Adama, 34

"Dr. Aviva, my PMS is awful. For almost a week before my period, every single month, I'm exhausted, moody, and depressed. My breasts hurt and I'm so tired. I also have heavy periods. I bark at my wife, I'm irritated by our kids—and am impatient with my customers. I crave sugar like crazy and before the end of my workday I'm already thinking about that bottle of red wine waiting for me at home. Once my period comes, I feel a little better for a few weeks. I get my workouts back on track and I eat better, but the fatigue just doesn't go away completely. Plus I get recurrent yeast infections."

Based on Adama's story and symptoms, I suggested we order basic lab work. She was low in vitamin D, iron, and B6. We began the Hormone Intelligence Diet, adding in nutrients and herbs for PMS support and for heavy periods, while doing the core plan with an emphasis on restoring her gut and vaginal ecology.

In just weeks she was gas, bloating, and constipation free, and in three months her PMS was, according to her report, 80% better—no more cravings and only mild mood shifts, but she learned that this was a sign to bump up her self-care. She also gained mastery over which foods she could eat freely, and which she was more sensitive to, and emphasized her feel-good foods in her diet. It's been years since she's had a yeast infection, and now she looks forward to the introspective, quiet time she's carved out for herself just before her period.

Cyclic Breast Tenderness

If your breasts are so achy and swollen the week before your period that you sometimes can't put on your bra—you're not alone. Millions of women experience monthly breast pain that interferes with sex, work, or school. Cyclic breast pain is a PMS symptom, so anything that helps relieve PMS (pages 264–65) may also help your "ladies" feel better. High estrogen levels are another trigger in some women. The recommendations in this section address both. You can expect to see moderate improvements in two cycles, significant improvements or complete resolution in as quickly as two to four cycles.

Lifestyle

- Wear a **properly fitting bra**; most women don't. It's so worth it.

- Take stock of **medications** that can cause breast pain: hormonal contraceptives, hormone replacement therapy (HRT), and some antidepressants.

- Apply a **heating pad** or hot water bottle.

- Eight weeks of **aerobic exercise**, 3 times weekly, for 60 minutes each time, can help reduce cyclic breast tenderness due to fluid retention.

Food

As part of the Hormone Intelligence Diet:

- Eat your **greens**—kale, collards, broccoli, Brussels sprouts, and broccoli sprouts contain compounds (page 232) that reduce and eliminate excess estrogen.

- Eat 2 tbsp. ground **flaxseeds** daily.

- **Ditch alcohol.**

- **Less coffee** = happier boobs.

Nutrients

- Try **krill oil** for 8 days each month before your period is due. Expect results in about 8 weeks.

- Take a multivitamin containing **iodine**.

- **Diindolylmethane (DIM)** derived from a compound in broccoli, kale, and cauliflower improves estrogen metabolism and cyclic breast tenderness.

Herbs

- Take **Vitex (chasteberry)** daily; expect effects in 1 to 3 cycles.

- Take **chamomile tincture** daily from the week after ovulation to the start of your period.

- **Ginkgo**, twice daily throughout the month, reduces breast pain associated with fluid retention. Expect results in 2 cycles.

Conventional Approach

- **SSRIs**, the most effective of the conventional PMS therapies, improve cyclic mastalgia as well.

Bloating

Premenstrual and period bloating can be due to prostaglandins affecting your digestive system or to hormonally triggered water retention. It's also a PMS symptom, so the recommendations under PMS are helpful (pages 264–65). If you generally have gas and bloating, or other digestive symptoms, prioritize gut healing.

Lifestyle

- **Aerobic exercise** for 8 weeks, 3 times weekly, for 60 minutes each time, improves PMS fluid retention and related bloating.

- **Constipation** a problem? See pages 199–200.

Food

As part of the Hormone Intelligence Diet for 3 days before your period:

- **Reduce salt and carbonated beverages.**

- Emphasize **potassium-rich foods** that reduce water retention: spinach, bananas, avocados, winter squash, lentils, raisins, baked russet potato, dried apricots and prunes, salmon, and kidney beans.

- Other **foods with natural diuretic properties**: asparagus, celery, cucumber, garlic, leeks, watermelon, and green tea.

- If gas is a problem, try a **low FODMAPs diet plan** (at www .avivaromm.com) for 3 to 5 days before your period.

Mind-Body

- We're conditioned to think a flat belly is sexy, so premenstrual belly bloating can be a big emotional or mental trigger. Practice **soft belly breathing** (page 194) to send your belly some healing, loving energy.

Herbs

- Sip **ginger tea**, 1 or 2 cups daily, for a few days prior to and during your period.

- Use **herbs for IBS** (page 202).

Conventional Approach

- The **same as for PMS**.

- **Pharmaceutical diuretics are not recommended** for water retention.

Marietta, 36

Marietta was tired of dealing with chronic gas, bloating, constipation, and recurrent yeast infections. She dreaded her period every month, when out-of-control rages turned her into someone even she didn't want to be around, and cramps had her popping ibuprofen! Then there were the sugar cravings, which she satisfied with anything she could get her hands on, and a couple of glasses of wine too many. Her eczema always flared before her period, making her itchy and irritable. She was often tired and her job as a nurse in a busy emergency department often left her stressed and depleted, and skipping meals in favor of sugary treats at the nurses' station. Her doctor diagnosed her with IBS and PMS, suggested an antidepressant, and gave her a prescription for the yeast infections. But she was tired of the endless loop of misery each month and found her way to my practice.

We uncovered that certain foods made her more bloated and tired, especially sugar. Digging deeper, I not only learned about the many stressors affecting her, but also about her long history of antibiotic use in her early twenties for urinary tract infections. So what did we do? We went to work nourishing Marietta's gut microbiome to health, along with adding in calcium, vitamin D, and magnesium, an herbal combination to help with her sleep, and recipes for easy meals she could bring to work and enjoy. Within a few months not only was her period pain resolved, but she stopped having eczema flares, her moods leveled out, her digestion was great, and she no longer hated her cycles—because they weren't making her miserable!

Hormonal Acne

Acne doesn't just affect teens; it affects about half of women between twenty and forty, 25% of women in their forties, and over 80% of all women experience a premenstrual flare. They're common in perimenopause, too. The two most common types of hormonal acne are cyclic or PCOS-related. You can have both types, and PCOS acne may also flare before your period.

Acne can take a toll on your mental well-being, so let's break that cycle—and start to heal your acne from the inside out by restoring hormone balance. It can take several months to see results, so be patient, and consider a combination of these natural approaches with a topical conventional approach for best results.

Lifestyle

- **Keep skin care simple.** Rinse with water and a gentle natural skin cleanser. Go minimalist with your cosmetics. I know this might be hard if you feel you need to cover your skin, but it can help.

- **Avoid exfoliating scrubs, abrasive cleansers, and antimicrobial soaps** that can damage the skin and its flora.

- Dry skin is more acne prone, so if you need it, **use a light, clean gentle moisturizer.**

- **Don't scrub, pop, or pick at pimples.**

- **Keep your hair clean and off your face** with a ponytail or headband.

- Bloating and constipation are 37% more likely with acne; so **heal your gut.**

- **Smoking is linked to acne** in women.

- **Treat PCOS** if you have it.

Food

As part of the Hormone Intelligence Diet:

- **Low intake of fruits, vegetables, and fish** is associated with a higher risk of acne—so bump it up.

- Keep **blood sugar and insulin steady.**

- **Avoid empty carbs** and refined sugar—they can worsen acne.

- **Skip dairy products** to avoid growth factors and hormones.

Mind-Body

- **Know you are beautiful.** Don't let the culture get into your head.

- **Get the emotional/psychological support** you deserve if needed.

- **Reduce stress** to break any vicious acne-stress-acne cycle.

Nutrients

- Low selenium, vitamin A, vitamin D, vitamin E, and zinc have been associated with acne and acne severity. **Take a multivitamin + vitamin D daily.**

- **Use a probiotic** with *Lactobacillus rhamnosus* GG (3 billion CFUs/day) for 12 weeks.

- **Take vitamin B6** to reduce cyclic and PCOS-related acne by reducing testosterone.

Herbs

- Daily use of **milk thistle and other bitters** (page 234) for 8 weeks in one study led to up to a 53% decrease.

- Mix 2 drops of a 5% solution of **tea tree oil** in a tsp. of coconut, avocado, or grapeseed oil and apply a dab as "spot treatment."

Conventional Approach

- **Topical retinoids** can dramatically improve acne, are generally safe, and can be used as needed. Drying occurs if overused.

- **Azelaic acid and benzoyl peroxide** are safe topical options.

- **Antibiotics** can reduce inflammatory acne but can damage your microbiome and lead to antibiotic resistance.

- The Pill can reduce androgen production, which controls sebum production. Use only a **low-androgen prescription** if you have PCOS or experience acne from the Pill.

Hormonal Migraines

Hormonal migraines are related to sharp declines in estrogen that occur in our cycles, triggering changes in serotonin and endorphins that affect our pain levels and our pain perception. They are also common after pregnancy (including after miscarriage or abortion), during perimenopause, and when coming off hormonal therapies (the Pill, on "placebo Pill" days, HRT). Hormone imbalances, lack of key nutrients, and other factors such as use of pain medication can trigger or worsen hormonal headaches.

Lifestyle

- Keep a **migraine journal**, noting when migraines occur and any related **triggers**: caffeine, red wine, alcohol, aged cheese, sugar, nitrites (found in hot dogs and deli meats), food additives, low blood sugar, stress, neck and shoulder tension, allergies leading to sinus congestion, medications, perfume odors.

- As you identify them, **remove triggers** and see if this makes a difference over weeks to months.

- Headache, pain, and migraine medications can cause medication overuse headache (MOH). As crazy as this might seem, **stopping all these medications** can reduce or eliminate migraines.

- If you're coming off the Pill or other hormonal therapies, **follow the post-Pill plan** on page 222. Give your hormones 6 to 12 weeks to adjust.

Food

As part of the Hormone Intelligence Diet:

- **Avoid migraine-triggering foods** (above).

- **Keep your blood sugar steady.**

- **Stay hydrated.**

- **Increase your intake of complex carbohydrates** (page 119) before your period to keep serotonin levels steady as estrogen drops.

Mind-Body

- **De-stress** with meditation or other relaxation techniques.

- Get **enough sleep**.

- Consider a **different pillow or mattress**.

- Get **massage or physical therapy** for neck tension.

Nutrients

- **Riboflavin (vitamin B2)**, daily, prevents migraines by as much as 50%. It may take a month for results.

- **Vitamin B6** (25 mg), **vitamin B12** (400 mcg), and **folic acid** (2 mg) reduced migraine-related impairment in 50% of migraine sufferers after 6 months of daily use.

- 500 mg daily of **calcium** may prevent and reduce premenstrual migraines by as much as 50%.

Herbs

- **Ginger** can nip migraine pain in the bud, even compared against sumatriptan.

- **Curcumin** may reduce frequency, severity, and duration, especially when taken with CoQ10 or omega-3 fatty acids.

- **Butterbur** (petasites), preventatively, reduces migraine frequency.

- **Feverfew,** a natural anti-inflammatory, prevents migraines and reduces severity.

- Apply 2 to 3 drops of **lavender or peppermint essential oil** "neat" or slightly diluted for relief within 30 minutes of migraine onset. Repeat as needed.

Conventional Approach

Only half of migraine sufferers achieve prevention with migraine medications, which also have side effects, including MOH.

- **NSAIDs** can be effective but can damage the gut and affect ovulation (see page 203).

- Abortive therapies, **medications that prevent migraines** when taken daily or at the earliest symptom, combined with NSAIDs, antinausea agents, and so on, can be used for when the migraine occurs anyway.

- **Hormonal contraceptive pills** are sometimes recommended but have risks and are contraindicated for increased risk of stroke if you have migraine with aura.

polycystic ovary syndrome (pcos)

ADVANCED PROTOCOL

The best treatment for PCOS focuses on the root problem with a total ecology approach for reducing inflammation, which you're doing by restoring blood sugar balance and insulin sensitivity, reducing stress and nourishing your HPA axis, optimizing your sleep, supporting gut health, reducing your environmental hormone exposures, and supporting your body's natural detox pathways. In short, the whole Hormone Intelligence Plan is perfectly designed to help you reverse PCOS. In this chapter you'll find the advanced protocols that, in addition to the core plan, will help you to not only reverse the root causes of PCOS but also start to fast-track improvements.

Give three to twelve months for a return to cycle regularity, regular ovulation and fertility, and improvement in androgenic hair loss. Hang in there—this plan can be life-changing.

All herb and supplement doses are listed in the
Botanical and Supplements Quick Reference Guide, starting on page 372.

Lifestyle

- Vitamin D deficiency, thyroid problems, and blood sugar problems are more common with PCOS so **get properly tested** for these and other risks like cardiovascular disease, sleep apnea (page 167), and depression screening.

- **Rev up brown fat.** Your body has 2 main types of fat: brown adipose tissue (BAT) and white adipose tissue (WAT). BAT is far more metabolically active, burning calories even while you're at rest, and women with PCOS seem to have less, which may explain why many have trouble losing weight and why lean women with PCOS tend to burn protein instead of fat while they're sleeping. Increasing BAT may shift this. Here are some ways to increase BAT:

  - **HIIT training, circuit training, or biking:** Engage in any of these activities for an hour a day, 4 times weekly. This can improve insulin sensitivity, reduce inflammation, and reset your hormones in just 6 months, including restoring ovulation and improving natural fertility and conception. Keep in mind that *overexercise* is a stressor that can worsen PCOS, so don't push beyond this sweet spot and listen to your body.

  - **Cold showers:** Dial your shower down to cool-to-cold and enjoy the "cold plunge" for 30 seconds to a minute before you get out.

  - **Sleep:** Brown fat activity increases when we're sleeping; get 7 to 8 hours a night to sleep your way to hormone balance!

  - **A healthy thyroid:** T3 (page 193) stimulates brown fat production. If T3 is low, starting thyroid hormone may help you get a handle on your PCOS.

- If your BMI is over 25, **reducing body fat by 5 to 7%** over a 6-month period can lower insulin and androgen levels. In one study, women with PCOS who lost an average of 13.9 pounds (6.3 kg) dropped their fasting insulin and testosterone levels, and 92% resumed ovulation, while 85% of those trying to conceive became pregnant.

Food

As part of the Hormone Intelligence Diet:

- **Balancing your blood sugar** reduces inflammation and reverses the insulin resistance often driving PCOS, leading to reductions in androgens and related symptoms.

- Even **a modest reduction in fast carbohydrates while increasing protein and healthy fats**, without even losing weight, decreases testosterone, improves insulin sensitivity, and reduces symptoms.

- Emphasize **buckwheat** in your diet—it's technically a seed not a grain, but cooks up like a tasty nutty flavored grain, and may be especially helpful in improving blood sugar balance and reducing insulin resistance. Enjoy the buckwheat recipes in Part Four, and that are included in the Hormone Intelligence menus.

- **Omega-3-rich fish** (page 116) 3 times weekly also reduces insulin resistance and inflammation.

- Add 2 tbsp. of **flaxseed** to your daily diet to lengthen your luteal phase, improve ovulation, and reduce testosterone levels.

- **Sesame seeds** are also a great addition for PCOS; they can reduce elevated androgen levels by improving DHEA-S and SHBG (sex-hormone-binding globulin) levels.

- **Legumes** (garbanzo beans, kidney beans, and non-GMO organic soy) are a rich source of inositol, which I discuss below; enjoy them several times a week.

Mind-Body

- **Support your HPA axis.** Elevated stress hormones make women with PCOS more susceptible to overwhelm, anxiety, depression, and chronic "fight or flight" symptoms.

- **Be patient with yourself.** Women with PCOS + insulin resistance have the opposite brain response to high-calorie, high-carbohydrate meals and foods: rather than triggering satiety in your brain, your brain becomes hyperactive and makes you crave even more sugar and carbs! Not fair, I know! What can you do? Balanced blood sugar can help reset these neurochemical pathways and give you more control over your food choices.

- **Make good sleep a priority**, and consider getting tested for sleep apnea (page 167) if you're exhausted during the day, can't lose weight, or have high blood pressure along with PCOS.

- **Don't go it alone.** Struggling with PCOS can be tough. Connect with women locally or in online groups who understand what you're going through, and work with a therapist if you need extra personal support. You deserve to feel happy and supported!

Nutrients

Insulin resistance and hormone balance:

- **Inositol** is a must for most women with PCOS. It reduces insulin resistance, testosterone, and AMH levels, restores ovulation, and improves fertility, egg quality, and pregnancy rates. It's also helpful for anxiety. Use a combination product containing myoinositol and d-chiro-inositol for maximum benefit.

- **Vitamin D deficiency** is tied to PCOS and symptom severity. Supplementing improves ovarian reserves, AMH levels, ovarian follicle health, and fertility, even if one isn't vitamin D deficient.

- **Omega-3 fatty acids**, taken for 2 to 6 months, can reduce testosterone levels and unwanted hair growth and improve insulin sensitivity, menstrual regularity, and weight loss.

- **N-acetyl-cysteine (NAC)**, in one study, was found to be comparable to metformin in lowering insulin and androgens and improving menstrual regularity.

- **Selenium** taken daily for at least 8 weeks can have beneficial effects on insulin metabolism in women with PCOS.

Ovulation and Fertility Support

- **L-carnitine** improves ovulation rates even in women in whom Clomid has failed to stimulate ovulation, and a combination of Clomid and L-carnitine outperforms either alone in inducing ovulating and increasing conception rate.

- In women with PCOS, 2 mg of **melatonin** daily for 6 months decreased testosterone levels and reduced menstrual irregularities.

- **Alpha-lipoic acid (ALA)** may improve insulin sensitivity, decrease waist circumference, and reduce inflammation.

Hair Loss with PCOS

- **Zinc and green tea extract** may reduce 5-reductase and improve hair loss. They're also effective for depression, even when medications haven't worked.

- **Reishi mushroom** also inhibits 5-alpha reductase and may be used for hair loss.

Herbs

Hormone balance / ovulation support:

- **White peony** reduces testosterone through its action on the aromatase enzyme in the ovaries, increases progesterone, and regulates estrogen and prolactin. The combination of white peony and licorice has been found to improve ovulation and fertility in PCOS.

- **Maitake mushroom**, an adaptogen, may also induce ovulation in PCOS, alone or as an adjunct to clomiphene citrate if you're trying to conceive.

- Two cups of **spearmint tea** daily for even just 30 days may lower testosterone levels and reduce hirsutism with PCOS.

- **Vitex (chasteberry)** reduces elevated prolactin, lengthens the luteal phase, and increases progesterone and pregnancy rates. It theoretically may exacerbate hormonal imbalance in women with high LH, so discontinue if there's any symptom increase, though this is uncommon.

Blood Sugar Balance

- **Adaptogens** like ashwagandha, holy basil, reishi mushroom, and maitake mushroom help reduce stress and cortisol, improve blood sugar metabolism, and reduce insulin resistance. A must with PCOS.

- **Berberine**, an extract from goldenseal and related herbs, is used to improve blood sugar and cholesterol. In the first study to look at its impact on PCOS, women taking 400 mg 3 times daily for 4 months had improvements in menstrual cycle regularity and ovulation.

Conventional Approach

If you don't see any changes in 6 months or your periods have been AWOL for more than 6 months, conventional therapies may be needed.

- **Oral contraceptives** are the first-line treatment for hyperandrogenism and menstrual cycle irregularities in women with PCOS. Must be low in progestins so they don't cause/worsen androgenic hair loss.

- **Metformin** increases insulin sensitivity, reduces androgen levels, and induces ovulation; commonly used as an "off label" treatment. Studies show contradictory results.

- **Antiandrogenic agents** (i.e., Aldactone) are used for symptoms such as acne and hirsutism. Study results are mixed; may be helpful for hair loss.

- **Estrogen agonist-antagonist medication** (i.e., Clomid) induces ovulation for women trying to conceive; it has a significant side effect profile, including ovarian hyperstimulation syndrome. Concurrent use of myoinositol may reduce this complication.

- **Gonadotropins** are used to induce ovulation.

endometriosis
ADVANCED PROTOCOL

The experience of living with endometriosis can be so overwhelming that it's no wonder so many women with it also struggle with depression and hopelessness. Even if your symptoms are mild, you may fear that over time, they'll become severe (good news, often that's not the case at all—not all endometriosis progresses!). If you have symptoms but no diagnosis, you may be feeling incredibly anxious about what's going on in your body—as well as terribly frustrated if one doctor's appointment after another hasn't gotten you closer to meaningful answers or help. The Hormone Intelligence Plan explains the many factors that lead to this complex condition—and gets to the root causes that can turn it around.

This protocol will provide you with a next-level range of nonpharmaceutical and nonsurgical options that you might not have heard of, that your medical provider likely doesn't know about, and that can be used as alternatives or adjuncts to your medical therapies, ideally putting endometriosis into remission, including a reduction in endometrial implants. Physical therapies can also improve pain from adhesions. These approaches can also be helpful if you struggle with chronic pelvic pain (CPP) due to chronic inflammation. Be patient; give three to twelve months to see dramatic improvement.

All herb and supplement doses are listed in the
Botanical and Supplements Quick Reference Guide, starting on page 372.

Lifestyle

- Redouble your efforts to **eliminate plastics, pesticides and herbicides, and hidden ingredients** in household and body products.

- **Emphasize the plan for gut health** to reduce higher levels of gram-negative bacteria in your pelvic fluids that produce an inflammatory toxin, lipopolysaccharide (LPS), involved in endometriosis and CPP.

- Recurrent vaginal infection doubles the risk of endometriosis and increases CPP. **Heal your vaginal ecology** as a key part of reducing "endo."

- **Calm your immune response** and inflammation to reverse lesions and pain.

- **Break up adhesions** with Arvigo massage or pelvic floor physical therapy.

- Try the **OhNut** if sex hurts. This wearable device fits on the penis or a sex toy and allows you to control and customize penetration depth, increasing your comfort and allowing you to enjoy sex.

Food

As part of the Hormone Intelligence Diet:

- **Reduce red meat, eat omega-3-rich fish** 3 times per week, and **consider going vegan** one day each week.

- Get a daily serving of **berries**, rich in resveratrol, which may help to "starve out" blood flow to endometrial lesions.

- Eat **citrus**. Women eating one or more servings of citrus daily, in one study, had a 22% lower endometriosis risk.

- Enjoy **WomanWise (Better Than Ibuprofen) Carrot-Apple-Ginger Juice** (page 370) to reduce inflammation throughout the month.

- A **gluten-free diet** for a year led to relief of 75% of symptoms in women with endometriosis. A small sacrifice for potentially impressive results!

- A **low FODMAPs diet** (at www .avivaromm.com) may provide relief if you also have IBS. It's restrictive, so I only recommend it if you're symptomatic after 3 months on this plan. But you can go FODMAP "lite" now. Avoid these foods, a few of which are in this book, but are easy to omit or swap out for other recipes: legumes, onions, cauliflower, apples, pears, stone fruit (i.e., peaches), watermelon, and prunes.

Mind-Body

- **Empowerment** improves success in treating endo, from getting a diagnosis to taking charge of your care. See Chapter 5 to become the CEO of your health.

- **Doctor shop** (page 89) if your doctor doesn't take your symptoms seriously. It's not all in your head.

- Endo can cause depression and anxiety for many reasons. Give yourself the gift of support through **friends, a support network, or professionally.**

- **Track your symptoms** to identify triggers and when in your cycle pain days occur so you can anticipate them and plan ahead whenever possible.

- Endo and CPP are tough! **Be gentle with yourself.**

- Strive for **better sleep and less stress.** Pain is exhausting. But fatigue and stress worsen pain and our ability to cope with it.

- **Hypnotherapy and self-hypnosis** can help with pain.

- **Massage, myofascial release work, and pelvic floor therapy** can all help to relieve chronic pain.

- In a study conducted at Harvard Medical School, 4 weeks of **acupuncture** led to 62% less pain compared in women with confirmed endometriosis versus the control group.

- While it's tempting to take up residence on your sofa, **gentle, regular movement** is beneficial for pelvic and endometriosis pain. **Luna yoga** (page 261) is great, and consider **belly dancing**, an ancient practice to help women with pelvic pain and facilitate childbirth.

Nutrients

- **Take a multivitamin.** Endometriosis is associated with low zinc, vitamin C (ascorbic acid), vitamin E, and selenium; the lower the levels, the worse the severity.

- **B-vitamins** can help with methylation (page 236) and healthy estrogen levels.

- **Use omega-3 fatty acids.** In one study, women were able to decrease pain medication after just 3 months of omega-3 use. Use 2 to 3 g of combined EPA/DHA, daily.

- **N-acetyl cysteine (NAC)** has been shown to reduce endometriosis lesions, including on the ovaries, enough to cancel surgery, and may improve pregnancy rates.

- **Melatonin**, 10 mg daily, significantly reduced chronic pelvic pain due to endometriosis, with an 80% reduction in need for pain medication. In animal studies, it's led to regression of endometriosis tissue.

- A **daily probiotic** containing *Lactobacillus gasseri* (10 billion CFUs), in one study, led to significant reduction in pain in just 12 weeks.

Abdominal Self-Massage Feels So Good!

1. Lie in a comfy place in a warm room.

2. Warm your hands and apply lavender, rose, or clary sage massage oil.

3. Place your palms down on either side of your navel, and begin taking slow deep breaths into your belly.

4. Now with your hands gently on your belly—or for extra pressure, with one hand on top of the other—use the pads of your fingers to massage in a clockwise direction, in a spiral starting at your navel and moving outward.

5. Repeat eight times, slowly, lovingly, and intentionally, going slightly deeper, but never uncomfortably so, each time.

6. Move back to any tender spots, repeat the same motion, slowly and not too hard. You can also use the palm of your now warm hand over any tender areas, pressing evenly and firmly.

7. Optionally, finish your session with a hot water bottle on your belly, or a hot bath or shower.

Repeat daily for optimal benefits, or as needed for pain.

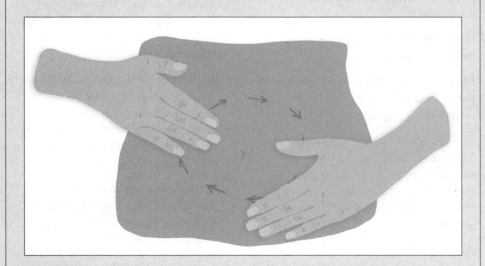

Herbs

- **EGCG**, an anti-inflammatory compound in **green tea**, may reduce endometrial implant growth. You can't get enough just drinking tea, so supplement with an EGCG green tea extract.

- **Pycnogenol**, an extract from pine bark, 30 mg twice daily for 48 weeks, led to a 33% reduction in pain and severe pain, not as well as hormonal treatment, but results persisted without relapse, unlike with medication. Five women in the pycnogenol group became pregnant.

- **Curcumin** regulates the immune system and reduces inflammation; use to reduce endometrial tissue.

- **Gingerroot** has been shown to reduce pain equal to the effects of ibuprofen; use over time to also reduce pain frequency.

- **CBD** may have a uniquely important role not just in endometriosis pain, but in treating and reversing endometriosis through complex mechanisms that include halting the replication and migration of endometriotic cells, calming hyperreactivity in the immune system, "starving" the cells out, and reducing pain in the uterus and pelvis, even in cases of deep infiltrating endometriosis. Use CBD oil orally, topically in the form of vaginal suppositories, or a combination of both.

Conventional Approach

Whether—and to what extent—you choose medical care for your endometriosis is a personal choice, and also depends on the severity and location of endometriotic lesions. Keep in mind that seven out of ten women with endometriosis experience unresolved pain despite medication use. Use the Hormone Intelligence Plan to reduce endometrial lesions and pain, and only progress on to hormonal therapies if this strategy doesn't provide adequate relief while you continue to address the root causes.

Options include:

- **Pain management:** Provides symptom relief only, but this may be very welcome.

- **NSAIDs:** This is probably the lowest risk of all the medical options, so I generally recommend using these for 6 months or so, if needed, while using the natural therapies and core Hormone Intelligence Plan.

- **Opioids:** These have mixed effectiveness and are a dangerous slippery slope; opioids are highly addictive and many women are also prescribed benzos for anxiety, a cocktail that can increase your risks of opioid overdose tenfold.

- **Danazol:** An androgenic drug, danazol is effective for treating endometriosis pain, but has numerous side effects.

- **Hormonal therapies** suppress ovulation, suppressing the hormones that "feed" endometrial tissue and helping to shrink it.

- **Combined (estrogen and progestin) contraceptives** are a first-line hormonal treatment for pain; they can be helpful but have some risks (page 218). **Progestin-only options** are also available.

- **GnRH analogues** suppress ovarian hormone production; their effectiveness is mixed. The best doses and length of use are unclear.

- **Aromatase inhibitors** suppress ovarian hormone production and are for severe, refractory endometriosis pain only; they can cause primary ovarian insufficiency (POI).

- **Surgery:** If you're at the end of your rope with pain, are struggling to get pregnant, or have exhausted yourself with alternative plans—don't let anyone judge you for choosing surgery. It's your business. It's essential to find a surgeon with an excellent track record of success and happy patients. When done by an unskilled provider, the recurrence rate of endometrial lesions can be as high as 50% in a couple of years, and as many as 20% of women experience no relief after initial surgery, leading to repeated surgeries. A skilled surgeon, however, can improve your outcomes and reduce your need for repeated procedures. The type of surgery is important:

  - **Excision surgery** is the most effective choice and should be the one used 99% of the time.

  - **Ablative vaporization** may be needed for lesions on the ovaries, and adhesiolysis for breaking up adhesions caused by endometriosis.

Helen, 26

"I've had very painful periods my whole life. They became unbearable in graduate school, forcing me to take a leave of absence. Then the pain became continuous, and severe, so dizzying it required ibuprofen—which sometimes doesn't even cut through. Not only have my periods become a nightmare, sex has become so painful it's impossible. Taking the Pill has barely helped and my doctors said this was normal for women—so have some of my friends. Recently, I finally received a diagnosis of endometriosis, but my initial relief has become fear: What if I have to have a hysterectomy and freeze my eggs to have children one day? I'm too young for this!"

Laparoscopic exploration showed that Helen did indeed have endometriosis. She decided to come off the Pill, and instead followed the Hormone Intelligence Solution, adding in the Endometriosis Advanced Protocol. Within a semester Helen's pain went from severe to moderate then to generally minimal. She was able to jump back into her classes and excel, and she was finally able to experience greater pleasure in her body, including her sex life.

fertility
ADVANCED PROTOCOL

Most women spend a decade or more trying not to get pregnant, then for so many women, when they're finally ready, the path to getting pregnant is anything but easy. Fertility specialists, while they can bring miracles into lives, are all too eager to tell women they're "over the hill," have "fried old eggs," or should "just start fertility treatment before it's too late." Even women in their late twenties and early thirties hear this! Incidentally, only 40% of the causes of infertility are even attributable to the woman and many are due to "unknown reasons"—

Conscious Conception

Whether you're wondering if you'll be able to get pregnant when you start trying and want to do everything you can now to support your reproductive health, you've hit a speed bump on your baby-making journey, you're deep into a fertility challenge, you're over forty and wondering if you can get pregnant, or you've experienced miscarriage and are worried about getting and staying pregnant, I invite you to take a journey with me into the world of natural fertility, optimal preconception self-care, and conscious conception in a full program at www.avivaromm.com.

All herb and supplement doses are listed in the
Botanical and Supplements Quick Reference Guide, starting on page 372.

hidden causes that conventional medicine doesn't recognize or address.

If you're here because you're facing a fertility challenge, I know it's not been easy and it may be pervading every aspect of your life: emotional, interpersonal, financial, and physical.

In Chapter 11 I walk you through a complete plan to optimize ovarian function and egg quality, including "First Aid for Your Ovaries" (page 248). The Fertility Advanced Protocol offers you additional tools to support and nourish fertility and have a healthy pregnancy.

There's no one answer to how long it will take to get pregnant, but there's a very good chance that it will happen! I've absolutely had couples get pregnant within one or two cycles, but it's preferable to give threee to six months to first nourish your total well-being—even if you're ready to get started on IVF or are feeling the crunch because of your age. It will optimize your results!

Lifestyle

- **Act "as if"**—make the choices you'd make if you knew you were already pregnant.

- **Go clean and green** with your foods, body products, home, and lifestyle. I can't overemphasize this enough.

- **Get into your best weight zone.** Being underweight increases the risk of anovulatory infertility—so gain enough to bring your weight up; being slightly overweight is not a problem, but a BMI over 25 may increase fertility challenges.

- **Too little or too much exercise** can impact fertility. Between 1 and 5 hours of moderate exercise weekly improves the likelihood of conceiving by nearly 20% while overexercising can cause hypothalamic amenorrhea (page 153). Find your sweet spot.

- **Toss the trackers and have hot sex.** Learn to use your cycle sense (Chapter 3) and put the pleasure back into baby-making—even if you're going down the route of assisted reproductive support!

- **Floss regularly and treat tooth and gum problems.** Gum inflammation can be a hidden factor behind fertility problems and miscarriage.

- **Smoking** reduces the likelihood of conceiving naturally by as much as 60%.

Food

As part of the Hormone Intelligence Diet:

- **Keep it whole.** In one large study, 39% of women who generally avoided fast food conceived within one month of starting to have unprotected sex, while women who included fast foods regularly in their diets had double the likelihood of still not having conceived at 12 months.

- **Eat less animal protein, eat more plants.** In the largest ongoing study of women's health and their diets, higher animal protein intake was associated with a 32% higher likelihood of ovulatory infertility, while women who consumed less animal protein, and instead ate even more plant-based protein (beans, legumes, nuts, seeds), had a 50% *decrease* in ovulatory infertility. Swapping even just one serving of animal protein for a serving of whole grain daily reduced ovulatory infertility by 43%.

- **Eat healthy fats.** Just 2% of your total daily calories in trans fats (one small donut or a medium serving of fast-food fries) increases infertility by as much as 70%. Healthy fats, on the other hand, bump up fertility.

- **Omega-3-rich fish** increases fertility and reduces all the gyn causes that can interfere with it. Keep it low mercury (page 117).

- **Avocados** contain the best kind of monounsaturated fat for fertility—try to include half of one daily.

- **Pass on the gluten.** Celiac disease, and possibly even nonceliac gluten

Having doubts about whether you can get pregnant?

Keep these stats in mind:

- Even with no treatment, 30% of women conceive within one month, 50% within four months, 70% within eight months, and by eighteen months, 90% of women will get pregnant.

- Even couples in their late thirties have a 91% chance of conceiving naturally within two years, and recent studies estimate that an average of 25 to 40% of women give birth without treatment during the three years after the first infertility consultation.

- At least 85% of women who experience a miscarriage go on to a healthy, full-term next pregnancy, and even after two miscarriages, which only happens in 5% of women, you have a 75% chance of having a full-term, healthy pregnancy next time.

- The term *infertility* sounds so final. But this is very different from being sterile, which means unable to get pregnant. Most women are actually experiencing subfertility—a differentiation that can create an enormous shift in your fertility mind-set!

- And here's a cool fact: fertility is yet another powerful vital sign; women who conceive naturally after thirty-five are four times more likely to live past age ninety, so getting your fertility vitality on is good for your overall longevity.

I've seen natural strategies work countless times over the past three decades, and there are even a few Avivas (and Avis) out there, named after me by happy new parents.

intolerance, can affect fertility, increase miscarriage risk, and affect your thyroid health.

- **Eat eggs.** It's no wonder eggs are a symbol of fertility. They're the richest source of choline, essential for baby's brain development. Eat up to 2 eggs daily. That's not a cholesterol risk!

- **Blood sugar balance** and insulin sensitivity are essential. Women with a diet high in processed, refined foods have nearly twice the risk of ovulatory infertility as women with low-glycemic diets.

- **Drink enough water** to improve cervical mucus (page 114).

- **What about alcohol and coffee?** Most studies have not found conclusive evidence that either a small occasional glass of wine, or even a cup of coffee now and then, interferes with fertility. The sweet spot seems to be keeping caffeine to less than 100 mg per day, which is typically what you'd get in an 8-ounce cup of regular, home-brewed dark roast coffee.

- **Skip the soda.** Soft drinks pose a specific fertility risk. According to the

Elena, 30

When Elena came to me for fertility treatment, she'd all but given up on getting pregnant naturally, but she really wanted to try. "I've been trying to get pregnant for eighteen months and it just hasn't been happening the way I thought it would. Several of my girlfriends got pregnant no problem and being around them, even though I'm happy for them, is hard. It's affecting my self-confidence. Sex is now all about getting pregnant, and it's stressing out our relationship; I find it hard to not think about my fertility 24/7. Every month is filled with anxiety—anxiety around sex, then the waiting to see if I'm pregnant followed by crushing disappointment when my period comes. My husband's sperm seems fine, so my doctor is recommending fertility treatments, but I'm just not ready to go down that road; it's expensive and I just don't have the bandwidth for the crazy emotions that I hear come with hormone treatment right now."

A review of Elena's history of irregular periods, severe acne, struggles with her weight, and moods since she was a teenager pointed to PCOS, and when I explained more of the symptoms, she nodded her head and said, "I suspected that's what it might be, but my doctor said don't bother with that—just start Clomid!" Agreeing to put fertility treatment on hold for six months, Elena readily embraced the Hormone Intelligence Plan and also followed the PCOS Advanced Protocol, and to her delight, she is now the mother of a healthy little boy.

Harvard Nurses' Health Study, women who consumed 2 or more sodas a day were up to 50% more likely to experience ovulatory infertility than women who drank less than one soda a week.

Mind-Body

- **De-stress.** I know it's hard because fertility challenges are so stressful. But HPA axis overdrive can dial down your fertility. Higher levels of stress hormone and chemicals may double infertility risk, and stress has been found to reduce egg fertilization. Stress can also cause hypothalamic amenorrhea, blocking ovulation.

- Good news! **Mind-body practices** that increase relaxation and positive beliefs can increase fertility and conception. A study of 54 women who completed a relaxation response program had decreased anxiety, depression, and fatigue, and 34% of the women

became pregnant within months of completing the program. Meditation, CBT, and other mind-body practices can get you out of fertility challenge survival mode, and improve fertility in as short as 3 to 4 months.

- **Cultivate belief in your body** and clear out emotional burdens about loss, failure, and doubt through conscious awareness, journaling, or therapy.

- I ask my patients to **shift the focus from getting pregnant to optimizing health**. I also ask them to take a big leap of faith and suspend "trying" so hard to get pregnant, and let it happen. Sometimes we have to step back from trying so hard, hit the pause button on the goal, and be in the moment. Not only does this give you more inner peace, but weirdly, it's one of my most important fertility success tips. I can't tell you how many of my patients have come back from a prescribed fertility vacation—where they just let it go and

Treat These Obstacles to Fertility with Hormone Intelligence

Healthy conception requires a whole lot of things to go right, in a specific sequence: healthy ovum, healthy cervical mucus, healthy sperm, patent fallopian tubes, receptive uterus with a healthy lining, adequate hormone levels, healthy chromosome transcription when sperm and egg meet, adequate nutrition, appropriately responding immune system, the right insulin and cortisol levels, and a host of other factors that must conspire to support the healthy growth of this new life. Make sure to address your root causes and concurrent conditions that can get in the way of fertility ease, including thyroid problems, PCOS, endometriosis, or recurrent UTIs or vaginal infections.

reconnect—and then find themselves pregnant.

- **Don't skimp on sleep.** As with the rest of your hormone health, there's a strong link between circadian rhythm and fertility. Sleeping less than 7 hours each night can interfere with ovulation as well as egg quality, can worsen pelvic pain interfering with sex, and can aggravate blood sugar problems with PCOS.

- A "ticking clock" mind-set makes you feel that you're running out of time, especially if you're in your early forties or mid-forties. **Step back and have perspective.** Women have always given birth at or in their forties; think of the celebrities who've done this: Salma Hayek, Halle Berry, Gwen Stefani, Tina Fey, and Eva Mendes to name a few. I've midwifed many healthy first babies and beyond to forty-and-over mommas, not a few who were told by a gynecologist or fertility doctor that they'd never be able to get pregnant naturally at their age.

- **Cultivate creativity.** Fertility manifests in so many ways—deepen your connection to your own creative force with dance, painting, or gardening, or other "flow" activities that create a highly attuned, relaxed state to enjoy your fertility dance more and create harmony between your brain, ovarian, thyroid, and adrenal axes.

Nutrients

- Take a **prenatal vitamin** with methylfolate (800 to 1,000 mcg), choline (400 mg), iodine (200 to 250

Cala, 36

"Four years ago my doctor told me that there was nothing I could do about my fertility except start fertility treatment. He told me my age was too much of a risk factor (I was thirty-two!) and that I'd probably never conceive naturally given that we'd been trying for a year. Nobody had ever told me to get my thyroid levels checked until I met Dr. Aviva. When we did, my TSH was high (5.2) and my antibodies were elevated into the hundreds. She started Hormone Intelligence living, along with a low dose of Armour Thyroid, and within just a few months not only was my TSH at an optimal level for conception, and my antibodies down to the double digits, but I felt great. I didn't even realize how much I was tired and dragging, or how low my sex drive was, until my energy perked up. And the best part of that wasn't just better sex, but I started ovulating regularly, had great cervical mucus—and I got pregnant—without (expensive and stressful) fertility treatments!"

mcg), zinc (15 to 45 mg), and iron (27 mg). It increases your chance of getting pregnant and having a healthier pregnancy. For example, methylfolate increases fertility, reduces miscarriage risk, and is important for baby's neural development; a prenatal vitamin containing 27 mg of iron reduces ovulatory infertility; zinc plays a role in ovulation, supports healthy estrogen and progesterone levels, and protects the developing egg against oxidative damage, and low zinc is associated with lower fertility. Many "prenatals" fall short on these nutrients, also needed for baby's optimal health when you do become pregnant, so choose one that includes these nutrients in as close to these amounts as possible.

- **Vitamin B6** supports progesterone production and can improve implantation. Take the active form, pyridoxal-5-phosphate (P5P), for best results. If you've been on an OCP, B6 is even more important.

- **Ascorbic acid (vitamin C)** promotes ovulation in hypothalamic amenorrhea and may improve progesterone due to anovulation, as well as improve ovulation in women undergoing IVF.

- **Omega-3 fatty acids** play an essential role in conception, and the formation and development of the oocyte and embryo. Higher intake is associated with better ovarian reserve and higher conception rates.

- **Vitamin D3** boosts progesterone levels, supports ovulation, and is specifically important for women with PCOS and endometriosis. With IVF, higher vitamin D levels are associated with 35% higher pregnancy rates and healthier embryos.

- Take a **probiotic** containing a broad spectrum of *Lactobacillus* species, including *L. rhamnosus*, *L. reuteri*, and *L. crispatus* for a fertility advantage.

Herbs

- **Vitex (chasteberry)** is a classic fertility herb. In a Stanford University School of Medicine study, taking chasteberry for 6 months improved fertility in women with low progesterone by 32% compared to 10% in the placebo group. It promotes regular ovulation, lengthens the luteal phase, and corrects progesterone deficiency. It's also helpful in restoring your cycle post-Pill. Take for 3 to 6 months.

- **FertilityBlend** contains chasteberry, green tea, L-arginine, folate, B-vitamins, magnesium, selenium, iron, and zinc. In one study, 93 women aged 24 to 42 years, who had tried to conceive for 6 to 36 months were pregnant after 3 months of use.

- **White peony**, used to regulate ovulation, is an herb commonly used in both Western and Chinese herbal medicine to support fertility.

- **Adaptogens**, including shatavari, can reduce stress, balance HPA axis health, balance hormones, and support fertility.

Advanced Protocol: **FERTILITY**

Conventional Approach

If after 12 to 18 months of trying you're still not pregnant, you might choose to do one or more of the commonly available treatments, usually suggested in the following order:

- **Ovarian stimulation** with a medication called clomiphene (i.e., Clomid) or hormone injections

- **Intrauterine insemination (IUI)**, a treatment usually combined with clomiphene or hormone injections

- **In vitro fertilization (IVF)** if other treatments have not worked

In addition to the high emotional and financial costs, invasive treatments carry substantial risks, and success rates are lower than might be expected given the costs—about 30% across all ages, with the least success in women over 35. An integrative approach combining nutritional and natural remedies with conventional treatments may improve your success with assisted reproduction and have lower risks (e.g., using inositol with Clomid may reduce ovarian hyperstimulation)—and for so many women, they work beautifully together.

uterine fibroids
ADVANCED PROTOCOL

It is possible to significantly reduce or even eliminate small fibroids—and to reduce symptoms and size of moderate-sized fibroids—naturally, by applying this protocol along with the core Hormone Intelligence Plan. Three to six months time following the full plan is a realistic window in which to see symptom improvement, the most important goal with treating fibroids. Symptom improvement is a likely sign that fibroid size is shrinking, in which case I recommend continuing the plan in this chapter and your Hormone Intelligence lifestyle indefinitely.

This protocol is meant to eliminate fibroids or, at the least, reduce their size enough to eliminate symptoms and the need for medical intervention, which is only necessary when fibroids are causing heavy bleeding or bothersome symptoms, or are getting in your way of getting pregnant. Even if large or symptomatic fibroids require surgery, a root cause approach is still important to address why they developed.

All herb and supplement doses are listed in the Botanical and Supplements Quick Reference Guide, starting on page 372.

Lifestyle

- **Achieve a healthy weight.** While you can be overweight and absolutely healthy, significant overweight and obesity means more circulating estrogen and growth hormone, both a risk for fibroids.

- **Improve estrogen levels** with a special emphasis on gut healing and detoxification.

- **Increased exercise** can lead to a substantial decrease in fibroids; women who exercise 7 hours or more per week reduce their risk.

- **Hip circling, pelvic thrusts, and belly dancing** can improve pelvic circulation and reduce discomfort as well.

Food

As part of the Hormone Intelligence Diet:

- **Eliminate red meat and ham.** Both have been associated with a higher rate of fibroids.

- Increase to the full 3 servings each week of **healthy fish** (page 116), which is protective against fibroids.

- Increase **green vegetable and fruit** intake to 8 to 10 servings daily, with an emphasis on leafy greens to reduce excess estrogen.

- Eat **citrus fruit**, which has been specifically found to be protective against fibroids, once daily.

- Consume 2 tbsp. of **ground flaxseed** daily.

- Include **legumes** in your diet 2 to 3 times weekly.

Catherine, 46

After a diagnosis from her ob-gyn of uterine fibroids that were "too many to count" and "the size of oranges," who then tossed out the word *hysterectomy*, Catherine decided to try a natural protocol. "I looked four months pregnant," she said, "but I wasn't sure I was done having babies, and either way, I didn't want major abdominal surgery unless I tried everything else first!"

She began eating for Hormone Intelligence, addressing her personal root causes, and added in daily flaxseeds and EGCG (green tea) extract. Within a few months she began experiencing symptom improvement, and in less than a year, not only had her belly flattened and her nagging fibroid symptoms were gone, but a repeat ultrasound, much to her ob-gyn's (and her own!) surprise, confirmed the fibroids were largely gone. Not only did Catherine avoid the hysterectomy, she gained a new sense of wonder for her body's ability to heal. Her doctor, fascinated by the solid scientific evidence—and patient proof—behind this approach, decided to make it a part of his plans for patients in the future, before a hysterectomy.

- Diets high in food sources of **vitamin A**, including carrots, broccoli, spinach, cantaloupe, sweet potatoes, and winter squashes, may be protective; supplementing vitamin A doesn't have the same benefit.

- **Alcohol**, especially beer, is associated with an increased risk of developing fibroids.

Mind-Body

- There is a suspected connection between stress hormones and uterine fibroids; it's always important to **tend to the stress in our lives**. Pressure to have a hysterectomy (page 17) can also cause stress, so take a step back to see if there are ways to reduce stress and, ideally, find a provider who will not pressure you.

Nutrients

- Lower **vitamin D** levels increase fibroid risk. Take vitamin D3 daily.

- Try either **indole-3-carbinol (I3C) or diindolylmethane (DIM)** daily for 6 months, or longer if needed, to support healthy estrogen levels.

Herbs

- **Green tea extract** (with EGCG) has been found helpful for reducing uterine fibroid size and symptoms, including heavy bleeding. In one study, women who took green tea extract daily for 4 months had a 32.6% reduction in fibroid volume and a 32.4% reduction in severity of fibroid symptoms.

- **Curcumin** supplementation has been shown to inhibit fibroid cell growth.

- In a small 2014 study, women who took 40 mg of **black cohosh** daily experienced an average decrease in fibroid size of 30.3% after a 12-week treatment period. Remifemin, a commonly available product, can be used.

- **Dr. Aviva's Uterine Fibroid Tincture:** A number of traditional herbal remedies can help to shrink uterine fibroids; these work on the principle of "toning" the uterus and acting as astringents. Combine the following tinctures (you can purchase these individually). Take 5 mL (about 1 tsp.) daily in ⅛ cup of water, for 3 to 12 months:

  - Yarrow 28 mL

  - Red raspberry leaf 28mL

  - Nettle leaf 20 mL

  - White peony 14 mL

  - Ginger 10 mL

Conventional Approach

Fibroids that do not cause symptoms, are small, or occur in a woman who is nearing menopause often do not require treatment. If fibroids aren't causing any troublesome symptoms or problems, then it's best to leave them alone, take a natural approach, and observe for changes over time.

- For aching and discomfort, pain medications such as **acetaminophen and nonsteroidal anti-inflammatory drugs (NSAIDs)** can be used.

Advanced Protocol: UTERINE FIBROIDS

- **Mirena IUD** is an option for women with fibroids that do not distort the inside of the uterus. It reduces heavy and painful bleeding but does not treat the fibroids themselves. Possible side effects: acne, spotting (vaginal bleeding between periods), weight gain, abdominal pain, and breast tenderness.

- **Birth control pills** have hardly any research on them for fibroid treatment; they may reduce heavy menstrual bleeding and prevent anemia.

- **GnRH agonists (e.g., leuprolide) and ulipristal acetate** can reduce symptoms and fibroid size, but fibroids grow again after treatment is discontinued and have side effects, especially GnRH agonists.

- **Surgical options** include myomectomy, laparoscopic surgery, endometrial ablation, and hysterectomy. Between 15 and 30% experience fibroid regrowth after 5 years. Uterine scarring may occur from the procedure and affect fertility. If you do choose a hysterectomy for very troublesome fibroids, it's optimal and usually possible to spare the ovaries.

"down there" sexual and vaginal health
ADVANCED PROTOCOL

Healthy, happy vaginas are not just important for our daily comfort, they're also a "sixth vital sign": our hormones affect our vaginal and cervical health, and in turn problems in our vaginal microbiome can contribute to symptoms and conditions that brought you to this book: pelvic pain, endometriosis, fertility, vaginal dryness, or perhaps pain with sex, and more obviously to the topic, vaginal discharge, odor, or recurrent vaginal infections.

Similarly, while everyone has a unique version of what sexual health is for herself, in some cases, low libido and other challenges to our sexual satisfaction can be due to underlying causes that can be impacting your health generally as well.

And of course, sexual and vaginal health are intimately interrelated. So let's take a look at both. There's no advocacy group for keeping our vaginas healthy or our sex lives happy. I hope this chapter inspires you to become an advocate for your own.

All herb and supplement doses are listed in the Botanical and Supplements Quick Reference Guide, starting on page 372.

Vaginal Health Advanced Protocol

While we've come to accept that vaginal infections "just happen" and the only solution is yet another round of a medication, there is a great deal you can do to prevent common infections, reverse mild ones naturally, and nip recurrence in the bud. Getting an accurate diagnosis from your health care provider is important. All the preventative steps in this Advanced Protocol apply and can help prevent recurrence.

Here are the most "down there" problems, which are addressed in this chapter:

- **Vulvovaginitis**—a catchall term for inflammation and irritation of the vulva, vagina, or both, causing itching, burning, or pain. It's usually due to some type of local irritation or trigger.

- **Yeasts infections**—a fungal infection in the *Candida* family, yeast infections cause a whitish or yellowish "curd-like" discharge, yeasty odor, and lots of itching.

- **Bacterial vaginosis**—not caused by a single organism, but a form of vaginal dysbiosis in which your good local flora aren't keeping the more annoying species at bay, allowing them to proliferate. Bacterial vaginosis (BV) can lead to increased vaginal discharge, a spoiled fish odor, itching, redness, burning, and irritation. BV affects nearly a third of women and can make us more susceptible to sexually transmitted infections. It's also associated with abnormal Pap smears and pelvic inflammatory disease (PID). In pregnancy, it can increase risk of second-trimester miscarriage or preterm labor.

Lifestyle

- **Low estrogen** is associated with vaginal dryness, burning, irritation, pain with sex, and more frequent vaginal and urinary infections, and can be a sign of perimenopause or POI. See page 315 for healing vaginal dryness.

- **Estrogen-containing oral contraceptives** can increase yeast infections, so you might want to switch to a low-estrogen product (or get off the Pill completely, page 222).

- **Vaginal ecology disruptors**, including antibiotics, steroids, scented sanitary products, synthetic tampons or pads, and douches can affect your vaginal pH and flora; reduce or avoid these triggers (page 232).

- **Don't douche**, ever. Clean your vulva with water only, or gentle soap, when desired.

- **Wipe front to back** when you poop, not the other way around (you'd be amazed at how many women don't know this).

- **Say goodbye to thongs (a.k.a. bacteria tightropes).** Wear boy shorts, briefs, or bikinis instead.

- **Go green with your period products**, change them regularly during your flow, and wear a pad instead of a tampon overnight.

- **Sex impact: avoid anal-to-genital sexual contact** (including with toys) to avoid bacteria ending up in the wrong place. If **receiving oral sex** is causing itching or infections, it's a pH thing; rinse afterward and pass on the fun for a couple of week to let your flora rebalance if you're symptomatic.

- **Choose a natural lube brand.** Chemically laden vaginal lubes can individually or collectively disrupt the vaginal flora and pH and increase your susceptibility to vaginal infections.

- **Condoms** can prevent BV; even if you've got your birth control otherwise covered, having your man "wrap it up" can help. Skip the spermicides and choose a natural brand.

Food

As part of the Hormone Intelligence Diet:

- **Keep your vaginal tissue healthy** with plenty of phytonutrients.

- **Nourish your vaginal and gut flora**, and include lacto-fermented foods in your diet.

- **Balance your blood sugar.** Troublemaking gut and vaginal microorganisms thrive on sugar, so keeping sugar intake low and blood sugar balanced can support healthy vaginal ecology.

- **Keep alcohol intake low.**

Nutrients

- **Repopulate your gut** and your vagina with a probiotic that includes *Lactobacillus reuteri*, *Lactobacillus rhamnosus*, and *Lactobacillus crispatus* for at least 6 weeks but up to 24 weeks depending on your infection severity and frequency.

- Optionally, in addition to taking a probiotic, **insert one capsule of the same probiotic vaginally**, nightly before bed.

Herbs

- Try the **herbal suppository** on page 300 or purchase a suppository online (i.e., Vitanica Yeast Arrest Vaginal Support). Repeat every other night for 10 days, alternating with a probiotic capsule as a suppository.

- Despite some OBs' protestations that it's ineffective, **unsweetened, organic yogurt** as a vulvar cream and vaginal "gel" provides symptom relief within a day or 2 for many women. Continue for 3 days after the last symptoms have cleared up.

Conventional Approach

The mainstay of treating vaginal infections is antifungals and antibiotics, which are quick and effective. Unfortunately, some organisms are resistant and recurrence is as high as 50%, especially with BV.

Advanced Protocol: "DOWN THERE" SEXUAL AND VAGINAL HEALTH

Vaginal Relief Suppository

This is one of my classic herbal remedies, now in use by midwives around the world. These can be stored in the refrigerator for 2 weeks, or in the freezer for 6 weeks, defrosting them in the fridge for use as needed. This recipes makes about 24 suppositories.

Ingredients

1 cup cocoa butter

½ cup coconut oil

3 tbsp. calendula oil

⅛ tsp. thyme essential oil

⅛ tsp. lavender essential oil

⅛ tsp. tea tree oil

To prepare

1. Melt the cocoa butter and coconut oil together in a saucepan.

2. When melted, remove the pan from the burner.

3. Add the herbal ingredients and stir well.

4. Pour into the suppository mold (see below).

5. Refrigerate until firm.

Insert one suppository vaginally each night before bed, for 14 days. Always wear a sanitary pad while you sleep with the suppository in place. It will melt and will otherwise stain bedding or undies! Results are typically seen within several days; however, you may treat up to a week and repeat if necessary.

A suppository mold can be purchased online or you can fashion your own with the instructions you'll find over at avivaromm.com, along with many other women's health and herbal solutions.

Sexual Health Advanced Protocol

Sex can be one of life's greatest pleasures and sources of relaxation. But if you're not feeling it, you're not alone. Literally millions of women—and women of all ages, including in their twenties and thirties—struggle with concerns and questions about their sex lives, "performance," orgasms, and their libido.

There's no technical definition of what constitutes "normal" libido or how often you "should be" wanting to have sex. It's up to YOU to decide what's normal for YOU. Some women are completely happy with not having sex at all. There are no wrong answers here—the important thing is that you discover your own sexual needs. Unfortunately, a very profitable medical industry has sprung up around convincing women that our libido is low, that we should be orgasming within minutes, that vaginal intercourse is enough to have us hollering, and then when we don't experience that—which most women don't—medications will fix our problems! This is reinforced by movies and other media including women's magazines with the myth of the hour-long orgasm, pressure to have multiple orgasms, and ejaculation—all of which are remotely possible, but for most women as common as a unicorn—and aren't necessarily meaningful goals.

Hormonal changes throughout our cycles and lives do impact our sexual interest and responsiveness in predictable ways as I discussed in Chapter 3. And of course, hormone imbalances can play a role: low testosterone can keep your sex drive dialed down to practically nothing, low estrogen can lead to vaginal dryness making sex uncomfortable, if you're not ovulating you won't likely get that mid-cycle surge of sexual desire, and cortisol due to high stress can crash the whole system. However, hormones may be just one small part of the libido story for most women. But sexual function and a satisfying sex life don't happen in a vacuum—like the rest of our hormonal health it happens in the context of a culture. And in this one, the messaging we receive can be counterproductive to a healthy sex life—and very confusing.

Women's sexual response is a complex interplay of psychological, emotional, visual, "scentual," tactile, and physiologic stimuli. Erotic feelings are coupled with vascular changes that are characteristic of female sexual excitement. Libido is profoundly influenced by our sense of personal well-being, our physical health, hormones, stress levels, and relationship happiness and is less commonly caused by an actual medical problem. Interestingly, there's also little to no connection between having a low sex drive—that is, you're not thinking and fantasizing about sex on a regular basis—and enjoying sex when you do have it.

Common factors that affect sex drive, response, and desire include:

- **Medical conditions:** fatigue, physical pain (endometriosis, chronic pelvic pain, etc.), depression, diabetes, heart disease, hypothyroidism, chronic fatigue syndrome, and even cancer

- **Medications:** including antidepressants, antihypertensives, sedatives, antipsychotics, and beta-blockers

- **Emotional challenges:** stress, worry, history of trauma (including physical or emotional birth trauma), taboos around sex, history of threat or violence, relationship betrayals, or negative body image or self-esteem

- **Life factors:** busy lives, demands of breastfeeding and motherhood, changes in attraction to you partner

- **Partner factors:** your *partner* is depressed, struggles with anxiety, drinks even a little too much alcohol (a couple of beers can inhibit erectile function, for example), is taking medications, or is uninterested in a vigorous sex life, grew up with taboos about sex, or is emotionally unavailable

So what's getting in the way of a satisfying sex life for most women? There can be a gauntlet of obstacles. But there are many positive ways you can take charge of your sexual health. Let's get you started.

Lifestyle

- **Get a diagnosis and proper treatment** for any symptoms you might have of a medical condition (see above). Proper treatment may be all it takes to restore your sexual wellness.

- **Maximize your health** by keeping your condition and symptoms as well controlled as possible; for example, if you have diabetes, keep your blood

sugar steady; if you have high blood pressure, follow a careful diet, exercise, and stress reduction plan.

- **Minimize medications** that could be dampening your drive. Ask your medical provider which are truly essential and which aren't, seek alternatives with fewer side effects, and see if you can reduce medication doses. Improving your health will increase the likelihood you'll be able to do this.

- **Set realistic expectations.** Sex in real life, for most people, isn't like it is in the movies. A lot of women, as a result, think they have a problem that they don't. Most women need warm-up time and intimacy, as well as clitoral stimulation to get turned on and to achieve orgasm. Our arousal is tied into emotional and cognitive pathways.

Mind-Body

- **De-stress.** Stress pretty much always hits the brake on your brain's sexual accelerator; so does fatigue. So go deep into self-care and stress reduction.

- **Digitally detox your sex life.** In a 2015 study of nearly 150 married women, 70% said that technology was interfering with their sex lives. It's also one of the biggest reasons 20- and 30-year-olds are having less sex. Set boundaries around digital devices. Instead, make time for talking, touching, and eye contact.

- **Get physical.** Just 20 minutes of exercise can increase your arousal and responsiveness. Get a jump start: put on some music and dance, go for a bike ride or a run, or anything that gets your heart rate up a bit and your blood moving, alone or with your partner.

- **Make intimacy a priority** from early on in your relationship. Spend time touching, massaging, or enjoying something pleasurable together. Sex may happen, or it may not, but putting intimacy into your emotional bank account as a couple is always a win for relationship health—and ups the ante on having great sex.

- **Talk about it.** Connect with your partner about what you think is getting in the way of your sex life, and also be open to hearing what your partner has to say.

- **Reinvigorate desire.** Things can get stale in long-term relationships but for women in long-term relationships, desire is more likely to be triggered by your partner's desire for you, and them getting the party started with intimacy, romance, or gifts. Great info to pass on to your partner!

- **Make your bedroom a sensual space** with candles, dim lighting, sensual scents (vanilla, sandalwood, and amber, for example, are aphrodisiac), and soft bedding.

- **Practice tantric breathing together.** Tantra is an ancient practice designed to enhance unity and ecstasy. Tantric breathing, coordinated, deep, rhythmic breath, can be done alone or with your partner and helps you to focus in and turn off the external and internal noise, directing these toward areas of your body as you engage in pleasure. It also increases neurochemicals involved in sexual pleasure—nitric oxide, dopamine, and oxytocin—while reducing stress and, with it, lowering cortisol.

- **Reconsider Hollywood imagery.** Chances are your partner isn't Brad Pitt, Idris Alba, J Lo, Penelope Cruz, or whoever floats your boat. He or she may just be a regular human being, one who has even gained a little weight or has less hair than when you first met. Love is seeing the beauty within; and if gravity has started to take a toll, weight crept on, and so on, consider starting a wellness program together—which can also create connection that revs things up in the bedroom, too.

- **Individual and/or relationship counseling,** or **working with a sex therapist** can help when a relationship has lost its vitality and can help open blocks in finding pleasure together. And if the relationship is over, counseling can help with peaceful resolution. The Association of Sexuality Educators, Counselors and Therapists is a respected organization (www.aasect.org).

- **Healing from trauma** is not a one-and-done thing; it's a process. Starting on the journey is the first step to resolving old hurts and wounds that can be affecting your sexual wellness now.

Herbs

- **Adaptogens:** Maca and shatavari may play a helpful role in low libido associated with depression and low sexual function caused by SSRI antidepressants, particularly in menopausal women. Red ginseng is associated with improved sexual health and may be especially helpful during menopause. It may affect sleep, though, so do not take it if it's overstimulating you; stick with one of the previous options.

- **St. John's wort** can be used to enhance a feeling of sexual well-being.

- **Spicy foods** can spark up the heat.

- A study conducted at Stanford University School of Medicine found that **ArginMax**, a combination product containing L-arginine, ginseng, ginkgo, damiana, multivitamins, and minerals, increased sexual desire, sexual satisfaction, and clitoral sensation, and increased the frequency of orgasms in women close to or during menopause.

- While the jury is out on whether **cannabis** is an aphrodisiac, many women find it enhances pleasure and reduces inhibition. A Stanford University study published in the *Journal of Sexual Medicine* found a positive association between marijuana use and sexual frequency across all demographic groups. There's a reason it was called the Summer of Love!

- While, surprisingly, studies haven't found **chocolate** to be aphrodisiac, it's an undeniably sensual food that does increase feelings of relaxation and pleasure, so I often recommend it as a lead-up to sex or even during foreplay. Try a variety with some chili or other spices for a little extra heat.

When Sex Hurts

As more than one patient has said, "Sex should not be this hard." If sex is painful for you, you're *not alone*. About 30% of women in the US report pain during intercourse, including many in their twenties and thirties, not just during menopause! Centuries of stigma surround women's sexual pain, so it remains underdiscussed and undiagnosed. A large 2012 study found that 60% of women who sought medical care for pain with sex had to see three or more doctors to get a diagnosis. Most are told it's normal or psychological, to relax more, try foreplay, or use lube—but it's more complex than that.

Common Causes of Painful Sex Include

- Endometriosis
- Interstitial cystitis
- Vaginitis
- Vaginismus, painful vaginal spasms
- Pelvic floor dysfunction
- IBS
- Vulvodynia, a chronic pelvic pain condition that affects the vulva
- Uterine fibroids
- Vaginal dryness
- A retroverted uterus
- Surgeries that affect nerve sensation in the pelvis or vagina, such as a prior hysterectomy
- Sensitivity or damage from cancer treatments (surgical, radiation)
- History of trauma

Pain with sex is very often accompanied by anticipatory anxiety for the woman, shame, a sense of being broken, embarrassment, self-doubt, or relationship stress—many women have shared stories of breakups associated with the sexual tension around this issue.

What You Can Do

- **Speak up** and keep seeking until you find a practitioner who will listen; you may have more success with a CNM or NP, especially a woman.

- **Use a water-soluble lubricant** if you experience vaginal irritation or sensitivity.

- **Set aside a relaxed time for sex** when you and your partner aren't tired or rushed; start with foreplay. **Talk to your partner** about where and when you feel pain, as well as what activities you find pleasurable. **Try sexual activities—and positions—that don't cause pain.**

- **Before sex**, empty your bladder or take a warm bath; **after sex**, apply ice or a frozen gel pack wrapped in a small towel to the vulva.

- If endometriosis or period pain get in the way of penetrative sex (or any form that hurts), **track your symptoms and cycles** to avoid those times. And of course, use the plan in this book, or therapies best for you, to heal your endometriosis.

You Can Get Satisfaction

Mae West said it best, "Good sex is like good bridge. If you don't have a good partner, you'd better have a good hand."

As women, we're not given a pleasure playbook. Women have fewer orgasms than any other demographic (men, gay men, trans men), and straight women have fewer than women having sex with women.

We've been taught to give more than receive, to not ask for what we want or need (or even explore what that might be); we associate hot sex with something "wrong" or "dirty"; we are "slut shamed" if we do step into our sexual power; we're taken less seriously when we're sexual (executives and professors don't dress like pole dancers in movies); and you may have been raised to believe that sex is embarrassing, taboo, or something to hide, or that pleasure is selfish, dirty, unholy. It's none of these. It's like a vitamin. Vitamin P (for pleasure!)!

So on the road to learning how to experience, receive, and give yourself pleasure, you might have some unlearning to do and rules to let go of to get to where you have true confidence, empowerment, and comfort as a sensual, sexual being with ownership over your pleasure and satisfaction.

What You Can Do

- Explore the beliefs that you grew up with. Did you grow up believing sex was healthy, positive, safe? Nurture and reframe healthy beliefs about sex.

- Do at least one thing every day that makes you feel sexy!

- Read *Come as You Are* by Emily Nagoski or *Women's Anatomy of Arousal* by Sheri Winston, alone or with a partner.

- Practice giving yourself or asking your partner for what you want sexually.

- Get comfortable *receiving* pleasure.

- The days of masturbation shame are over. Fifty percent of American women from their twenties into their sixties own *at least one* vibrator (and married women are even more likely to own one!). Several companies now make state-of-the-art, anatomy-friendly designs.

Long-Term Solutions

- Try **pelvic floor physical therapy** for pain due to pelvic floor dysfunction, vaginismus, vulvodynia, and also postpartum perineal trauma.

- **Treat medical causes**, that is, vaginal infection, endometriosis, uterine fibroids, vaginal dryness, and so on.

- If you have a history of sexual trauma, **trauma healing** is so, so important.

- **Talk with women you trust, or join a support group** where you can share your story and hear others; when we suffer and isolate, we internalize the trauma; when we talk with others, we realize we're not alone, it wasn't our fault or something wrong with us, and that healing is possible.

- **Birth trauma** is a very real phenomenon, though often unacknowledged. If you think or know you've experienced it, please join my Mama pathway at my website avivaromm.com for resources and support for healing.

- **OhNut** is an intimate wearable device that can help you manage and potentially reduce pain during sex, particularly if deep penetration hurts; it allows you to customize penetration depth.

Conventional Approach

Like most everything else, conventional medicine pathologizes women's sexual experiences, focusing on pharmaceutical solutions without considering the whole woman. Treatments include antidepressants, hormone replacement (estrogen, testosterone), and sildenafil—a "female Viagra"—for arousal problems. These may all be helpful, but some of these treatments are not supported by adequate evidence, and hormonal therapies can have adverse effects. For example, long-term use of testosterone in women has not been thoroughly investigated; it can lead to symptoms of masculinization over time. So weigh the pros and cons, and make sure to look at the totality of your experience before hopping on a medication.

What Matters Is a Healthy, Satisfied YOU

A pleasurable sex life is an important part of overall health. But remember, there is no external measure of what counts as a healthy sex drive. What counts is what is healthy and satisfying to YOU. Similarly, there's no one time frame for improvement; it largely depends on the underlying challenges—irritation from a vaginal infection might clear up in days; vaginismus associated with past sexual trauma may require deeper physical therapy and trauma healing therapy, while relationship challenges may take their own time to sort out.

perimenopause
ADVANCED PROTOCOL

Puberty. Becoming a mom. Perimenopause. Our lives are full of BIG transitions. Welcome to the one that's been the least celebrated—perimenopause.

While each of us experiences menopause uniquely, the idea that this natural shift in our hormones signals some kind of slowdown is simply ludicrous. Internalizing the message that we're irrelevant, dried up, or past our prime holds us down and keeps us from claiming our authority and strength, so right here, right now, I invite you to reject that noise entirely. By the time we reach our mid-to-late forties and early fifties, we're smarter, sexier, and more badass than ever, with more wisdom, maturity, and life experience, and often a whole new level of freedom in our lives that can make us more productive, energetic, and in my opinion, downright sexy. Own your strength. You've earned it.

While perimenopause is a completely natural process, like all our women's cycles, there are very real symptoms women experience as a result of the very same multi-ecosystem imbalances we've covered in this book, with inflammation playing a major role in how well and easily we age, and with it, how we experience this new hormonal transition. Reframing our view can also radically shift our attitudes about our symptom approach; rather than seeing our bodies—failing and needing to be fixed, we can use Hormone Intelligence to support optimal well-being in each of our ecosystems and our total health. Chapter 11 is particularly important to

All herb and supplement doses are listed in the
Botanical and Supplements Quick Reference Guide, starting on page 372.

emphasize—maintaining and optimizing ovarian function can support an easier perimenopause.

If you're not having any symptoms of perimenopause, and you're experiencing it at an age-appropriate time in your life, your mid-forties to your mid-fifties, there's no need to do anything to support your wellness beyond the foundational Hormone Intelligence program. If you are having symptoms, this chapter will help you to navigate this transition so that you can embrace it as a new and amazing phase of your life, with a power you've never known, and with natural options to make the ride as smooth, healthy, and even as pleasurable, as possible.

Natural Protocols for an Easier Transition to Menopause

Lifestyle

- **Keep moving.** The benefits of exercise for perimenopausal symptoms are powerful; it prevents bone loss, protects heart function and cognitive health, improves sleep, prevents and reduces depression, improves sex drive, reduces hot flashes, and prevents the notorious menopausal weight gain. Aim for an hour, 4 times weekly, of aerobic (cardio) exercise with 20 minutes of weight training each time.

- **Support your adrenals.** Stress is often overlooked as a factor that contributes to perimenopausal symptoms, including irritability, panic attacks, fatigue, and night sweats. Revisit your goals and priorities—you've earned not having to live in constant overwhelm and overdrive, and the right to be choosier over who and what you say yes to—and nourish your adrenals.

- **Massage**, with or without aromatherapy essential oils, 1 or 2 times per week, for 4 to 8 weeks, has been found to be helpful, even in women with severe symptoms, especially hot flashes and sleep and mood challenges. Your insurance might even cover it!

- I know that perimenopause sometimes comes with a prescription for more red wine, but alcohol can tank your sleep and it's a huge hot flash trigger! It can also make you feel depressed. **So skip the booze, or keep it to a bare minimum.** Red wine is the worst culprit; vodka the least.

Food

As part of the Hormone Intelligence Diet:

- **Increasing your fiber** keeps your bowels moving daily, your microbiome nourished, your inflammation in check, and your hormones optimized.

A healthy microbiome also nourishes your brain. Can't beat that!

- **Fruits and veggies** keep inflammation and oxidative stress (a.k.a. cellular aging) at bay, so get your daily 6 to 8 servings!

- **Omega-3-rich fish** is invaluable for brain and vascular health. Three times weekly is not too much.

- **Flaxseeds**, 2 tbsp. daily, can support healthy estrogen levels, and also provide fiber.

Mind-Body

- **Reframing** this time in our lives can make it not only easier, but pleasurable and liberating. You can embrace this as a whole new time of freedom: sex is thought to be the best in our lives after fifty; we have more confidence in our careers, social lives, and money; and at some point you realize you don't have to give a shit about what anyone else thinks about you—pretty amazing and liberating all in all!

General Nutrients and Herbs for Perimenopause Support

- *Pueraria mirifica*, a safe, nonhormonal alternative to HRT, may reduce hot flashes, vaginal atrophy, and dryness; improve bone density; and reduce general symptoms. Take for at least 6 months for optimal results.

- **Adaptogens** help us respond to stressful times and transitions. I especially love these for perimenopause symptoms.

- **Shatavari or maca:** to improve sex drive and mood.

- **Ashwagandha:** for sleep, stress resilience, anxiety, and libido, and to reduce cellular damage.

- **Reishi:** to protect against cellular damage and promote sleep.

- **Motherwort** helps to balance mood, promote sleep, calm anxiety, and, with lemon balm, reduce hot flashes.

When Menopause Happens Too Early: Primary Ovarian Insufficiency

If you're entering menopause because of primary ovarian insufficiency (POI, page 83), it may make you suddenly feel very old, but having POI doesn't mean that *you* are aging prematurely—it means that your ovarian function is challenged. It can be devastating to hear if you haven't had or finished having children. Is a natural approach even possible? Hormone Intelligence, with an emphasis on the plan in Chapter 11, may help prevent ovarian decline, while the therapies in this next section, both natural and hormonal, can support you through symptoms while protecting your bones, heart, and brain should menopause be inevitable.

Help in a (Hot) Flash

About 75% of perimenopausal women in the US experience hot flashes; 87% have them daily, 33% have ten or more each day, and 15% have severe symptoms. They may overcome you like a wave of heat, leaving you drenched, only to get a chill after. Night sweats are hot flashes that wake you up, sometimes with soaked bedding. *Embarrassment, discomfort,* and *fatigue* are common words women use. Hot flashes usually last one to two years (no small amount of time if you're having them!) but may persist for as long as ten years. About 40% of women report that hot flashes and night sweats negatively affect their quality of life, interfering with work, leisure, mood, concentration, sleep, and even their sex life—so getting a handle on them can spare you a lot of discomfort and distress.

Lifestyle

- Wear **breathable natural fibers** and layer your clothes.

- Keep a **small fan** in your work area.

- Sleep with your **bedroom temperature** no higher than 67°F, use layered natural bedding.

- **Acupuncture** may relieve hot flashes, reduce sleep disturbances, and improve quality of life.

Food

- **Avoid low blood sugar, spicy foods, hot beverages, and alcohol.**

Mind-Body

- Hot flash severity increases with stress. Use **mindfulness practices** to significantly reduce the frequency and severity of hot flashes and improve quality of life, sleep quality, anxiety, and perceived stress.

- Fatigue is also a contributor, so **get your good sleep on**, practice hitting pause during the day, and reprioritizing so you're not exhausted.

- A technique called **"paced breathing"** is easy and can help you cool flash frequency and severity by as much as 40%. Simply inhale for 5 seconds and exhale for 5 seconds, for 15 minutes, twice daily (i.e., when you wake up and go to sleep).

- **Sweat through your clothes** at that board meeting? Own it. Fuck it. You're a wisewoman boss goddess! It happens.

Nutrients

- Make sure you're getting a **daily multi**.

- **Pycnogenol** may help with hot flashes, night sweats, and also fatigue, insomnia, concentration, memory, depression, and irritability.

Herbs

- **Valerian root** can reduce hot flash severity and frequency—day and night—and may also improve sleep. Best taken before bed. All the better combined with **lemon balm** and **hops**.

- **Chinese (Siberian) rhubarb** can help with hot flashes, night sweats, sleep quality, anxiety, and depression. It's in a number of products for peri-meno women.

- **Black cohosh** can offer some relief for day and night flashes; it's not very potent but some women report excellent results.

- **Sage lavender aromatherapy mist** calms your nervous system, promotes sleep, and may help reduce hot flashes. Put 20 drops of each essential oil and a cup of water into a mister. Keep beside your bed or desk and spritz the air around you every few hours during the day, or before sleep. Shake well before using.

- **Vitex (chasteberry)** can reduce frequency and severity of hot flashes. It may take 4 weeks to notice improvement.

Claire, 51

"I'm a mess, Dr. Romm! I'm having hot flashes ten times a day. I've broken a sweat giving a presentation at work in front of my whole team! And they're waking me up at night. Sex hurts; this is upsetting—I was divorced for eighteen years and I'm just recently remarried but feel I can't enjoy my husband. Not to mention I'm having these insane cravings for cookies and candy and I've packed on fifteen pounds in the past six months. The only thing that gives me pleasure is a couple of glasses of red wine in the evening."

Claire readily started the Hormone Intelligence Diet, giving up gluten, sugar, and dairy. She added more fiber—and flaxseeds—to her diet, which helped her start to move her bowels each day. She replaced the wine with melatonin, magnesium, and an herbal plan with ashwagandha, valerian, passionflower, and lemon balm before bed. I also suggested lube and foreplay and prescribed low-dose vaginal estrogen gel, which she applied twice weekly. Within six weeks she was sleeping much better, her cravings had disappeared, and she was down to a few mild hot flashes a day, and she and her husband, well, all she said one day in my office was "Ooh la la!" Within a few months she'd lost ten pounds and was feeling clearer and more energized.

Insomnia

If there's any fountain of youth, it's good sleep. But 40 to 50% of perimenopausal women experience sleep problems. Patterns include waking up in the middle of the night unable to fall back to sleep, being woken by night sweats and hot flashes, or waking up too early and still feeling tired. A combination of hormonal changes and changes in the stress response system are responsible; addressing these can help restore restful sleep. If hot flashes are waking you up, see above.

Lifestyle

- Emphasize the **evening wind-down** (page 175) and other strategies for better sleep.

- Keep your **bedroom temperature** no higher than 67°F at night.

Food

- **Avoid spicy foods.**
- **Avoid all alcohol**; even a small amount can seriously tank a good night's sleep.

Mind-Body

- Use **mindfulness and self-care practices** to calm the mind and support healthy sleep.

Nutrients

- As we get older, our **melatonin** levels decline slightly; supplementing may improve sleep.

- **Calcium and magnesium** can improve sleep quality and reduce anxiety and muscle tension.

Herbs

- **Ashwagandha** calms the nervous system, promotes restful sleep, and is especially helpful if you're "tired and wired." Reishi mushroom is another option.

- **Hops** has mildly estrogenic effects and can reduce night sweats and improve sleep.

- **Valerian** can improve sleep quality, sometimes immediately, with more significant benefits after 4 weeks of use. Combine with **lemon balm** for added benefit for sleep, hot flashes, and anxiety, or with **passionflower and hops**, a combination found comparable to Ambien, without the risks or side effects.

- **Relora**, a combination of tradition Chinese herbs, magnolia and phellodendron, reduces stress and anxiety, improves sleep and energy, reduces cortisol, and improves DHEA, calming an overactive stress response.

Vaginal Dryness

The constellation of perimenopausal symptoms affecting the vagina and urinary system (urethra, ureters, and bladder) is called genitourinary syndrome of menopause (GSM) and includes vaginal or vulvar dryness, burning and irritation (ouch, right?), bleeding after sex, decreased lubrication, discomfort or pain with vulvovaginal touch or penetration, and reduced arousal or orgasmic response. Urinary symptoms can include a sense of urgency, pain when you pee, and even recurrent urinary tract infections (see page 316). Not all women experience vaginal dryness or urinary problems. But if you do, there's plenty that can rehydrate yourself "down there"!

Lifestyle

- Check your **medications**—some can dry up vaginal and cervical secretions.

- Having **sex more often** may prevent vaginal changes, even without taking estrogen. So, whether you have a partner or please yourself, keeping it juicy in your life can help keep things juicy down there, too.

- Make **foreplay** an extended part of lovemaking, and **use lube**—but make sure it's a vagina-friendly brand because some ingredients can dry your vagina. Vitamin E or other natural, commercially available **vaginal suppositories and gels** can be like moisture from heaven.

Food

- **Stay hydrated**—when you're dehydrated, so is your cooch and your pee gets concentrated, too, increasing your risk of UTIs.

Herbs

- *Pueraria mirifica* may improve vaginal lubrication after 12 weeks of daily use, and restore vaginal wall lushness after 24 weeks of use, also relieving pain with sex.

- **Hops** may increase estrogen and progesterone levels and improve the thickness of the vaginal tissue lining, helping with vaginal dryness and pain.

Advanced Protocol: PERIMENOPAUSE

Recurrent Urinary Tract Infections (UTIs)

Urinary tract, and especially bladder, infections are super common—over half of us will have at least one at some point in our lives, up to 20% of all women have some urinary discomfort or a bladder infection every year, and as many as 20% of us gals will have a recurrence six months after a bladder infection. That's a lot of bladder infections! During perimenopause and beyond, the same hormonal changes that cause vaginal dryness can cause chronic or recurrent urinary tract infections. Both the gut flora and vaginal ecology play a key role in preventing UTIs by keeping bacteria that can migrate from either place to the urethra in check. *Lactobacillus* species naturally present in the vagina specifically prevent *E. coli* from proliferating. These recommendations help prevent recurrent UTIs at any age.

Lifestyle

- Emphasize **healing your gut and vaginal ecology** if you experience recurrent UTIs.

- Stay **well hydrated**.

- **Pee** as soon as you feel the urge rather than putting it off, and pee right after sex.

Nutrients and Herbs

Take the following daily for at least 3 months (or ongoing) to prevent recurrent UTIs recurrence:

- **Cranberry/D-mannose:** 500 mg twice daily; increase to 2 g daily if you feel a UTI coming on.

- A **probiotic** with *L. rhamnosus*, *L. reuteri*, and *L. crispatus*.

- Optionally, include an herbal product containing **Uva ursi and marshmallow root**, for up to 3 months.

Urinary Incontinence

While hormone replacement therapy is usually the first urinary incontinence treatment recommended by a gynecologist, and surgery is usually the first approach recommended by urogenital surgeons, neither should be frontline treatments unless symptoms are severe. I always recommend starting with pelvic floor physical therapy and exercise: studies show that at least 60% of women, even with more significant stress incontinence, can avoid surgery and get dramatic symptom improvement this way—and there's no side effect risk!

Mood Changes

Depression, anxiety, irritability, and mood swings are common in perimenopause due not just to hormonal shifts, but to what is, beyond doubt, a major, undercelebrated life cycle change. Fears about the future and financial security, accompanied by loss or grieving for our younger self, may surface or dominate, and simultaneously, kids may be leaving for college, divorce is more common, and you might be caring for an older parent (or a partner). Women with more hot flashes may also experience more depression, a sign of more dramatic estrogen fluctuations and lower progesterone, and possibly, disturbed sleep. Here's how to make this time easier.

Lifestyle

- **Acupuncture** was compared with the antidepressant Venlafaxine for anxiety and hot flashes and created a longer-lasting sense of well-being, sex drive, and energy.

Food

As part of the Hormone Intelligence Diet:

- Strive for **rock-steady blood sugar**.
- Eat plenty of **healthy fats and omega-3-rich fish** up to 3 times weekly.

Sex in Perimenopause and Beyond

Loss of interest in and pleasure from sex are not inevitable as we get older. In fact, a spate of studies over the past fifteen or so years have shown just the opposite—that our sex lives can improve well into our eighties, and that we have the best sex of our lives not in our twenties and thirties as we might think, but after our fifties! According to *The New Hite Report* older women are more likely to enjoy more multiple orgasms than younger women. The Pennell study found that women's sexual arousal or capacity to orgasm actually increases with age.

It's thought that as we get into our forties and beyond, sex gets better because we're more confident, and more adventurous about positions and locations; we're having sex with partners who are also older and more concerned about pleasing their partner; having sex with younger/older partners becomes less taboo; and sex in longer-term relationships has been found to be more satisfying.

However, numerous menopausal factors can interfere with sex life, including lower hormone levels, fatigue from sleep disruption, vaginal dryness, reduced clitoral sensitivity, pain from prior pelvic or bladder surgery, changing body image, and even the belief that you're less sexual because you're not fertile. See page 301 for more on sex and sex drive.

- Consume plenty of **veggies and fresh fruit** to reduce inflammation.
- **Ditch the alcohol**, even high-quality red wine. It may feel good now, but it probably won't tomorrow.

Mind-Body

- **Get more/better sleep** and draw deeply on your **mindfulness tools**.
- **Honor this major life transition** with self-care, ritual, or a special gift to yourself, and be patient with yourself—it's a big deal!
- **Connect with women** going through this transition, read supportive books and articles. Humor helps!
- **Do something you've always wanted to do or learn but haven't**—take that trip, get that graduate degree, invest in yourself.
- And **don't give a shit what anyone thinks about you**! It's liberating!

Nutrients

- **Supplement:** A multivitamin, vitamin D3, B-complex, fish oil, extra calcium and magnesium, and a probiotic are all beneficial for daily mood support.

Herbs

- **Adaptogens** can improve your sense of well-being.
- **St. John's wort** will alleviate depression in about 60% of women who take it for perimenopausal symptoms, a much higher rate than for antidepressants.
- **Black cohosh + St. John's wort** may offer even more benefit when it comes to depression. Results may take 4 weeks to 4 months to be noticeable.
- **Lavender oil** is helpful for sleep disrupted by anxiety.
- **Kava kava** has been associated with significant improvements in anxiety after 4 weeks of use, reduction in depression, and improvement in overall perimenopausal mood symptoms.

Can't I Just Take Hormones?

No and yes. **Hormone replacement therapy (HRT)** has been a standard treatment—and has been touted as a panacea for menopause-related symptoms for decades, based on the premise that menopause is a hormonal deficiency state, a "failure" of our ovaries, and a sign of declining womanhood. Hormones were "God's (or medicine's!) answer to women." Medicalized menopause became a cash cow. But even as early as 1975, medical reports documented an increased risk of endometrial cancer. Finally, in 2002, the largest study on HRT to date was canceled three years ahead of time because the women in the group taking it had so many serious adverse outcomes.

There are **four areas in which HRT has clear benefits**, and for which the benefits are felt to outweigh the risks when used properly. These are:

- **Vasomotor symptoms**, which include sleep problems, hot flashes, and night sweats. Progesterone can make a huge difference.

- **Genitourinary symptoms** including vaginal dryness, discomfort during sex, and recurrent urinary tract infections. Estrogen is used, starting with a vaginal suppository (DHEA is another option), progressing to a patch or topical cream or oral medication if needed.

- **Prevention of bone loss** is treated usually with an estrogen or an estrogen-progesterone combination if you still have your uterus.

- **Low estrogen caused by primary ovarian insufficiency (POI), or medical or surgical menopause** is treated with an estrogen or an estrogen-progesterone combination, if you still have your uterus.

HRT is considered safe for healthy women under age sixty who are within ten years of menopause. For women age sixty and over, or who are ten to twenty years postmenopause, the benefits may not outweigh the very real risks for heart disease, stroke, deep vein thrombosis, and even dementia.

One of the greatest areas of confusion in treating menopause is **bioidentical hormones**. Bioidentical hormones have been the rage since Suzanne Somers put them on the map. They're promoted as a safer, more natural alternative to HRT—but they, too, may be synthetic and can contain inconsistent amounts of hormones, and there's no evidence that they have fewer side effects. Their greatest advantage is that they can be customized to your individual hormonal needs and may be used when conventional HRT doesn't meet your needs for symptom relief. They should only be used for the same conditions as conventional HRT and with the same precautions.

All hormone therapies, including bioidentical hormones, are **best used as a temporary measure** for symptom relief; the long-term changes in the Hormone Intelligence Plan are the most sustainable way to reach hormone balance, symptom relief, and long-term health and vitality.

hormone wisdom

A woman in harmony with her spirit is like a river flowing.
She goes where she will without pretense and arrives at her
destination prepared to be herself and only herself.

—Maya Angelou

When you picked up this book, you may have believed that your body was betraying you, that there was no hope for meaningful solutions, or that you were defective, abnormal, or very alone in what you were going through. I hope you now have a bold new awareness of just how powerful and intelligent you—and your hormones—really are! You now also know that you are absolutely not alone—nor are you defective—that what you're experiencing is your body's natural response to a world that presents no end of challenges to your body's innate desire to keep your hormones in a gorgeous, dynamic flow. Our hormone imbalances are not solely individual problems; they are reflective of much larger social and environmental problems that we're all facing. They are a reflection of a culture that continues to devalue and disrespect women and that has systemically disenfranchised us from understanding our bodies while at the same time teaching us, from our earliest ages, to see ourselves with shame and self-blame.

Getting Radical About Our Health

What you've learned in this book may be completely new to you and may even feel radical. Radical means roots—and that's what this book is about: understanding the roots of how we have arrived, collectively, as women, where we are in the moment, historically and health-wise. And in understanding these roots, we find the path to healing, wholeness, and empowerment.

This book is also a return to our roots in another way—the information I've shared with you is a modern adaptation of a knowing and wisdom that is ancient, with a lineage that can be traced far back in women's history. It just gets buried in a world that denies the power of the feminine and elevates stereotypically masculine traits that are often diametrically opposed to the needs of the female body. And this is exactly what's been happening for a few consecutive centuries now as women's wisdom, and the Earth's wisdom, are overridden. We're seeing the impact of this on our personal health—and planetary health. Indeed, healing one is connected to healing the other—the roots of the wounds are the same. Women's consciousness is once again rising, and with this, the need for an entirely new understanding of our bodies, our health, and medicine.

The awakening of my own Hormone Intelligence came initially from books, like this one, written by women committed to not only preserving women's wisdom, but to awakening it in the next woman, and the next, while also giving women permission to reclaim sovereignty over their bodies. I started learning about my body, my cycles, and my hormones when I was fifteen years old. I built on the knowledge of the women who had come before me; the founders of the self-help movement, who wrote books like *Our Bodies Ourselves*, *A New View of a Woman's Body*, *Hygieia: A Woman's Herbal*, and *Spiritual Midwifery* that showed me there was a whole new way to think of my body—and to own my sovereignty on how my body is treated; and the historians who reminded me in their books, for example, *When God Was a Woman*, that there was a time when the power of women's wisdom—and medicine—was respected, even revered.

Like those books, this one is not part of a *trend* in women's wellness; this is a powerful tradition, and one that is the answer to the gaping hole in what conventional medicine has to offer us in terms of not just health solutions, but care of us as whole women, whose well-being is the result of a breadth and depth of factors that go far beyond what a pill or surgery alone can solve—factors like cultural (and medical) misogyny and threats against women and our fundamental right to control our bodies, and the belief that our bodies are not just machines to be disassembled and reassembled on a medical assembly line, but whole human beings in whom reality influences biology, and our biological experience can shape, and even determine, our reality.

Living in the Flow

Now in my fifties, my body continues to offer me a lifelong adventure of self-discovery. When I began writing this book three years ago, I was fifty-one and still cycling regularly. Over the past year my periods dwindled down to just a scant flow for a day or two, once every few months. After a full forty years of enjoying a healthy, regular flow, beautiful conceptions, pregnancies, and births of my four babies, I've had enough hot flashes to know that I'm close to menopause. These heat waves are a powerful reminder of the fire in our woman-souls, the inevitability of change, and the incredible transformative power that we embody. At first, like getting my first few periods, or the contractions of early labor, these new sensations in my body caught me off guard, made me feel out of control, and at moments, were uncomfortable, but I learned to ride these new waves, too.

Our hormones are dynamic. They shift daily, cyclically, and throughout our life cycles. Staying open to how my body has changed over time, and how my needs have shifted as well, and what life brings has kept me flexible and has allowed me to stay in tune with my own cycles and seasons, while helping me keep my hormones in optimal balance, or get back quickly at those times I've felt that they were calling for my attention.

Owning Your Hormone Wisdom at Any Age

Helen Mirren said, "At seventy years old, if I could give my younger self one piece of advice, it would be to use the words 'fuck off' much more frequently." I couldn't agree more. But none of us should wait until we're seventy to claim our power, to live in more harmony with our own rhythms, or to allow ourselves to honor our own unique strengths—and weaknesses—with confidence. Hormone wisdom is the step into doing exactly all of those things, starting now. And it's more: it's trusting and loving ourselves, which means trusting and loving our bodies, and being "hormonal," wherever you are on the journey.

Perhaps the greatest lessons paying attention to my Hormone Intelligence has brought me is to be more loving to myself, kind to myself, patient with myself, and to stop judging or comparing. This is not easy. We are so deeply engrained to not feel beautiful enough, thin enough, smart enough, and okay with who we are—we're fed a single ideal of a woman, and spend our lives not measuring up in our own eyes—and it's an exhausting and impossible quest: we cannot be someone else. But in the process, we lose our self-love, our delight in our own uniqueness, and with it the con-

tribution of our particular strengths to the world. In always feeling "less than" we give up our power. This relinquishment of power also makes us vulnerable to a medical system that thrives on our insecurities and a culture that has been shutting us out and keeping us down for so long.

And that's where I believe hormonal wisdom starts: it's in truly, deeply, profoundly, unwaveringly trusting our instincts, that deep yes or no we feel in our bones, and allowing ourselves to give less of a fuck about what anyone thinks about us. Here are ten ways you can start to step into your Hormonal Wisdom, right now:

1. Listen to your body, inner Wise Woman, intuition, gut—or whatever you call it—no woman has ever regretted doing that. When we lose trust in our bodies, we lose trust in ourselves. What we have been led to believe are weaknesses—the ebbs and flows of our hormones, our cycles, our moods—are in fact strengths that give us deepened intuition, creative reserves, the ability to connect with others, and tremendous social advantages.

2. Take stress and overwhelm seriously. Give yourself ample permission to pause, get quiet, retreat, cave, be alone, and simply listen inward. Listen to, learn to trust, and begin to live in harmony with the flow of your cycles and seasons, daily, monthly, and throughout the bigger arc of your life. Make your own natural timing, ebbs, and flows your touchstone for what to take on, when to say yes and no, and how to spend your precious time and energy.

3. Put down the need to prove anything to anyone and let go of the race to perfection—you're already there.

4. Own your self-worth and realize you have a right to achieve your wants, needs, and dreams. Within that, determine what feminine power means to you, and live from that place (hint: it's usually not the same as masculine power). When you are able to reconnect to your power on all levels, you are able to start to take more control over your life—starting with the self-respecting basic choices to make time to eat well, sleep enough, play, love, and be loved.

5. Recognize that you are the author of your story—and start writing it! When we lose confidence in the creative functions of our bodies, we lose confidence in our own creative power. How would your life be if you were free from symptoms right now? Who would you be if you felt confident to do that one thing? What would you do with the time you had if you weren't always working on healing your body? Reconnect with these thoughts and see how this shifts your consciousness and ease.

6. Intentionally practice embodiment— move, dance, enjoy pleasure. Reconnect with your wild girl self, that small girl who I hope roller-skated to music, danced with abandon, jumped rope with glee, or rode a bike with the wind in her hair; find the freedom you had before shame and discomfort set in.

7. Heal trauma and shake off the wounds of patriarchy: There are so many ways women hold trauma in our bodies and psyches, and it can keep us from fully living and enjoying our lives. This trauma could be from physical and sexual violence, chronic exposure to microaggressions, or postpartum abandonment and isolation. Seek the support and practices that will help you be free from the grip of trauma so you can live your life fully, not held back. Practice releasing shame, self-blame, and self-loathing. One powerful way to do this is to share your story with other women and listen to theirs. Women all have stories, and many are kept locked up tight in the deep, dark places, sometimes to which the key has been thrown away. But the way out is to shine a light on those places, to speak of these things— the abortion or miscarriage you never talked about with anyone, the sexual assault you might even blame yourself for or feel so ashamed about that you buried it deep inside of you, the violence happening in a marriage with a shiny veneer, the postpartum depression you feel embarrassed about because you think it meant you were a bad mom or hurt your child (it means neither), and the list of secret suffering goes on. Holding on to these in silence and secret only causes us harm. It's amazing what you can feel— and accomplish—when you release the energy bound up in those thoughts, in your body, and in those feelings.

8. Be a force of nature—after all, you literally are! You are part of something bigger, something wild, something powerful, something innately intelligent. Remember this often by spending copious time outdoors: walk barefoot, sit on the earth and feel your body connect vibrationally to the Earth's, learn from her seasons and cycles, and consider how your decisions impact the health of the planet because planetary healthy decisions are usually also personally healthy decisions.

9. Remember that you have parts of your body made solely for pleasure. This is a powerful statement about letting pleasure into your life—not just sexual pleasure—but playfulness, downtime, joy, and physical ease.

10. Celebrate in circles of women, as often as you can. To move forward we have to support each other, elevate each other, bear witness to each other's stories, and hold space for each other's experience.

Where to Find Circles of Women—and More Answers

I hope that the results you're seeing are also giving you a sense of respect and awe for the power of your amazing body, an awareness of how your hormones are talking to you—and how you can respond. I also hope that in this six or twelve weeks together you've seen that this isn't just a plan; it's a whole new way of living in alignment with your inner knowing, of paying attention to your needs. But if you're not there yet, that's okay, too. There is no one perfect timing any more than there's one perfect menstrual cycle. We each have our own unique biorhythms—and healing time. Sometimes it takes more than just what a book can offer you. And I know that, so there's more.

Some of the most powerful healing stories I've witnessed and have had the privilege to be a part of have come not only from my medical practice and the 1:1 care I give, but in online groups of women who have a shared story or experience. Further, a book only allows an author space to convey so much. I want to help you to access both the power of community and the wealth of thirty-five years of experience in women's health I have to share with you, beyond what I could fit in these pages. So on my website, you'll find many more helpful resources specific to the conditions addressed in this book, and to supporting the root causes affecting women's health today, including many free resources, as well as a thriving online community that you can join for free, or at a membership level that meets your needs.

Even if by now, at the end of our time together in this book, you're feeling pretty damn fabulous, I invite you to join me, because this is more than a plan, more than a lifestyle; it's a women's healing revolution, and the most powerful way we can make change is with small steps in our own lives and by creating a revolution together.

the hormone intelligence kitchen

getting started on the hormone intelligence diet

One of my big goals for this book is to help shift your relationship to food so that you see it as a healing tool that you can use to transform how you feel on any given day, time of your cycle, or season in your life. I know, though, that for busy women, eating a healthy diet can feel like a major chore or even an obstacle—especially when it comes to food prep. I've got one simple principle for cooking and eating for Hormone Intelligence: Keep It Simple, Sister (KISS). Real food is simple, satisfying, and delicious—and there are so many options that can often be prepared relatively quickly. Most importantly, it leaves you feeling nourished, satisfied, light, and energized.

I'm not kidding when I say you can make a great meal in fifteen minutes. For example, a fantastic salad with toasted pumpkin seeds, garbanzo beans, and leftover salmon takes just minutes. One-pan frittatas can be prepared in thirty-five minutes start to finish—including prep and clean up. Serve with a mixed field greens salad; not only do you have a complete breakfast, lunch, or dinner, but you've got leftovers. None of the recipes in this book require elaborate, complicated, fancy, or gourmet tools or techniques. But they do require a commitment to your health!

In this section, you'll find all the recipes you need for six weeks of meals, and a lifetime of possibilities and enough suggestions for variations on many of the meal options so you can recombine any number of them to create more meal plans for a long time to come. I've created five meal plans for you to rotate through, use as they are, or pick and choose from to create your own menus. There's a plant-based vegan meal plan and also a quick-and-easy menu to enjoy as is, or select from.

It takes thinking ahead to eat well, even more so if your job takes you out of the house or if you work night shifts with all the temptation and fatigue that lead us to nosh on this and that. I've created meals that are simple enough that you can knock most of them out in thirty minutes. Many of the meal plans make use of leftovers to enjoy as a complete meal or to repurpose as part of other meals—so you get more deliciousness with less prep. Always look ahead to the next day's lunch to plan ahead for extra. That's all part of KISS. To your health!

Quick Tips

1. Do your shopping at the beginning of the week, or at least at one consistent time each week, and have your shopping list with you. No time to shop regularly? Let your local grocery store deliver your food to you, or order from an online market, for example, Thrive Market. Their motto? Healthy food is not for the rich. And it's not.

2. Prep ahead: Wash your veggies, and even cut some that you'll be using early in the week, and store those in glass containers ready for use. Or buy prewashed and precut, as long as they look fresh.

3. Shortcuts like canned or frozen are fair game: I keep about four cans of all the beans I use regularly, stocked in my pantry. Most of your fruits and veggies should ideally be fresh, but frozen vegetables and fruits retain much of their nutrition and can be used in smoothies, soups, and frittatas, for example. I keep several bags of my favorite frozen berries, frozen spinach, and other veggies in the freezer for quick use or when they're not in season. Just make sure they have no added sugar, salt, or other ingredients.

Pantry Essentials

Having a pantry and fridge stocked with the basics makes meal prep much easier—you never have an uh-oh moment where you're missing something. These are the staple ingredients you'll want to have in your pantry and refrigerator specifically for these meal plans. This does not include the produce, meat, and so on, which you'll want to buy fresh at the beginning of each week and create your meals around.

Bulk Grains

- Brown basmati rice
- Brown short-grain rice
- Buckwheat (soba) noodles—look for 100% gluten free
- Millet
- Old-fashioned rolled oats
- Quinoa
- Rice noodles

Nuts, Seeds, and "Butters"

- Almond butter
- Chia seeds
- Flaxseeds
- Nuts: almonds, pecans, cashews
- Sesame seeds
- Sunflower seeds
- Tahini

Legumes/Beans

- Black beans—canned
- Garbanzo beans (chickpeas)—canned
- Miso paste: chickpea (mellow, white, or yellow) and rice (red, brown)
- Red lentils—bulk

Oil and Vinegar

- Balsamic vinegar
- Butter or ghee

- Champagne vinegar
- Coconut oil
- Extra-virgin olive oil
- Red wine vinegar
- Rice vinegar

Herbs and Seasonings

- Black pepper
- Cardamom powder
- Chili powder
- Cinnamon powder
- Cumin
- Curry powder
- Garlic powder
- Oregano
- Red chili flakes
- Sea salt or Himalayan salt
- Thyme
- Turmeric powder
- Vanilla extract
- Optional but recommended: za'atar, adobo powder, chili paste, garam masala, red sumac powder

Condiments

- Dijon mustard
- Honey (raw, wildflower)
- Maple syrup
- Tamari (gluten free, natural soy sauce)
- Optional: organic salsa and/or Sriracha for enjoying with bowls or on eggs, or wherever you like

Other

- Coconut milk
- Coconut sugar
- Dried wakame or alaria seaweed
- Nori seaweed sheets
- Unsweetened dark baking chocolate
- Unsweetened shredded coconut
- I always keep lemons, limes, and ample fresh garlic, fresh ginger, a couple of jalepeños (or other hot peppers) and two ripening avocados in my kitchen.

Kitchen Tools

Even as an active, daily cook, I have a very simple, low-tech kitchen. Here are the basics you'll want to have, all available affordably online or in major stores.

- A small whisk is ideal for sauces and dressings, but optional
- Blender or food processor
- Box grater
- Citrus squeezer
- Garlic press
- Ideally, a medium cast-iron skillet (Lodge company skillets are affordable and last forever!)
- Measuring cups
- Measuring spoons
- Microplane (important for grating ginger!)
- Set of stainless-steel pots and pans
- Vegetable peeler (if you have any waxed cucumbers, for example, that need the skin removed)

Six Weeks of (Scrumptious!) Meals

Enjoy these meal plans laid out for you as is, or feel free to move menu items / meals around. In the spirit of Hormone Intelligence, each meal provides you with the essential ingredients that optimally nourish each of your ecosystems: you'll find gut-friendly fiber, detoxification-supporting phytochemicals, and ovary-, adrenal-, and thyroid-nourishing vitamins and minerals, all in the form of healthy proteins, good healthy fats, a rainbow of veggies and fruits, an assortment of greens, healthful nuts and seeds, and more.

You can also take it one step further for hormone healing, moving menu items around per the eating for cycle sense guidelines on page 133. So, for example, move any dishes with red meat to just after your period when you want to replenish iron you might have lost; eat lighter menu items, especially salads and bowls, around ovulation; and eat heartier warming curries, soup, and bowls in the days leading up to your period. This is totally optional—but fun to play with and see how you feel.

While all these menus serve all women eating for Hormone Intelligence, you'll also find a 100% plant-based vegan menu; you can use this if you're vegan or vegetarian, along with the many additional vegan options you'll find in the recipes section, but it's also an anti-inflammatory plan that you can use perhaps one week of the month premenstrually if you struggle with period, endo, or chronic pelvic pain.

A Typical Day

Start Your Day: Begin with an anti-inflammatory hot beverage (coffee alternatives provided in the recipes!) or lemon water.

Breakfast: Eat breakfast within an hour of waking (unless you're trying intermittent fasting, see page 173) to keep your energy steady through the morning, maintain your focus and clarity, and avoid blood sugar crashes that send you heading for a sugar fix. Breakfast should always be high protein and have a healthy fat; even the menu items that have a wee bit of sweet or grain, which I've sprinkled in to keep things interesting for you and to provide options to eggs if you don't love them, meet this criteria. But if you love eggs, you can sub out any egg dish for muesli, millet

Remember Your Daily Supplement Dose

Remember to take your supplements, including your daily doses of:

- Multivitamin
- Vitamin D
- Essential healthy fatty acid (i.e., fish oil)
- Any additional supplements per your root causes as you identify these going through the six weeks and/or your particular Hormone Intelligence Advanced Protocol, as needed

porridge, etc. Buckwheat is fantastic, too. It's technically a seed not a grain, but cooks up like a tasty nutty flavored grain, and may be especially helpful in improving blood sugar balance and reducing insulin resistance. Try the buckwheat crepes recipe on page 349.

Lunch: This is where you can up your game, especially if your lunch is typically something quick from a less-than-healthy menu. I've given you a wealth of lunches that repurpose menu items from the previous night's dinner—so look ahead each day to make sure you make any called-for leftovers by doubling recipes as needed.

Afternoon: This is a good time to get a half cup or so of berries into your diet. If you tend to need an afternoon snack, check out the options on page 155, or consider light, nourishing items from the recipes—a Hummus Wrap, an Avocado Mash lettuce cup, etc.

Dinner: This is where you get to shine—and also think ahead. These meal plans are suggested menus only; you can have the same dinner twice in a row by doubling up the previous night; you can make four poached chicken breasts on a Sunday instead of one (if you're just feeding yourself) and cluster all the meals that use chicken together—and use the extra poached chicken breast; ditto that on fish or other menu items. The goal is to eat well, bump up your nutrition, fiber, and food variety, achieve healthy blood sugar and insulin—and still KISS. But yes, food prep does take some

work. So make it fun—music, boogie around, experiment; or make it a meditation. Truly, we have to take back our kitchens to take back our hormones. It's a bizarre twist—but it's a kick-ass feminist thing to do.

Evening: Have tea, wind down, and reflect on what you did well today.

The Meal Plans

These five meal plans can be used exactly as is or as a guide that allows you to mix and match and also move menu items around using your cycle sense. The main thing is that these menu items meet the criteria for the Hormone Intelligence Diet, and the menu, overall, provides most of your nutritional needs. There are enough recipes and variations in the meal plans, to trade out items you're not keen on. Because I want you to Keep It Simple Sister (KISS), you'll see I rotate similar menu items so that preparing them becomes easier as you get familiar with this way of eating and food prep. You can also swap in easy items; for example, if you have a great gluten-free bread or crackers you already use, love, and know are healthy enough for this plan, use those; if you can find premade salmon burgers, by all means use those, and above all, relax, play, have fun, experiment, and make your food your own.

Enjoy!

The Basic Hormone-Balancing Menu

	Monday	Tuesday	Wednesday	Thursday	Friday	Saturday	Sunday
Morning Ritual	Golden Milk Chai Latte	Lemon water (optional with fresh ginger juice)	Ginger Lemon Tea	Golden Milk Chai Latte	Ginger Lemon Tea	Lemon water	Golden Milk Chai Latte
Breakfast	Quick Fried Egg Tartine over Seed Bread with Avocado Mash + mixed field greens	Super Seed muesli with berries and almond milk	Egg and Guac Bowl	Overnight Oats—your choice	Quick Pan Omelet or Fried Egg on Tartine with Seed Bread + Avocado Mash and mixed field greens	Savory Buckwheat Crepes with your choice of Sautéed Greens and Pulled Poached Chicken Breast with your choice of sauce	Super Seed muesli with berries and almond milk
Lunch	Hummus Wrap (or on Seed Crackers) + Bright Citrus Arugula Salad	Quick Chopped Salad with added Pulled Poached Chicken Breast, top with your choice of dressing	Chickpea Turmeric Curry + Cauliflower Rice	Best Fish Tacos + Not Your Mama's Slaw + Roasted Sweet Potato Rounds	Za'atar Chicken over Quick Chopped Salad and Hummus	Goddess Ova Bowl + Avocado Mash on Sakara Seed Toast or Seed Crackers	Frittata Cups + mixed field greens with toasted pumpkin and sunflower seeds
Dinner	Chicken and Black Bean Soup + Roasted Sweet Potatoes + Quick Chopped Salad	Chickpea Turmeric Curry + Cauliflower Rice	Best Fish Tacos + Not Your Mama's Slaw + Roasted Sweet Potato Rounds	Za'atar (or your way) Chicken + Curry Baked Cauliflower + Lemony Quinoa	Thai Steak (or Chicken) salad + roasted kale or steamed broccoli	Maple Dijon Salmon over quinoa (or Simple Baked Sweet Potato) + Steamed Greens Your Way	Broccoli Sesame Noodle Bowl + Salmon Burgers
Evening Ritual	Sleepy Time Chai	Chamomile tea	Mint tea	Chamomile tea	Sleepy Time Chai	Chamomile tea	Mint tea

The Love Your Gut Menu

	Monday	Tuesday	Wednesday	Thursday	Friday	Saturday	Sunday
Morning Ritual	Golden Milk Chai Latte	Lemon water (optional with fresh ginger juice)	Ginger Lemon Tea	Golden Milk Chai Latte	Ginger Lemon Tea	Lemon water	Golden Milk Chai Latte
Breakfast	Eggs and Guac Breakfast Bowl with kimchi	Millet Breakfast Porridge with chopped apricots, flaxseeds, and pumpkin seeds	Quick Fried Egg Tartine over Seed Bread with arugula, Avocado Mash, and kimchi	Super Seed Muesli with berries and coconut yogurt or nut milk	Omelet with Avocado Mash + Gingery Lemon Green Juice	Savory Buckwheat Crepes with sautéed greens and chicken (or protein of your choice) topped with sauerkraut	East Meets West Frittata + berries + optional WomanWise Carrot-Apple-Ginger Juice
Lunch	Hummus Wrap (or on Seed Crackers) + Bright Citrus Arugula Salad	Macro Bowl with Lemony Tahini Sauce with Cauliflower Rice and picked vegetables or sauerkraut	Za'atar Chicken over Quick Chopped Salad with hummus and flaxseeds	Chickpea Turmeric Curry + Cauliflower Rice	Thai Lettuce Wraps (with salmon) + optional kimchi + Avocado Mash on Seed Crackers	Asian Breakfast Egg Scramble + Bright Citrus Arugula Salad	Burrito Bowl with Cauliflower Rice
Dinner	Mediterranean Lemon Salmon + Roasted Squash and Kale with Lemony Tahini Sauce and chopped walnuts	Za'atar Chicken over Lemony Quinoa + sautéed collard greens or roasted asparagus	Chickpea Turmeric Curry + Cauliflower Rice + optional steamed broccoli	Miso-Glazed Salmon over Napa Citrus Salad with Tangy Ginger-Lime Dressing or Peanut Sauce + Roasted Sweet Potato Rounds	Ginger Rice or Chickpea Miso Soba Noodle Soup with Pulled Poached Chicken Breast + optional Easy Seaweed Salad	Quinoa, Black Bean, Sweet Potato, and Fajita Burrito Bowl with Cauliflower Rice	No-Fail Veggie Stir-Fry with steak, chicken, or tofu, topped with cashews and kimchi + brown rice
Evening Ritual	Sleepy Time Chai	Chamomile tea	Mint tea	Sleepy Time Chai	Chamomile tea	Sleepy Time Chai	Mint tea

The Detox Menu

	Monday	Tuesday	Wednesday	Thursday	Friday	Saturday	Sunday
Morning Ritual	Golden Milk Chai Latte	Lemon water	Ginger Lemon Tea	Golden Milk Chai Latte	Ginger Lemon Tea	Lemon water	Golden Milk Chai Latte
Breakfast	Frittata Cups with toasted pumpkin and sunflower seeds	Super Seed Muesli with berries and almond milk	Quick Fried Egg over Seed Toast with Avocado Mash + mixed field greens salad	Overnight Oats—your choice	Quick Pan Omelet Tartine with Seed Bread + Avocado Mash and mixed field greens	Millet Breakfast Porridge with chopped apricots and nuts	Vegan Buckwheat Crepes with your choice of Sautéed Greens and Pulled Poached Chicken Breast with your choice of sauce
Lunch	Brown rice + Roasted Squash and Kale with Lemony Tahini Sauce	Asian Pulled Chicken Salad or Wraps (see Wraps)	Green Tara Lentil Bowl	Spicy Salmon Sushi Bowl (with salmon)	Hummus Wrap (or on Seed Crackers) + Quick Chopped Salad	Goddess Ova Bowl + Avocado Mash on Seed Toast or Seed Crackers	Mediterranean Lemon Salmon + baby green or your choice salad with roasted sunflower seeds and half an avocado
Dinner	Ginger Rice or Chickpea Miso Soba Noodle Soup with Pulled Poached Chicken Breast + optional Easy Seaweed Salad	Green Tara Lentil Bowl	Rice or Chickpea Miso-Glazed Salmon with Scallions and Sesame Seeds + quinoa + lemon-drizzled steamed carrots and broccoli	Asian Breakfast Scramble + Bright Citrus Arugula Salad with Chili-Lime Dressing	Quinoa, Black Bean, Sweet Potato Bowl + Fajita Chicken, or Steak or salmon	Mediterranean Lemon Salmon + brown rice + Roasted Squash and Roasted Kale with Lemony Tahini Sauce	Chicken and Black Bean Soup + Roasted Sweet Potato Rounds + Quick Chopped Salad
Evening Ritual	Sleepy Time Chai	Chamomile tea	Mint tea	Chamomile tea	Sleepy Time Chai	Chamomile tea	Mint tea

The Quick & Easy Menu

	Monday	Tuesday	Wednesday	Thursday	Friday	Saturday	Sunday
Morning Ritual	Lemon water	Ginger Lemon Tea	Lemon water	Ginger Lemon Tea	Lemon water	Ginger Lemon Tea	Lemon water
Breakfast	Eggs your way, topped with avocado + side of berries	Overnight Oats—your choice	Almond Butter Cup Smoothie or build your own	Quick Fried Egg over arugula topped with chopped tomatoes + splash of champagne vinegar	Turmeric Ginger Relief Smoothie or build your own	Overnight Oats—your choice	Egg Scramble + avocado + side of berries
Lunch	Build Your Own Salad with spinach, cherry tomatoes, chickpeas, pumpkin seeds, avocado, and olive oil/vinegar dressing	Macro Bowl (with salmon, quinoa, and broccoli), your choice of fresh lemon juice or Lemony Tahini Sauce	Black Bean Soup (Vegan Version)+ mixed field greens salad	Quick Chopped Salad with chicken, top with your choice of dressing	Best Fish Tacos + Not Your Mama's Slaw + Roasted Sweet Potato Rounds	Mixed field greens salad with salmon, walnuts, and ½ avocado	Hummus Wrap + Quick Chopped Salad
Dinner	Maple Dijon Salmon + Lemony Quinoa + steamed broccoli	Black Bean Soup (Vegan Version) + mixed field greens salad	Pulled Poached Chicken Breast (with optional Peanut Sauce) + Cauliflower Rice + Simple Baked Sweet Potato	Best Fish Tacos + Not Your Mama's Slaw + Roasted Sweet Potato Rounds	Mediterranean Lemon Salmon + brown rice + sautéed spinach	Omelet + your choice of Roasted Veggies (broccoli, kale, sweet potato, squash)	Bright Citrus Arugula Salad with Pulled Poached Chicken Breast + optional quinoa
Evening Ritual	Chamomile tea	Mint tea	Chamomile tea	Mint tea	Chamomile tea	Mint tea	Chamomile tea

The Plant-Based Vegan Menu

	Monday	Tuesday	Wednesday	Thursday	Friday	Saturday	Sunday
Morning Ritual	Golden Milk Chai Latte	Lemon water	Ginger Lemon Tea	Golden Milk Chai Latte	Ginger Lemon Tea	Lemon water	Golden Milk Chai Latte
Breakfast	Super Seed muesli and berries with Nut Milk	Tofu Scramble with sautéed spinach	Sakara Seed Bread with Avocado Mash + Roasted Kale	Super Seed muesli and berries with Nut Milk	Millet Breakfast Porridge + Seed Bread with almond butter	Goddess Ova Bowl + Avocado Mash on Seed Toast or Seed Crackers	Vegan Buckwheat Crepes with your choice of Sautéed Greens and your choice of sauce + optional tofu, dahl, or beans
Lunch	Goddess Ova Bowl + Avocado Mash on Seed Toast or Seed Crackers	Chickpea Turmeric Curry + Cauliflower Rice	Green Tara Lentil Bowl	Hummus Wrap (or on Seed Crackers) + Quick Chopped Salad	Burrito Bowl + Roasted Sweet Potato Rounds	Vegan Nori Wrap with brown rice and veggies	Broccoli Sesame Noodle Bowl with Peanut Sauce or Creamy Cashew Dressing
Dinner	Chickpea Turmeric Curry + Cauliflower Rice	Green Tara Lentil Bowl	Brown rice + Roasted Squash and Kale with Lemony Tahini Sauce	Quinoa, Black Bean, Sweet Potato, and Fajita Burrito Bowl (vegan style)	Build Your Own Stir-Fry Goddess Bowl with Tofu	Napa Citrus Salad Bowl with Lemony Tahini Sauce or Peanut Sauce + Ginger Rice or Chickpea Miso Soba Noodle Soup	Black Bean Soup + Roasted Sweet Potato Rounds + Easy Steamed Veggies drizzled with lemon juice
Evening Ritual	Sleepy Time Chai	Chamomile tea	Mint tea	Chamomile tea	Sleepy Time Chai	Chamomile tea	Mint tea

the recipes

Eat a Rainbow Salad Basics

Simple Tossed Baby Green Salad with Toasted Seeds

Provides 2 servings of veggies, 2 of healthy fat, and 1 seeds + protein

2 cups mixed field greens or other mixed field greens—prewashed is totally fine

2 tbsp. Anytime Vinaigrette, using lemony olive oil or champagne olive oil

Optional: add ½ cup chopped avocado, slices of grapefruit, some fresh berries, or 1 tsp. toasted seeds (pumpkin or sunflower) or a tsp. of ground flaxseeds

Toss the above ingredients together. Serve immediately—enjoy!

Make it a meal: Fantastic with Pulled Poached Chicken Breast (page 356), Mediterranean Lemon Salmon (page 355), chickpeas, or a hard-boiled egg. And the perfect side with most meals as is.

5 minutes: 1 serving

Quick Chopped Salad (with toasted almonds)

Provides 2 servings of veggies, 1 of healthy fat + protein

Use 4 cups total of mixed veggies:
   Romaine lettuce
   Carrots
   Celery
   Red onion
   Red pepper
   Red cabbage
   Cucumber
   Apple

Wash your veggies and cut into smaller than bite-size pieces. Mix together. Top with your choice of dressing.

Make it a meal: Fantastic with Pulled Poached Chicken Breast (page 356), Mediterranean Lemon Salmon (page 355), chickpeas, or a hard-boiled egg.

10 minutes: 2 servings

Bright Citrus Arugula Salad (with pumpkin seeds)

Provides 2 servings of veggies, 1 fruit, 1 healthy fat, and 1 seeds + protein

Bitter. It's a taste we often neglect but it's so important for our digestive and detoxification systems. Here's a favorite easy salad that's packed with flavor—the avocado and grapefruit soften the slight bitter-spicy flavor of the arugula, and toasted pumpkin seeds round the whole salad out with a nutty deliciousness that will delight your taste buds.

1 cup arugula
½ avocado, sliced
½ grapefruit, peeled and sectioned
2 tbsp. toasted pumpkin seeds (see Nuts and Seeds)
Oil and champagne vinegar dressing (see Anytime Vinaigrette in Sauces and Dressings; page 359)

Put arugula on a plate or in a bowl, layer on avocado and grapefruit slices, top with seeds and dressing.

Make it a meal: Add a hard-boiled or fried egg, Pulled Poached Chicken Breast, smoked salmon, Mediterranean Lemon Salmon, or sardines.

5 minutes: 1 serving

Napa Citrus Salad (with sesame seeds) with Chicken, Steak, Salmon, Egg, or Tofu

Provides 4 servings of veggies, 1 healthy fat, and 1 nuts + protein

1 small napa cabbage sliced very finely crosswise
2 grated carrots
4 chopped scallions
1 finely chopped red pepper
1 cup chopped fresh basil
¼ cup fresh chopped cilantro
¼ cup bean sprouts
1 cucumber
¼ cup toasted cashews, almonds, or peanuts
Your choice: vegan (as is or with tofu)
Tangy Ginger-Lime Dressing

Put cabbage on a plate or in a bowl, layer on remaining vegetables, and top with nuts and dressing.

Make it a meal: Pulled Poached Chicken Breast, or Rice or Chickpea Miso-Glazed or Ginger-Lime Salmon, or hard-boiled or fried egg.

10 minutes: 2 servings

Build Your Own Salad

Greens (pick 1 or more)	Vegetables (pick 3–4)	Protein (pick 1–2)	Healthy fat (pick 1)	Dressing (pick an oil, vinegar, and seasonings)
Romaine lettuce Kale Butter lettuce Mixed greens Spinach Green/red leaf lettuce Arugula	Cucumber Cherry tomato Bell pepper Broccoli Beets Bean sprouts Alfalfa sprouts Sweet potato Red onions	Chickpeas Black beans Grilled, baked, or sautéed chicken Grilled, baked, or sautéed steak Whole or diced hard-boiled eggs Fried egg or poached egg	Avocado Toasted sunflower or pumpkin seeds Toasted nuts (almond, walnut, etc.) Olives	Olive oil Sesame oil Avocado oil Dijon mustard Lemon juice Lime juice Cilantro Basil Red wine vinegar Balsamic vinegar Apple cider vinegar Honey Chili pepper Black pepper Sea salt Shallot

Not Your Mama's Slaw

Provides 2 servings of veggies, 1 healthy fat

½ red and ½ green cabbage, chopped fine or minced in the food processor
2 carrots, grated or minced in the food processor
2 tbsp. finely minced red onion
½ jalapeño, finely minced
1 bunch cilantro, finely chopped
Juice of 1–2 limes, to taste
¼ cup olive oil
¼ tsp. salt
¼ tsp. chili powder
¼ tsp. cumin

Mix cabbage, carrots, red onion, jalapeño, and cilantro together. In another bowl, whisk lime juice, olive oil, and seasonings. Toss with the veggies.

Make it a meal: Serve on a gluten-free tortilla, lettuce cups or bed, or as a bowl with Best Fish Tacos and guacamole.

10 minutes: 2 servings

Easy Seaweed Salad

Provides ½ serving of veggies, ½ healthy fat, and ½ seeds

¼ cup dried wakame or alaria seaweed
1 cup cold water
1 scallion, chopped
½ small organic unwaxed cucumber, thinly sliced
½ tsp. rice vinegar
1 tsp. toasted sesame oil
1 tsp. tamari
1 tsp. sesame seeds, toasted

Soak the wakame or alaria in 1 cup of cold water for an hour. Strain and chop into bite-size piece. In the meantime, toss all the other ingredients (except sesame seeds) in a bowl and let marinate. Then mix the seaweed in and toss again. Top with toasted sesame seeds.

1 hour to soak alaria, 10 minutes to prepare salad: serves 1 or 2

Keeps in the fridge for 2 days.

The Ultimate Goddess Bowls

Goddess Bowls (my spin on Buddha bowls) are basic one-dish meals that contain all you need for a healthy meal in one place. They are some of my favorite quick meals, are universally healthy, and will probably become a staple for you, too. They are also one of the best ways to repurpose leftovers. Always look ahead to your next day's lunch when making dinner, so you make leftovers for the bowl.

And hey, if you don't want to eat any of these as a bowl, simply arrange the various ingredients on your plate, and use the toppings and sauce on the grain and veggies.

A bowl typically contains:

- **The Base:** a prepared grain OR a base of finely chopped ribbons of lettuce, kale, or napa cabbage, for example.

- **The Veggies Layer:** Stacked on top of the base. This can include the protein: sautéed or grilled beef, chicken, fish, OR a vegan option, for example, grilled tofu, red lentil dahl, or hummus, or an egg your way—or any of these together that appeals to you.

- **The Sauce:** It's your call as to which of the many sauces you drizzle over your salad; it all depends on your ingredients and the flavor vibe you're going for. I give you lots of examples in Dressings and Sauces. This is where you get a healthy fat into the bowl. Avocado is a great topping in this layer, too.

- **The Crunch:** A few tbsp. of chopped raw veggies as a topping, for example, mung bean sprouts or chopped cilantro, and toasted nuts or seeds.

Here are the bowls in the meal plan—the ones I return to again and again in my own diet.

Eggs and Guac Breakfast Bowl

Provides 2 servings of veggies, 2 healthy fat + protein

½ avocado
4 cups baby spinach or mixed field greens
2 hard-boiled eggs, peeled and sliced in half, or fried eggs
2 tbsp. thinly sliced red onion
½ lemon, juiced
Sea salt and black pepper, to taste
1 tbsp. extra-virgin olive oil

Make Avocado Mash or chop the avocado in half. Put greens into a bowl and top with avocado, egg, red onion, lemon juice, salt and pepper, and olive oil. Optional: You can also top this with a few tbsp. of warm black beans, salsa, and serve with an organic sprouted corn tortilla.

10 minutes: 2 servings

Goddess Ova Bowl

Provides 4 servings of veggies, 2 healthy fat, 1 seeds, 1 grain + protein

This is a great meal to think ahead to; you can use leftover Roasted Sweet Potato Rounds, roasted kale, and hummus, or hard-boiled eggs you've made.

½ cup cooked brown rice, quinoa, or millet
2 cups kale prepared any way
1 cup roasted sweet potatoes or delicata squash
½ cup grated carrot
¼ cup thinly sliced red pepper
½ avocado, diced
¼ cup canned chickpeas OR ¼ cup of Classic Hummus AND/OR sliced hard-boiled egg
2 tbsp. toasted sunflower seeds (or ¼ cup sunflower sprouts) OR toasted walnuts
Dressing: Lemony Tahini Sauce (page 360) or any of your choice
More protein: Add Pulled Poached Chicken Breast (page 356), tofu, or your choice of fish.

Layer all the ingredients in the order listed above.

10 minutes if using leftovers, or 40 additional minutes if making from scratch: 1 serving

Macro Bowl with Lemony Tahini Sauce (vegan, egg, salmon, or chicken)

Provides 2 servings of veggies, 1 healthy fat, 2 seeds, 1 grain + protein and fermented veggie

½ cup cooked brown rice, quinoa, or millet
2 cups your choice steamed veggies
Select one of these sauces: Lemony Tahini (page 360), Spicy Thai (page 360), Creamy Cashew (page 360), Rice or Chickpea Miso-Tahini (page 360), Peanut (page 360)
1 tbsp. toasted pumpkin and/or sunflower seeds
Side of sauerkraut or kimchi
More protein: Add your choice of fish, salmon, chicken, tofu, egg, or adzuki beans
Layer all the ingredients in the order listed above.

10 minutes if using leftovers, or 25 additional minutes if making from scratch: 1 serving

Spicy Salmon Sushi Bowl (fish or other variations)

Provides 2 servings of veggies, 1 healthy fat, 2 seeds, 1 grain + protein and fermented veggie

½ to 1 cup cooked quinoa, brown rice, pink rice, or rice noodles
4-ounce Rice or Chickpea Miso-Glazed Salmon (page 355)
2 cups mixed sautéed or roasted greens
¼ cup sautéed shiitake mushrooms
1 tbsp. grapeseed or sesame oil
2 tbsp. chopped scallions
2 tbsp. chopped fresh cilantro
Your choice Spicy Thai Sauce (page 360), Tangy Ginger-Lime Dressing (page 360), or Peanut Sauce (page 360)
Optional: fresh avocado to garnish

Layer all the ingredients in the order listed above.

10 minutes if using leftovers, or 35 minutes if making from scratch: 1 serving

Broccoli Sesame Noodle Bowl with Peanut Sauce (vegan, egg, salmon, or chicken)

Provides 3 servings of veggies, 1 healthy fat, 1 seeds, 1 grain + protein and fermented veggie

½ package buckwheat soba noodles (can use rice instead)
1 cup broccoli, steamed or raw
1 cup red bell pepper, steamed or raw
¼ cup bean sprouts
1 cup snow peas
2 tbsp. coconut oil

Build Your Own Goddess Bowl

Base	Veggie Layer (pick 3–4)	Protein (pick 1–2)	Dressing	Toppings
Brown rice, wild rice, quinoa, millet, rice or buckwheat noodles AND/OR Ribbons of lettuce, kale, collards, or napa cabbage	Chopped greens if not already used for the base Lots more veggies, often in a medley of varieties and colors, in a combo of steamed, sautéed, roasted or raw. For example: Roasted sweet potato or winter squash Roasted or steamed beets Cucumber Bell pepper Broccoli Broccoli rabe Brussels sprouts Cauliflower Zucchini Asparagus Carrots Green beans Spinach Dandelion greens Mushrooms	Chickpeas Black beans Grilled, baked, or sautéed chicken Grilled, baked, or sautéed steak Tofu Fried or hard-boiled egg Hummus Dahl	See Dressings and Sauces (pages 359–60) for options Fresh lime or lemon juice	Avocado Toasted seeds or nuts Chopped scallions, shallots, or red onion Sunflower or other sprouts Chopped basil or cilantro

1 tbsp. tamari
1 tsp. fresh grated ginger
1 bulb garlic, minced
1 tbsp. sesame seeds
More protein: Serve with a salmon burger, a soft-boiled egg, add your favorite Asian-style chicken recipe and layer in between noodles and veggies, or top with Peanut Sauce (page 360).

Cook noodles or rice according to package instructions, and sauté veggies in coconut oil. Add the tamari, ginger, and garlic, and sauté for 1 minute. Put rice or noodles into individual bowls, then layer on broccoli, bell pepper, bean sprouts, and snow peas. Layer on your added protein; sprinkle with toasted sesame seeds.

30 minutes: 2 servings

Green Tara Lentil Bowl (vegan)

Provides 2 servings of veggies, 1 healthy fat, 1 grain, 1 legume

The classic, soothing Ayurvedic bowl; to make it even more delicious, add 2 tbsp. of shredded coconut to your rice when cooking!

½ cup cooked brown basmati rice drizzled with 2 tsp. coconut oil and a pinch of salt
¼ cup green or red lentil dahl (You're a [Lentil] Dahl; page 352)
1 cup Curry Baked Cauliflower (page 347)
½ cup Roasted Sweet Potato Rounds (page 346)
Fresh cilantro
Fresh chopped cucumber
Sea salt and black pepper, to taste
Optional: dollop of coconut yogurt or Lemony Tahini Sauce (page 360)

When all the ingredients are done cooking, place the cooked rice into a bowl, add a healthy scoop of the lentils, then layer on the veggies and herbs. Sprinkle on salt and black pepper to taste and enjoy. Optionally drizzle with Lemony Tahini Sauce.

45 minutes: 1 serving

Quinoa, Black Bean, Sweet Potato, and Fajita Burrito Bowl (vegan, chicken, or steak)

Provides 3 servings of veggies (2 with cauliflower rice), 2 healthy fat, 1 grain (unless omitting cauliflower), 1 bean/legume + protein

½ cup cooked quinoa (or Cauliflower Rice; page 346)
½ cup warmed-up can of black beans (seasoned with ¼ cup cumin, chili powder, and salt and black pepper, to taste)
1 serving of chicken or steak fajita
Chili roasted sweet potato wedges
1 cup chopped romaine lettuce
Chopped tomato
¼ red onion, finely minced
1 ripe avocado, sliced thinly, or 2 tbsp. Guacamole Mash (page 345)
Toasted pumpkin seeds (1 tbsp. per bowl)
¼ cup chopped cilantro per bowl
Chili-Lime Dressing (page 360) or fresh lime juice

In a meal-size bowl, layer all the ingredients in the order listed above, topping with Chili-Lime Dressing or lime juice.

10 minutes (with leftovers) or 40 minutes from scratch: 1 serving

Burrito Bowl

Provides 3 servings of veggies, 2 healthy fat, 1 grain, 1 bean/legume + protein

½ cup cooked brown rice or quinoa
½ cup Not Your Mama's Slaw (page 341)
½ cup Roasted Sweet Potato Rounds (page 346)
½ cup seasoned black beans (see Quinoa, Black Bean, Sweet Potato, and Fajita Burrito Bowl; page 344)

¼ cup Guacamole Mash (page 345) or ½ diced
  avocado
Chopped cilantro
Add protein from: Best Fish Tacos–style tilapia
  or salmon (page 356), Fajita Chicken or Steak
  (page 357), Pulled Poached Chicken (page 356),
  sliced hard-boiled or fried egg, or keep it vegan
  with just the black beans.
Top with Chili-Lime Dressing
Optional: diced red onion or scallion, chopped
  tomato, toasted pumpkin seeds

*Assemble by layering all the ingredients in the order
listed above in a meal-size bowl.*

*10 minutes (with leftovers) or 40 minutes from
scratch: 1 serving*

Ginger Rice or Chickpea Miso Soba Noodle Soup

*Provides 3 servings of veggies, 2 healthy fat, 1 grain,
1 bean/legume + protein*

A lovely simple classic for any meal, soothing
and easy on the digestion, and packed with
healthy buckwheat.

⅓ package buckwheat soba noodles (or 2 servings as
  indicated on package)
2 tbsp. rice or chickpea miso
2 cups water
1 tbsp. grated ginger
1 tbsp. tamari
1 tbsp. sesame oil
1 cup bok choy, quartered
1 medium carrot, julienned
1 cup snow peas
½ lime
More protein: Add a cooked salmon fillet, tofu
  steaks, edamame beans, or chicken.
No soba noodles? Use rice noodles instead.

Bring a medium pot of water to a boil. Add
the soba noodles and cook for 6 to 7 minutes,
until done. Drain and rinse with cold water until
completely cooled. Set aside. In a small bowl
combine rice or chickpea miso with just enough
water to form a paste. Add the paste to a small
saucepan along with the water, ginger, tamari,
and sesame oil. Bring to a gentle simmer but be
careful not to boil. Rice or chickpea miso is a
probiotic food and should not be boiled. While
the broth is warming, divide the cooked noodles,
bok choy, carrots, and snow peas between bowls.
Pour the rice or chickpea miso soup broth over
the veggies to warm everything. Squeeze lime
over each bowl and enjoy!

25 minutes: 2 servings

Greens and Other Veggies

These are the perfect veggie accompaniments
to round out any meal and make it easy to get
your Hormone Intelligence servings of veggies
to support your health in every way.

Avocado Mash 2 Ways

Provides: ½ avocado = 1 healthy fat

Simple Lemon Mash

Mash ½ of an avocado, mix with a pinch of salt
and a squeeze of lemon. Spread on toast or
crackers. Top with any of the following: broccoli
or sunflower sprouts, thinly sliced radish. Serve
as is or drizzle with a small amount of olive oil.

A few minutes to prepare: 1 serving

Guacamole Mash

1 ripe avocado
Juice of ½ to 1 lime, to taste
2 tbsp. chopped and destemmed cilantro
1 clove garlic, crushed

Pinch of salt

Optional: minced hot pepper to taste (wash hands after cutting pepper)

Cut the avocado in half lengthwise, scoop out the pit, and scoop the avocado into a bowl. Mash avocado with a whisk to a smooth and creamy consistency (or you can use a food processor).

Add remaining ingredients and mix together. Serve with crunchy veggies, tortilla chips, gluten-free crackers, or my personal favorite, jicama! Keeps for 2 days in the fridge, may turn brown on the surface, but it's still good—stir well before serving.

10 minutes: 2 servings

Cauliflower Rice

A delicious substitute for grain, each serving provides a "daily dose" of leafy greens!

Provides 1 serving of veggies, 1 healthy fat

½ of a small cauliflower

Sea salt

1 tbsp. olive oil, coconut oil, ghee, or your choice of oil

Put cauliflower florets in the food processor. Pulse until the cauliflower has a rice-like consistency. You may need to do this in batches. For cooked cauliflower, rice prepare in either of these two ways:

Steamed: Put ¼ inch of water in a medium skillet on medium heat. Cover and cook for 5 minutes, or until cauliflower is soft and warm. Drain out the water in a mesh strainer. Add 1 tbsp. oil if desired, and salt/season to taste.

Sautéed: Put your choice of oil in a medium skillet on medium heat. Sauté for 3 to 5 minutes and serve. Salt/season to taste.

10 minutes: 2 servings

Simple Baked Sweet Potato

Provides 1 serving of veggies, 1 healthy fat

1 medium sweet potato

Butter, ghee, or coconut oil

Sea salt

Preheat oven to 400°F. Wash and dry sweet potato. Puncture lightly with a fork in several places. Place on a baking rack. Place a cookie sheet or foil on the lowest oven rack. Place sweet potatoes on the rack above it. Bake for 30 to 40 minutes, until soft to the touch. Remove. Let cool for 5 minutes. Serve plain or slice open and serve with a little butter, ghee, or coconut oil and sea salt.

Roasted Veggies

Roasted Squash or Sweet Potato Rounds

Provides 1 serving of veggies, 1 healthy fat if adding oil

Your choice:

1 small butternut squash

1 small delicata squash

2 medium sweet potatoes

1 tbsp. olive oil

Optional seasonings: sea salt, ginger and lime, adobo chili powder, roasted paprika

Preheat oven to 400°F. Cut your choice of above veggie into rounds. (If using squash, cut it in half widthwise and scoop out the seeds first.) Place in a bowl, drizzle with olive oil, and toss with your seasoning choice until well coated. Spread out onto a sheet tray covered with parchment paper and roast until tender and slightly browned, 15 to 25 minutes. Turn slices over once, halfway through cooking.

30 minutes: 2 servings

Roasted Greens

Provides 2 servings of veggies, 1 healthy fat if adding oil

We tend to think of steaming and sautéing greens, but a quick, easy, overlooked way to prepare them is by roasting them. This is done simply by placing your washed and cut greens onto a cookie sheet or into a cast-iron skillet, drizzling with olive oil, sprinkling with salt and baking in a 425°F oven for about 12 to 15 minutes, until soft and lightly roasted. This technique works beautifully for kale, broccoli, broccoli rabe, cauliflower, and Brussels sprouts. If preparing kale this way, stir every couple of minutes and remove when the kale looks wilted but still bright green.

If I'm cooking more Italian, I'll toss with a drizzle of balsamic vinegar when done; if more Asian style, with toasted sesame oil, tamari, and a dash of lime juice or rice vinegar.

15 minutes: 2 cups of raw veggies per person

Curry Baked Cauliflower

Provides 2 servings veggies

1 small head cauliflower, cut into bite-size pieces
2 tbsp. coconut oil
1 tbsp. curry powder
1 tsp. ground cumin
Salt, to taste

Preheat oven to 400°F

Toss all the ingredients in a bowl, transfer to a cookie sheet.

Bake for 15 minutes, or until cauliflower is golden and tender.

20 minutes: 2 large or 4 small servings

Sautéed Greens

2 cups cooked provides 2 servings of veggies, 1 healthy fat if adding oil

This is the classic way to eat spinach, chard, kale, collards, napa cabbage, and bok choy. Lightly heat 2 tbsp. of olive oil, coconut oil, or ghee in a skillet. Optionally add 1 to 2 cloves crushed garlic and stir for 1 minute. Add 1 bunch of chopped greens, and sauté for 3 to 5 minutes for spinach and chard, 5 to 7 minutes for the other greens, and then splash with a couple of tsp. of tamari. Alternatively, you can use salt and lemon.

No-Fail Veggie Stir-Fry

2 cups cooked provides 2–3 servings of veggies, 1 healthy fat if adding oil

My secrets to a great, no-fail stir-fry are: never use more than five types of veggies per stir-fry; quickly blanch the longer-cooking veggies before stir-frying to soften them and cut down on stir-fry time—do this while you're sautéing the onions or scallions, ginger, and garlic; chop or cut all ingredients into roughly similar sizes; don't overcook or your stir-fry will be mushy; stir quickly and almost continuously; and ideally, use a wok, though any stainless-steel pan will also work.

Grapeseed or coconut oil
1 yellow onion cut into half-moons or 1 bunch of chopped scallions
1 tbsp. freshly grated ginger
2 cloves freshly crushed garlic
¼ tsp. red pepper flakes
4 cups of veggies to include: broccoli florets, napa cabbage OR bok choy, 1 large red bell pepper cut into thin slices, 1 large carrot cut into matchsticks
¼ cup roasted peanuts or toasted cashews
¼ cup chopped fresh basil leaves (optional)
1 tbsp. tamari

Heat oil in a large pan and at the same time, bring a medium saucepan of water to a boil. Sauté onion, ginger, garlic, and red-pepper flakes for 2 minutes, while blanching the broccoli and carrots in the water for 3 to 5 minutes until they are bright green and orange but not soft. Sauté the red pepper, and napa or bok choy for 3 to 5 minutes, drain the broccoli and carrots and add to the stir-fry. Sauté all for 5 minutes until veggies are tender but still crisp. Season with tamari. Serve over rice noodles or brown rice. Top with peanuts and basil (optional) and drizzle on an Asian-style sauce of your choice from the sauces suggestions.

To add meat, cut 2 chicken breasts or 8 oz. flank or other steak, sliced thin (put meat in freezer for 15 minutes before slicing to make it easier), and sauté for 5 minutes after adding onions, ginger, and garlic, then add the other veggies and stir-fry until the veggies are done. Marinate meat for at least 30 minutes prior to cooking, though this is optional. You can, instead, use cubed firm tofu.

30 minutes: 2 servings

Easy Steamed Veggies

You can use virtually any veggies you want for a steamed veggie dish. My personal standbys for decades have been a combo of 1 sweet potato cut into ½-inch rounds, a yellow onion cut into 8 large sections (quarter it, then cut the quarters in half), 2 carrots cut into slices on the diagonal, butternut squash cut into chunks, and either 1 bunch of kale or a head of broccoli. Put water into a large soup pot, just enough to touch the bottom of a metal steamer basket that fits into the pot (you can get one at Target or any kitchen supply store). Layer the heartier root veggies into the bottom, then the onions, then the greens or broccoli.

Steam for about 8 to 12 minutes, until the root veggies are soft but not mushy. Transfer to serving bowls and then top with any of your favorite sauces. My favorite is a creamy tahini dressing. You can serve steamed veggies with any meal, but they go especially beautifully in Goddess Bowls and are a healthy, simple staple in my home.

Grains and Legumes

GRAINS

Overnight Oats

Provides 1 healthy fat, 1 grain, 1 fruit + 1 nuts and + protein if using nut butter

Simple Overnight Oats

½ cup old-fashioned rolled oats
¾ cup of water or nut milk of your choice (I prefer almond milk)
Optionally add to soaking: 1 tbsp. chia seeds or 2 tbsp. sunflower seeds
Combine all ingredients and place in fridge overnight.

For variety, stir any of the following into your oats after soaking and just before serving:

What a peach: Soak your oats in the water with 2 tbsp. sunflower seeds; add 1 ripe peach, diced, and a dash of cinnamon
Gone bananas: Chop in 1 small ripe banana, 2 tbsp. sliced toasted almonds, 1 tbsp. toasted coconut
Apple jacks: Chopped ½ apple, 1 tbsp. almond butter, ¼ cup toasted pecans, and ground cinnamon
Almond joy: ¼ cup shredded coconut, 2 tbsp. chopped almonds, 1 tbsp. dark chocolate chips (this one is dessert, not breakfast!).

5 minutes to assemble the oats, 2 hours for quick soaked oats, overnight for overnight oats. Makes 1 serving; you can increase portion size as needed; the oats keep for several days in the fridge, so you can make a couple of servings for yourself ahead of time.

Super Seed Muesli

Provides 1 healthy fat, 1 grain, 1 fruit, 2 nuts, 2 seeds + protein

2 cups rolled oats
½ cup cashews
½ cup almonds
¼ cup pecans
¼ cup sunflower seeds
¼ cup pumpkin seeds
¼ cup flaxseed
1 tsp. sea salt
1 cup shredded coconut
3 tsp. melted coconut oil
1 tbsp. vanilla extract
½ cup maple syrup

Preheat oven to 350°F. Mix all ingredients and spread in an even layer on a parchment paper–lined cookie sheet. Bake for 10 minutes, then stir. Bake for 10 more minutes and watch until golden brown. Cool on the cookie sheet.

25 minutes: 8 to 10 servings. Store in an airtight container for up to 10 days.

Vegan Buckwheat Crepes

Provides 1 healthy fat, 1 grain

1 cup un-toasted (raw) buckwheat flour
1¾ cups light (canned) coconut milk or almond milk
1 pinch sea salt
1 tbsp. coconut oil (plus a bit more for cooking)

Put ingredients into a mixing bowl, blender, or food processor. Mix until the batter is pourable but not thin or watery.

Heat a cast-iron or crepe pan over medium heat.

When hot, add a small amount of coconut oil, heat until hot and the oil coats the pan. Before adding batter, test to see if the oil is hot enough by dropping a drop of water onto the pan; if it splatters, it's ready.

Add ¼ cup of batter to the pan.

Cook until the top is bubbly and the edges are dry.

Flip carefully and cook for 2 to 3 minutes on the other side.

Repeat until all crepes are prepared. Add more oil to the pan only if it seems necessary.

Keep warm by placing on a plate and covering with a dish towel.

20 minutes to prepare. Leftovers keep sealed in the refrigerator for 2 days or frozen for about a month. Place between sheets of parchment paper before freezing to prevent sticking, and to make them easy to defrost as you want to use them.

Sakara Seed Bread

Provides 1 healthy fat, 1 grain, 1 fruit, 2 nuts, 2 seeds + protein per serving

Makes 1 loaf; you can double or triple this recipe.

2 cups gluten-free rolled oats
⅔ cup sunflower seeds
½ cup sliced almonds or chopped walnuts
½ cup flaxseed meal
⅓ cup psyllium husk powder
3 tbsp. pumpkin seeds
3 tbsp. pine nuts (or additional pumpkin seeds)
3 tbsp. chia seeds
3 tbsp. white sesame seeds
1 tsp. Himalayan salt

3 tbsp. extra-virgin olive oil, plus 1 tsp. for greasing the pan

1 tbsp. wildflower honey

4 cups water

In a large bowl, stir together the oats, sunflower seeds, almonds, flaxseed meal, psyllium husk powder, pumpkin seeds, pine nuts, chia seeds, sesame seeds, and salt. Fold in the oil and honey to coat, then slowly stir in 4 cups of water. Stir until the entire mixture is moistened. Cover the bowl with plastic wrap and let the dough rest for 30 minutes.

Preheat the oven to 350°F. Lightly grease an 8 × 4½-inch loaf pan with the oil and set aside.

Leaving about one inch at the top of the pan, tightly pack the dough into the prepared pan, using your hands to press it down firmly. Bake for 45 minutes, or until the crust is golden brown. Let the bread cool in the pan for 5 minutes, then turn out the loaf on a cooling rack to cool completely. Cut into ¼-inch thick slices and enjoy!

2 hours: 8 to 10 servings

Store leftover bread wrapped in waxed paper and foil in the fridge for up to 5 days, or in the freezer for up to a month.

Recipe courtesy of Danielle Duboise and Whitney Tingle, my friends at Sakara.

LEGUMES

Classic Hummus

Provides 2 healthy fats, 2 seeds, 1 bean/legume + protein

1 cup cooked garbanzo beans

¼ cup tahini

2 tbsp. olive oil

2 tbsp. water to the consistency you prefer (thick or thinner)

¼ cup fresh lemon juice

¼ tsp. roasted paprika powder

Blend all ingredients in a food processor on high speed until smooth. Optionally, add a dash of cumin powder.

How to Cook Quinoa

Rinse ½ cup of dry quinoa for 2 minutes in strainer under running water, place in a small pot with a lid, and cover with 1 cup of water. Bring to a boil, then turn heat down to lowest setting and cook covered for 15 minutes. Turn off heat and let stand, covered, for 5 more minutes. Fluff with a fork and *optionally* stir in 1 tbsp. of olive oil, coconut oil, butter, or ghee, depending on the meal you're cooking, to give it more body and energy balance. You can put the bowl in the fridge if you want it to cool thoroughly for salads or use warm. Because this is a seed and not truly a grain, it's very protein rich and shouldn't make you feel sleepy the way some grains can in the morning. Makes 2 servings.

For Lemony Quinoa: Add 1 tbsp. fresh lemon juice and 1 tsp. fresh lemon zest when cooking the quinoa. Stir in 1 tbsp. ghee, coconut oil, or olive oil. Serve warm.

Serve with a drizzle of olive oil and dash of the paprika on top as well.

10 minutes: 3–4 servings

Keeps 5 days in the fridge.

Chickpea Turmeric Curry (chicken or vegan)

Provides 1 serving of veggies, 1 healthy fat, 1 bean/ legume + protein

2 tbsp. coconut oil
1 large onion, diced
3 cloves garlic, chopped
1-inch ginger, peeled and minced
1 tsp. each of ground cumin, ground turmeric (and optionally, garam masala)
1 can of chickpeas, drained and rinsed (or 1.5 cups cooked chickpeas)
1 can of "lite" coconut milk
2 cups cauliflower florets
1 small sweet potato, diced into ½-inch chunks
½ cup organic golden raisins
Salt to taste
Fresh cilantro, for garnish
¼ cup roasted cashews

Heat the coconut oil in a medium pot. Sauté the onion, garlic, and ginger and cook until softened, 2 to 3 minutes.

Add all the spices, stirring for about 1 minute. Add the chickpeas, coconut milk, sweet potato chunks, raisins, and cauliflower.

Bring the temperature up so that the stew comes to a quick boil, then reduce heat to a simmer and cook for 25 minutes. Be careful when cooking as it can easily scorch, so stir regularly. Salt to taste. Serve over whole-grain rice with a topping of fresh cilantro and cashews.

35 minutes: 4 servings as a side dish, 2+ servings as a main protein

Keeps 3 days in the fridge.

How to Cook Millet

On a low flame, in a small skillet or saucepan that has a lid, toast ½ cup of millet for about 1 minute, stirring often. Cover the millet with 1½ cups of water. Turn up the heat, bring to a boil, reduce heat again to low, and cover the pan. Let cook for 20 minutes or until there is no more liquid in the pot and all the kernels are "open." Fluff with a fork.

You can also cook millet with chopped dried apricots or raisins, about 1 tbsp. for this amount of millet, and serve as a delicious breakfast cereal topped with chopped toasted nuts.

Millet Breakfast Porridge: Cook your millet with 2 cups of water and ⅓ cup chopped dried organic, unsulfured apricots (you could also use raisins, dried currants, or dried apple pieces). When done, top with 1 tbsp. coconut oil or ghee or a pat of organic butter, or stir in 1 tbsp. of almond butter or tahini. Top with chopped toasted nuts and, optionally, toasted shredded coconut. Because this is a seed and not truly a grain, it's very protein rich and shouldn't make you feel sleepy the way some grains can in the morning. Makes 2 servings.

You're a (Lentil) Dahl

Provides 1 healthy fat, 1 bean/legume + protein

1 medium onion, chopped
2 tbsp. coconut oil
2 tsp. curry powder
1 tsp. turmeric powder
½ cup red lentils
1½ cups water
¼ tsp. salt

Sauté onion in the coconut oil until translucent, about 2 minutes. Add spices and sauté for 30 seconds. Add lentils and stir until coated in oil, about 30 seconds. Add the water, cover, and simmer for 25 minutes.

Check and stir periodically to keep from sticking. Add salt at the end and stir.

25 minutes: 2 servings

Quick Spanish Black Beans

Provides 1 bean/legume + protein, 1 carb serving

½ yellow onion, minced
2 cloves garlic, crushed
2 scallions, finely chopped
4 tbsp. chopped red bell pepper
2 tsp. olive oil
1-15 oz. can black beans, drained
½ tsp. cumin powder
½ tsp. dried oregano
1 bay leaf
½ tsp. salt
Black pepper to taste
1 tbsp. chopped cilantro per serving for a topping
Wedge of ¼ fresh lime (optional) to drizzle on per serving

Sauté the onion, garlic, scallions and red bell pepper in the olive oil for 5 minutes, until the onions are translucent. Add black beans, cumin, oregano, bay leaf, salt, pepper, and water. Stir well and cook for 10 minutes, stirring to avoid sticking. Serve topped with fresh chopped cilantro and a drizzle of lime.

Serves 4 as a side, 2 as a main dish. Keeps well in the fridge for 2 days.

Fish, Eggs, Poultry, Meat, and Tofu

These are healthy choices for the animal-based proteins recommended for Hormone Intelligence.

EGGS, 4 EASY WAYS

Frittata Cups

Provides 2 servings of veggies, 1 healthy fat + protein

2 cups mixed veggies of your choice—see recipes below for ideas
Seasonings/spices of your choice
1 tbsp. olive oil for sautéing
10 free-range eggs
½ tsp. salt and a few dashes pepper or red pepper flakes

Preheat oven to 400°F.

Sauté all the vegetables and fresh seasonings (i.e., garlic, ginger, or variations below) in olive oil for 3 to 5 minutes, until glistening and just on the edge of tender and turn off the heat. In a bowl, crack the eggs and mix in the salt and pepper. Beat lightly for 30 seconds. Fill a muffin tray with dye- and bleach-free muffin liners, place a small amount of prepared veggies in each liner, then fill to three-quarters of the way full with the beaten eggs. Use a fork to lightly mix and disperse the veggies into the egg batter. Bake for about 20 minutes, until very lightly brown on top and firm to the touch.

East Meets West Frittata

2 cups small broccoli florets
¾ cup chopped shitake mushrooms
1 small bunch scallions, chopped
1 red bell pepper, diced
Coconut or sesame oil or ghee
2 tsp. freshly grated ginger
2 cloves garlic, minced
¼ tsp. black pepper
2 tbsp. gluten-free tamari or 1 tsp. sea salt
Dash of organic rice vinegar

Top the baked cups with extra scallions and if you like it, sriracha, and serve on a bed of mixed salad greens or as part of any Asian-style bowl or salad.

Latin Vibe Frittata

½ cup roasted sweet potato nuggets (optional if you have time or leftovers—incredibly delicious)
½ bunch cilantro, chopped
1 yellow onion, diced
1 green bell pepper, diced
½ cup frozen corn
Olive oil
½ tsp. chipotle pepper
½ tsp. cumin
Sea salt
Black pepper

Top the baked cups with avocado or guacamole and extra cilantro, optional salsa, or use in any Latin-style salad or bowl.

Italian-Style Frittata

1 yellow onion, diced
2 cups frozen spinach or 1 bunch asparagus cut into bite-size pieces
1 red bell pepper, chopped

Olive oil
1 cup chopped basil or 1 tsp. dried
½ tsp. dried oregano
¼ tsp. red pepper flakes
¼ tsp. black pepper
½ tsp. salt

Serve on a bed of arugula or mixed greens.

Serve plain, over salad, in a bowl, or with some of your favorite hot sauce.

35 minutes: 8 large or 12 small muffin cups, 2–3 muffin cups per serving

Quick Pan Omelet

Provides 1 healthy fat + protein

Beat 2 eggs, add sea salt and black pepper to taste. Other seasonings include za'atar, oregano, and thyme, or you can sauté some finely chopped scallion and add to the beaten eggs.

Heat your skillet. Pour the eggs into the skillet.

Let set and when you see the omelet "firm up," flip the whole thing over to cook on the other side.

Should be golden yellow and firm on both sides.

Slide onto a plate and top with your choice of veggies.

5 minutes: 1 serving

Quick Fried Egg

Provides 1 healthy fat + protein

One of my favorite meals, excellent for breakfast, lunch, or dinner, is simply a bed of about ½ cup arugula, 1 to 2 fried eggs (either over easy or over hard), topped with chopped tomatoes, a splash of champagne vinegar, salt, and pepper.

Egg or Tofu Scramble

Provides 1 to 2 servings of veggies, 1 healthy fat + protein

How to make a scramble:

Place 1 tbsp. of your oil of choice into a cast-iron or stainless-steel skillet and bring to a medium heat.

Sauté ½ cup mixed vegetables; if you use onions, sauté those first for 2 minutes until translucent, then add the remaining veggies, which should be sautéed for about 3 to 5 minutes until they are bright in color and coated in the oil.

Season the veggies with the recommended herbs and flavorings.

If you're using eggs, beat them and then add a dash of salt and black pepper, or other seasonings of your choice.

Either add in your tofu or remove the veggies and scramble 2 eggs in the skillet, adding the veggies back when the eggs are finished.

This makes a complete breakfast meal, or if having for lunch or dinner, serve over a bed of rice noodles, quinoa, or other grain, or a sprouted rice tortilla.

Asian Breakfast

¼ brick tofu or 2 eggs
½ cup mixed sautéed scallions or sliced yellow onion
Shitake mushrooms
Broccoli
1 tbsp. coconut or sesame oil, lightly heated
1 tbsp. gluten-free tamari
Optional: serve with ½ cup cooked brown rice or millet

Mexican Egg

2 eggs
¼ cup chopped red bell pepper
1 cup baby spinach
¼ cup finely chopped red onion
1 tbsp. olive oil, lightly heated
Minced cilantro
¼ to ½ avocado
Fresh salsa
Optional: serve with 1½ cup Roasted Sweet Potato Rounds

Hippie Tofu

¼ brick tofu
2 cups chard or spinach
¼ cup chopped red pepper
1 tbsp. olive oil or coconut oil, lightly heated
1 tsp. powdered turmeric
½ tsp. ground cumin seed
Salt and pepper to taste

To Make a Tartine

Spread Simple Lemon Mash (under Avocado Mash; page 345) on toasted Sakara Seed Bread (page 349), layer with arugula, mixed field greens, roasted kale, or sprouts (broccoli, radish, or sunflower), top with a fried egg or small pan omelet, sprinkle on a dash of champagne vinegar, and enjoy as an amazing complete meal.

Baked Salmon 4 Ways

Provides 2 healthy fats + protein

Preheat oven to 425°F. Lay two 4-ounce fillets of salmon on a parchment-lined baking sheet.

In a small bowl, whisk together one of the following sauces. Brush your fish with your preferred sauce and bake for 20 to 35 minutes, depending on how well done you prefer your fish.

25 to 40 minutes: 2 servings

Keeps for 2 days in the fridge.

Rice or Chickpea Miso-Glazed Salmon with Scallions and Sesame Seeds

Sweet white rice or chickpea miso
Toasted sesame oil
1 tsp. honey or maple syrup
Sesame seeds
Scallions, thinly sliced

Combine miso, sesame oil, and honey. Spread a thin layer of the mixture over each salmon fillet and sprinkle with sesame seeds. Garnish with scallions.

Maple Dijon Salmon

1 tbsp. maple syrup
1 tbsp. Dijon mustard
¼ tsp. sea salt and pepper

Combine all the ingredients and spread a thin layer of the mixture over each salmon fillet.

Mediterranean Lemon Salmon

2 tbsp. lemon juice
2 tbsp. olive oil
2 cloves garlic, crushed
½ tsp. each dried thyme and oregano
½ tsp. sea salt
Combine all the ingredients and spread a thin layer
   of the mixture over each salmon fillet.

Ginger-Lime Salmon

1 tbsp. grapeseed oil OR toasted sesame oil
1 tbsp. lime juice
2 tsp. tamari
1 or 2 tsp. peeled, freshly grated ginger
1 large clove garlic, crushed
¼ tsp. black pepper

Combine all the ingredients and spread a thin layer of the mixture over each salmon fillet. You can also replace the lime juice with freshly squeezed orange juice or do a combo.

Salmon Burgers

Provides 2 healthy fats + protein

8-ounce skinless salmon fillet cut into ½-inch chunks
¼ cup finely chopped cilantro
1 tbsp. peeled, finely grated ginger
1 tsp. tamari
1 tsp. lime juice
1 tbsp. olive oil

Freeze your salmon fillet for 15 minutes to make it easy to chop. In the meantime, mix the other ingredients in a bowl. Place the salmon pieces into your food processor. Pulse the salmon in the food processor until finely chopped—do not puree it. Mix the chopped salmon into the other ingredients and form into 2 to 4 patties. If too wet, refrigerate the mixture for 15 minutes. Heat the olive oil in a skillet. Cook the salmon burgers for 5 minutes on each side until slightly brown and firm to the touch. Serve over greens or over a noodle or other Goddess Bowl.

35 minutes: 2 servings

Keeps in the fridge for 2 days, but best served fresh.

Best Fish Tacos

Provides 2 servings of veggies, 2 healthy fats, + protein (+ 1 bean/legume if you add black beans)

A quick baked fish to include in your fish tacos, or as a protein dish for any meal.

2 tilapia fillets
1 tbsp. olive oil
Cajun spice (buy from a company that has no MSG, caking agents, or sugar)

Preheat oven to 400°F. Rub the fillets on both sides with olive oil, then sprinkle thoroughly on both sides with the Cajun spice. Place on a parchment-paper-lined cookie sheet. Bake for 20 minutes.

Serve with Not Your Mama's Slaw (page 341), Guacamole Mash (page 345), or sliced avocado with juice of ½–1 lime or Chili-Lime Dressing (page 360), and a side of Roasted Sweet Potato Rounds (page 346). Optionally, also top with black beans with Mexican seasoning (see Quinoa, Black Bean, Sweet Potato, and Fajita Burrito Bowl; page 344)

30 minutes: 2 servings

Pulled Poached Chicken Breast

Provides protein

2 skinless, boneless chicken breasts
2 cloves of garlic
2 tsp. sea salt
4 cups water or low-sodium chicken broth

Place chicken, garlic, and salt into a shallow saucepan. Add enough liquid to cover the chicken about halfway. Bring to a boil, turn heat down to medium, and simmer for 5 minutes. Turn off heat, cover, and let sit for 15 minutes. Remove from pot and shred ("pull") or slice the chicken for use in your favorite recipes.

20 minutes: 2 servings

Keeps in the fridge for 3 days.

Za'atar Roast Chicken Breast

Provides 1 healthy fat + protein

Juice of 1 lemon
2 tbsp. extra-virgin olive oil
2 tbsp. za'atar spice, plus 1 tsp.

To Make Pulled Chicken Salads

Pulled chicken beautifully takes up any dressing you mix it into. As a side to any dish, or in a salad, you can use seasoning to create endless varieties, for example:

Asian Pulled Chicken Salad
Combine 1 or 2 pulled chicken breasts with ¼ cup of Tangy Ginger-Lime Dressing (page 360) or Peanut Sauce (page 360).

Green Goddess Chicken Salad
Combine 1 or 2 pulled chicken breasts with ¼ cup Creamy Cashew Dressing (page 360). Place on top of noodles, a noodle bowl, or salad, or in lettuce or a nori sheet for a quick, easy wrap.

1 tbsp. sumac, plus 1 tsp.

1 tsp. cinnamon

2 tsp. roasted paprika

3 large garlic cloves, crushed

1 medium red onion, sliced

2 boneless, skinless chicken breasts

2 tbsp. pine nuts

½ cup freshly chopped parsley leaves

First, make the marinade: In a deep dish, mix the lemon juice, olive oil, 2 tbsp. za'atar, 1 tbsp. sumac, cinnamon, paprika, garlic, and red onion. Add the chicken, coat liberally, and place in fridge, turning the chicken over halfway through your marinade time.

Preheat oven to 400°F. Move the chicken and marinade to a cast-iron skillet, or if you don't have one, any baking dish. Toss on the remaining za'atar and sumac, add the pine nuts, and cover with a layer of chopped parsley. (Optionally, before adding the parsley, add ¼ cup golden raisins.) Bake uncovered for 45 minutes.

Make it a meal: Serve over quinoa and with a chopped mixed green salad with Anytime Vinaigrette (perhaps the lemon olive oil option; page 359), or just add whole or sliced chicken breast to your salad.

1 to 4 hours to marinade, 1 hour to prep and cook: 2 servings

Thai Steak or Chicken

Provides healthy fat + protein

Cut 2 boneless, skinless chicken breasts or 8 ounces of grass-fed steak (ideally skirt or hanger steak, but sirloin or round is okay if that's all you can get) into thin strips. Put in the freezer for 15 minutes before cutting to make it easier. Combine the following, pour over the sliced meat, and marinate for at least an hour:

2 tbsp. grapeseed oil

2 tbsp. lime juice

1 tbsp. tamari

1 tbsp. peeled, freshly grated ginger

2 large cloves garlic, crushed

½ tsp. black pepper

¼ tsp. red chili flakes (optional)

After the meat is marinated, preheat your oven to 400°F. No time to marinate? That's okay—skip that step and this recipe still works! Just mix the meat and marinade in a bowl and go onto the next step.

Toss in:

1 medium sweet red pepper, thinly sliced

1 yellow onion, cut into thin half-moons

Put the entire mixture into a cast-iron skillet and bake for 30 minutes, tossing once or twice. After 15 minutes of cooking, optionally mix in 1 cup broccoli florets.

4 hours to marinate, 10 minutes prep, 30 minutes cooking: 2 servings

Keeps 2 days in the fridge.

Fajita Chicken or Steak

Provides 1 veggie serving, 1 healthy fat + protein

Cut 2 boneless, skinless chicken breasts or 8 ounces of grass-fed steak (ideally skirt or hanger steak, but sirloin or round is okay if that's all you can get) into thin strips. Put in the freezer for 15 minutes before cutting to make it easier. Marinate for at least an hour in:

2 tbsp. olive oil

2 tbsp. lemon or lime juice

1 tsp. seasoned salt

1 tsp. dried oregano

1 tsp. ground cumin

1 tsp. garlic powder

1 tsp. chili powder

½ tsp. smoked paprika

After the meat is marinated, preheat your oven to 400°F. No time to marinate? That's okay—skip that step and this recipe still works! Just mix the meat and marinade in a bowl and go onto the next step.

Toss in:

1 medium sweet red pepper, thinly sliced
1 medium green pepper, thinly sliced
1 yellow onion, cut into thin half-moons

Put the entire mixture into a cast-iron skillet and bake for 30 minutes, tossing once or twice.

4 hours to marinate, 10 minutes prep, 30 minutes cooking: 2 servings

Keeps 2 days in the fridge.

Chicken and Black Bean Soup (+ vegan version)

Provides 1 healthy fat, 1 bean/legume + protein

½ pound boneless skinless chicken breasts, cut into 1-inch cubes
2 cans (14½ ounces each) reduced-sodium chicken broth, divided
1 can (15 ounces) black beans, rinsed and drained
1 can (10 ounces) diced tomatoes
1 jalapeño pepper, seeded and chopped
3 tsp. chili powder
½ tsp. ground cumin
2 tbsp. minced fresh cilantro for topping

Combine all the ingredients except cilantro in a stove-top pot and simmer for 30 minutes. For a vegan version, omit the chicken and double the black beans. Serve topped with chopped cilantro.

Quick Snack (or Lunch) Wraps

Provides 2 veggie servings, 1–2 healthy fats, 1 seed/nut if using one of the tahini sauces or Peanut Sauce, + protein

Wraps are a quick way to enjoy just about any of the Goddess Bowl ingredients in a light, easy-to-make package. I use buttercrunch or romaine lettuce or sheets of nori seaweed, but you can also use blanched napa cabbage or collard green leaves. To prepare your wrap, assemble the various ingredients and layer them onto the recommended wrap and then drizzle on some of the "secret sauce" of your choosing. A cool trick is to spread a light layer of your sauce, avocado, or hummus against the wrap, then layer on the grain, then on top of this, place your veggies. This layering technique holds everything nicely in place. For the lettuces, the roll is casual; with nori sheets you can quickly learn to make an even, tight roll with online videos.

Thai Lettuce Wraps

Pulled Poached Chicken Breast, or your favorite salmon, or tofu
Boston lettuce leaves
¼ cup sautéed shitake mushrooms
4 cups mixed raw mung bean sprouts
Fresh cilantro
Steamed matchstick or raw grated carrots
Scallions for layering
Spicy Thai Sauce

Hummus Wraps

Use a GF wrap or romaine or Boston lettuce
Hummus
Cucumber
Tomato
Sprouts
Red onion
Chopped Kalamata olives
Lemony Tahini or Spicy Thai Sauce

Cajun Lime Fish or Fajita Chicken "Tacos"

Boston lettuce leaves and a little rice or quinoa, or a
   sprouted corn tortilla
Best Fish Tacos or Fajita Chicken (or if you're vegan,
   tofu seasoned as for Best Fish Tacos or Spanish
   Black Beans)
Not Your Mama's Slaw
2 tbsp. guacamole per taco
Lime juice to taste
Optional: Salsa is terrific, too.

Vegan Nori Wraps

Roasted nori sheets
Brown rice or cooked quinoa
Tofu
Carrot
Avocado
Sprouts
Red onion
Spicy Thai Sauce

Dressings and Sauces

A simple salad dressing or sauce can transform and enliven a basic salad, bowl of rice noodles, chicken, and steamed veggies into a taste masterpiece. They're also an amazing way to get an extra healthy dose of high-quality oil, seeds in the form of tahini, and herbs into your diet.

As all the sauces and dressings are prepared similarly, here are the instructions for the whole lot:

- For recipes with only liquid ingredients, salt, and pepper, you can simply whisk them in a glass or bowl and serve—it's that simple.

- For recipes with seed or nut butters, or solid ingredients (i.e., garlic, cilantro, etc.), combine all ingredients in your blender or food processor. Blend on high speed until smooth, about 1 minute. Dressings typically store well in a glass jar for 3 days in the fridge.

- Separation of the oil and other ingredients is normal—just whiz back in your blender or give the dressing a whisk or shake before using.

- Use them on any of the salads, bowls, and wraps.

- These each take about 5 minutes, at most.

Here are my favorites.

Anytime Vinaigrette

The oil: ⅓ cup olive oil
The acid: 3 tbsp. of balsamic vinegar OR champagne
   vinegar OR fresh lemon juice
¼ tsp. salt or to taste
Optional: For variety also add 1 tsp. fresh or dried
   rosemary leaves, 1 tsp. fresh or dried oregano leaf,
   and a dash of black pepper.

Green Goddess Dressing

⅓ cup olive oil or ½ ripe avocado + 2 tbsp. water for a
   creamy dressing
½ cup cilantro leaves
1 clove garlic, minced
3 tbsp. fresh lime juice
¼ tsp. salt or to taste

Dijon Salad Dressing

¼ cup olive or grapeseed oil, or another favorite oil
2 tbsp. fresh lemon juice
½ tsp. Dijon mustard
1 clove garlic, peeled and grated or minced
½ tsp. sea salt

Peanut Sauce

½ cup unsalted creamy peanut butter or almond
   butter
2 tbsp. tamari
2 tbsp. lime juice
¼ cup water (or as needed to thin to your desired
   consistency)
1 clove garlic, crushed
Optional: 1 tsp. Thai chili paste, 1 tbsp. maple syrup
   (or other sweetener of choice)

Lemony Tahini Sauce

½ cup tahini
1 clove garlic, crushed
¼ cup fresh lemon juice
2 tbsp. water
¼ tsp. salt or to taste
For a spicy version, add an additional garlic clove and
   ¼ tsp. cayenne pepper.

Rice or Chickpea Miso-Tahini Sauce

¼ cup tahini
1 tbsp. white rice or chickpea miso
2 to 4 tbsp. water (to the thickness you prefer)
1 tbsp. peeled, freshly grated ginger
1 tbsp. rice vinegar
Optional: 1 tsp. maple syrup

Creamy Cashew Dressing

⅓ cup olive oil
⅓ cup raw cashews
1 clove raw garlic
⅓ cup water
¼ cup lemon juice
1 tsp. Dijon mustard

Spicy Thai Sauce

⅓ cup toasted sesame oil
¼ cup fresh basil leaves OR cilantro leaves
3 tbsp. lime juice
2 tbsp. tamari (or 1 tbsp. Bragg's Aminos if you don't
   use soy)
¼ tsp. salt or to taste
1 tsp. honey (optional)
¼ tsp. freshly grated gingerroot
½–1 serrano pepper, minced, depending on how
   spicy you like it; remove the seeds first

Tangy Ginger-Lime Dressing

¼ cup grapeseed oil
2 tbsp. toasted sesame oil
Juice of 2 limes
1 tbsp. tamari
1 tbsp. freshly grated ginger
1 tbsp. maple syrup (optional)

Chili-Lime Dressing

¼ cup olive oil
Juice of 1 to 2 limes (to taste)
¼ tsp. chili powder
¼ tsp. cumin
¼ jalapeño, finely minced, or 1 tsp. red chili flakes
¼ tsp. salt

For a creamy version, substitute olive oil for an
avocado, and blend until smooth.

Nuts and Seeds

Nut Milk at Home

I love the weekly ritual of preparing nut milk. It's a mindful reminder to think ahead about my food, and a wonderful alternative to the store-bought kinds, which are generally ecologically unfriendly, overly sweetened, and have guar gum or carrageenan as thickeners. It's surprisingly easy—enough so that once you make your own, you'll wonder why you ever bought it. The reality is, there's not a whole lot of nutrition in nut and seed milks, but they are a good alternative to dairy where you'd usually use it in your diet.

½ cup whole, organic, unroasted, unsalted nuts; my two favorites are almonds and cashews
2 cups cold water
Optional: Vanilla extract

Soak ½ cup of whole nuts in 2 cups water for at least 4 hours, or preferably overnight. Strain and rinse the soaked nuts, discarding the soaking water. Place the soaked nuts and water into your blender or Vitamix. Blend at high speed for about 2 minutes. Strain by pouring the blender contents through a mesh bag (or cheesecloth), catching the milk in a container or large measuring cup. Squeeze firmly to extract as much milk as possible. Add vanilla and store in the fridge.

For a thick and creamy version: If you like a little "cream" in your chai, you're making chai latte, or you'd like to add some cream to your overnight oats, make a concentrated cashew milk using 1 cup of water per half cup of soaked cashews.

For a quick version: If you forget or don't have time to soak your nuts the night before, no worries! You can use unsoaked nuts—just use raw nuts!

Prep time: 4 to 12 hours to soak the nuts. 5 minutes to prepare and clean up.

Makes about 2 cups. Keeps in the fridge for 5 days.

Not for the Birds Seed Crackers

Provides 2 servings seeds

You'll be amazed at making your own "gone crazy" kind of crackers! You'll need parchment paper for this recipe.

½ cup whole flaxseeds
6 tbsp. sesame seeds
4 tbsp. pumpkin seeds
2 tbsp. sunflower seeds
1 tbsp. millet
3 tbsp. sesame seeds
1 cup boiling water
¼ tsp. sea salt
Optional: cracked black pepper, onion powder, garlic powder, red pepper flakes

Preheat the oven to 325°F. In a small mixing bowl, combine all the ingredients. Let sit for 15 to 30 minutes to allow the flaxseeds to absorb the liquid. Put a piece of parchment paper on a medium cookie sheet, spread the cracker batter onto the parchment paper, then place another piece over the top of the mix. Roll it out with a rolling pin until about ¼ inch thick—thinner if you want a very thin cracker. Bake for 45 minutes, remove from oven, and allow to cool. Break into smaller pieces. Will keep for a week in an airtight container.

1 hour: Makes an 8 × 10-inch sheet cracker.

Toasty Savory Nuts and Seeds

Provides 1 to 2 servings nuts/seeds

Although you can purchase decent quality roasted nuts and seeds, it's easy to toast your own and they are much fresher.

Place ¼ to ½ cup of your choice of almonds, walnuts, or pecans, or sunflower, pumpkin, or sesame seeds into a cast-iron or stainless-steel skillet. Turn heat on low and toast, stirring occasionally, until the nuts or seeds start to brown. (Pumpkin and sesame seeds will begin to make a popping sound when ready.) Turn off heat and cool to room temperature. Store in a glass jar or container.

For a savory treat, when the seeds are just about done toasting, add ½ tsp. of any of the following, or a combination of more than one:

Tamari
Garlic powder
Chili powder, plus 1 tsp. lime juice and a dash of salt
Curry powder
Onion powder
1 sheet of toasted nori seaweed torn into bite-size
    pieces or ¼ cup toasted dulse seaweed pieces

Serving size: 2 tbsp. up to ¼ cup

10 minutes

Off the Beaten Trail Mix

Provides 2 servings nuts/seeds, 1 serving fruit (dried)

Pick several of any of the following. A good ratio to follow is: Mix and match nuts (½ cup total) + Mix and match seeds (½ cup total) + Mix and match dried fruit or chocolate (¼ cup)

Dry-roasted or raw cashews
Dry-roasted or raw almonds
Pecans
Walnuts
Sunflower seeds
Pumpkin seeds
Goji berries
Mulberries
Raisins
Currants
Dark chocolate chips or chopped dark chocolate
    (70% or darker)
Dried coconut chips
Cacao nibs
Unsweetened dried cherries

Mix together your favorites and enjoy! Can be stored in a container at room temperature for several weeks at a time, so make a big batch to grab and go when you need it.

5 minutes: 4–6 servings

Keeps months in an airtight jar.

Fermented Foods

Homemade Kimchi (Spicy Asian Fermented Vegetables)

Kimchi, a spicy Asian fermented "kraut," can be done in a glass jar and doesn't need any special equipment—just a cutting board and a knife. Making kimchi is fast, easy, inexpensive, and satisfying—and it keeps for a couple of weeks in the fridge. I enjoy it as a condiment to many meals and especially love a liberal amount of it atop a Goddess Bowl of steamed or stir-fried vegetables over rice or, when I can splurge on them, pure buckwheat soba noodles. I've tempered this one so it's not as spicy as the traditional fare, which I find too hot.

1 large head napa cabbage (remove the hard end, cut cabbage in half lengthwise and into 2-inch lengths)
¼ cup sea salt

4 medium carrots in matchsticks or cut on the
  diagonal
1 bunch scallions cut into thirds
2 tbsp. freshly grated ginger
½ tsp. cayenne pepper or red pepper flakes

Place the cut napa cabbage into a bowl and
sprinkle well with the sea salt. Mix well with your
hands until the leaves are well coated—this just
takes about 30 seconds. Let sit in the bowl for
2 hours, then place in a colander and rinse well
to remove the salt. Return the napa cabbage to
the now-rinsed-out bowl and add the remaining
ingredients. Refrigerate and start to eat after 24
more hours in the fridge.

*15 minutes; ferment time, 24 hours refrigerated: 10
or more servings*

Keeps 2 weeks in the fridge.

Simple Cultured Veggie Pickles

"Dill Style" Pickles

3 cups of the following veggies cut into bite-size
  pieces: cauliflower, broccoli, carrots
1 large clove garlic, minced
1 tsp. yellow mustard seeds
½ tsp. turmeric powder
2 large sprigs fresh dill or 1 tsp. dried dill
1 bay leaf

Eastern Medley

3 cups broccoli florets, thickly sliced cucumbers (½-
  inch rounds; remove the skin unless organic and
  unwaxed), and carrots sliced into matchsticks
2 inches fresh ginger, peeled and sliced into thin
  sections
1 tsp. turmeric powder
Optional: wakame seaweed or dulse pieces

The Brine

Place all your veggies into a clean, dry, quart-size
Mason jar. I like to layer them by veggie because
it looks so pretty.

Cover with brine and put the lid on your jar.

*20 minutes to prepare the pickles, 7 to 14 days to
ferment them*

Keeps 2 weeks in the fridge.

Green Juice and Smoothies for the Gal on the Go

Gingery Lemon Green Juice

This delicious green drink is simple to make
in a juicer or Vitamix and packs in 3 servings
of veggies; it's a nice addition to a healthy
balanced breakfast, or an energizing afternoon
pick-me-up.

To make, juice or blend a combo of:

2 cups of a combination of spinach, chard, parsley,
  or kale (keep kale to no more than once weekly if
  you have hypothyroidism)
½ cup frozen organic blueberries
Juice of ½ lemon
Optional but optimal: 1 thin slice of fresh gingerroot
  (or if you have access, add slices of fresh turmeric
  root or ½ tsp. turmeric powder)
1 cup water (for Nut Milk see page 361)
Optional: crushed ice

Enjoy!

Smoothies

You might notice the absence of smoothies in the meal plans; that's because while smoothies are great for an on-the-go meal or snack on occasion, it's not quite the same as having a regular meal. I don't emphasize them, but I do want you to have healthy options.

How to make a smoothie:

All smoothies contain a protein source, a healthy liquid that usually adds additional protein and a healthy fat, fruits or vegetables, and health "extras." Place the following ingredients into your blender:

1 scoop high-protein seeds or 1 heaping tbsp. nut or seed butter
½ cup total mixed fruit (frozen makes the smoothies so much creamier and more delicious, but you can use fresh)
¾–1 cup liquid (depending in the thickness you prefer) of choice (usually chilled almond milk, coconut milk, coconut kefir, goat's milk if you eat dairy)
Optional nutrient boosts

Blend all ingredients in a blender until smooth. Serving size 8 oz.

Provides 2 servings fruit, 1 serving nuts/seeds + protein

SMOOTHIE OPTIONS

Turmeric Ginger Relief

Anti-inflammatory and pain relieving

1 tbsp. hemp seeds
1 tbsp. almond butter
1 frozen banana
Coconut milk
¼ cup frozen pineapple pieces

1 tsp. turmeric powder (or 1 inch of fresh turmeric)
½ tsp. freshly grated gingerroot
¼ tsp. crushed cardamom seeds

Almond Butter Cup

Ovary-boosting nourishment

1 tbsp. hemp seeds
2 tbsp. almond butter
½ avocado
1 frozen banana
1 cup unsweetened almond milk
1 tbsp. raw cacao powder
Optional: 1 tbsp. ground flaxseed

Hot Zone Super Smoothie

Hormone supporting, sleep supporting, adrenal soothing

1 tbsp. hemp seeds
2 tbsp. almond butter
½–1 frozen banana
½ cup frozen black cherries
1 pitted Medjool date (optional for some sweetness)
Unsweetened almond milk
1 tsp. maca powder
1 tsp. ashwagandha powder
1 tsp. freshly grated ginger
1 tbsp. ground flaxseed

Healthy Indulgences

Okay, how could I do a book on hormones without being real? Even with the best balanced blood sugar, and healthiest diet in the word, we all want a little something sweet now and then, and with premenstrual hormone changes, even naturally, we want a "treat." Dark chocolate is always fair game—as long as it doesn't keep you awake at night, and you keep it to 2 ounces/

serving. Here are some other healthful options you can feel good about. Just keep it to no more than twice/week at most, and ideally not during the first two weeks of being on the plan.

Chocolate Avocado Mousse

Provides 2 servings healthy fat.

I grew up in the era of chocolate pudding from a box. My mom made it in green pudding bowls. From licking the spoon of warm pudding to opening the fridge every ten minutes to watch that skin form on top, to finally skimming that skin off the top and enjoying it and then the soft creamy chocolate below—the whole thing was heavenly. The problem is, it was filled with artificial ingredients. This one is a revelation: unlike the stuff of my childhood, it's actually good for you! So, enjoy and create a new healthier tradition for yourself.

2 ounces chopped semisweet chocolate or dark chocolate chips

2 large, ripe avocados, halved and pitted

2 tbsp. maple syrup

¼ cup coconut milk (light or regular)

1 tsp. pure vanilla extract

3 tbsp. organic unsweetened dark chocolate cocoa powder

⅛ tsp. Himalayan sea salt

Optional: strawberries or raspberries, and for a little extra exotic flavor, choose either a sprinkle of cinnamon or cardamom powder or a dash of chili powder

Place the chopped chocolate or chocolate chips in a saucepan or double boiler and melt, watching carefully to avoid burning. Scoop the avocado "meat" into a food processor with a steel blade or a Vitamix. Add the maple syrup, coconut milk, vanilla extract, melted chocolate, cocoa powder, and sea salt to the processor. Blend until very creamy.

Spoon into parfait cups or, my fave, mini Mason jars. (Lick the spoon!)

Chill for 1 to 3 hours depending on how thick you'd like it to be. Serve topped with a sprinkle of sea salt, strawberries, or raspberries, and for a little extra exotic "sexiness," either a sprinkle of cinnamon or cardamom powder or a dash of chili powder!

Serves 4 (about ¼ cup each). Don't let the small amount fool you—it's rich!

When You Want a Little Something . . .

Sweet: Dark chocolate, Dark Chocolate Sea Salt Coconut Almond Joys, Chocolate Tahini Date Fudge

Salty Sweet: Sliced apple with roasted almond butter and Himalayan salt, Dark Chocolate Sea Salt Coconut Almond Joys, roasted almonds and chocolate

Ooey-Gooey: Raw Cookie Bites, Chocolate Tahini Date Fudge

Creamy or Frozen: Chocolate Avocado Mousse, Frozen Banana Soft Serve, or frozen Raw Cookie Bites

Comfort Beverage: Golden Milk Chai Latte

Women's Bliss Bites

Provides 2 servings healthy fat, 1 nuts/seeds + protein and fiber

1½ cups walnuts

½ cup dates, pitted

2 (or so) tbsp. almond butter

¼ cup dark cacao powder (dark unsweetened), plus 1 tbsp. for dusting

4 level tbsp. maca powder

¼ tsp. cardamom powder

¼ tsp. cinnamon powder

¼ cup coconut flakes, finely ground

Optional: orange zest

Put the walnuts into your food processor and grind until they are close to finely ground. Add in the dates and grind to form a thicker blend. Add in the almond butter and mix until a dough forms. Sometimes you might have to add a little extra to get the dough to form nicely. Add in the ¼ cup of cacao powder, maca, cardamom, and cinnamon until well mixed. Remove your blade from your food processor, then form round balls using about 1 tbsp. of "dough" per ball. Roll these in your hands, then roll in the extra cacao powder, coconut flakes, and the orange zest, if using. Place on a platter or into a glass storage container for later enjoyment. These can be eaten straightaway or kept in the fridge and enjoyed over the next 3 to 4 days. They can be taken anywhere in a small storage container.

Makes 16. Serving size: 2 to 4 Bliss Bites per day

Seed Power Bites

Put the following ingredients into your food processor with a chopping blade in place:

⅔ cup of a combination of sesame, sunflower, and pumpkin seeds, plus optionally, your choice of almonds or walnuts

4 pitted Medjool dates OR 2 tbsp. high-quality honey

2 tbsp. tahini (sesame seed butter)

¼ cup or so of coconut flakes

Optional: 2 tsp. of any of your favorite adaptogen or medical mushroom powders, ground flaxseed, or dark cocoa powder

Blend all the ingredients until well mixed but you still see some bits of nuts and seeds. Remove from food processor, shape into balls using about 1 tbsp. of dough per ball, and roll in some extra raw or toasted coconut flakes or sesame seeds.

Serving size is 2 balls. These keep in a container in the fridge for 5 days.

Dark Chocolate Sea Salt Coconut Almond Joys

Provides satisfying goodness and some fiber.

My daughter Mima deserves credit for this recipe. You'll never belief how good—and easy—these are until you make and try them yourself. And they only contain five ingredients!

The Joys

2 cups unsweetened shredded coconut

2 tbsp. maple syrup

2 tbsp. coconut oil

A pinch of sea salt

8 raw almonds

Optional: 2 tsp. of ashwagandha or reishi powder to make these into Adaptogen Almond Joys

The Secret Sauce

4 ounces dark baking chocolate chips (65% cacao or more)

½ tbsp. coconut oil, melted (to mix in with the chocolate)

Extra sea salt for sprinkling on top

Put the shredded coconut, maple syrup, coconut oil, and sea salt in your food processor (and the adaptogens if you're going for the boost). Process until it starts to form a sticky "batter." Lay a piece of parchment paper on a cutting board or platter. Moisten your hands and use them to form oval "logs" using about 2 tbsp. of the mixture per log. Place these on the parchment paper as you form them. Place one almond on the center of each log. Next, in a metal bowl placed over boiling water, melt the baking chocolate or chocolate chips with ½ tbsp. coconut oil. Remove from over the water. Place one coconut log at a time in the chocolate bowl, spooning chocolate over it until it's coated. With a fork, lift the log, dripping off any excess chocolate. Place it back on the parchment paper and continue until all the logs are coated. I love to sprinkle a tiny bit of sea salt on each log for a grown-up elegance.

Place in the freezer for 20 minutes to harden.

Makes 8, serving size 1 (or okay, 2). These store in the fridge for 1 week.

Frozen Banana Soft Serve

Provides 1 serving fruit, 1 healthy fat

As my four-year-old grandson said, "It's nice to have a little something cold once in a while," his way of saying, "Biba (that's what he calls me), it's ice cream time." Let's face it. We all love ice cream. But it's just one of the unhealthiest things we can do to our body—and if you've ever experienced healthy fatigue or an outright ice cream coma after indulging beyond a bite, you know what I mean. This is a nice alternative that is completely unsweetened aside from the naturally occurring sugar in the fruits you'll use.

4 frozen bananas (peel and freeze bananas in a glass storage container at least one day before)

4 tbsp. full-fat coconut milk
Optional: 1 cup frozen fruit (I love frozen strawberries, black cherries, or mixed tropical fruit including mango), cacao nibs or dark chocolate chips, 1 tsp. fresh mint leaves, vanilla extract, coconut flakes

Place frozen bananas and coconut milk into a Vitamix for best results, or place half of these ingredients at a time in your blender, and blend/mix at high speed until creamy. Add additional optional ingredients to your preference if desired, and whiz again for 30 seconds. Put back into your glass container and freeze again for about 30 minutes, then serve. If you freeze for longer, allow to soften to your liking at room temperature before serving.

Sample Combos: Banana-Mango Coconut, Banana Chocolate Chip, Mint Chip, Chocolate Cherry Nib

10 minutes (assuming bananas are already frozen): 4 servings

Raw Cookie Bites

Provides 2 servings healthy fat, 1 nuts/seeds + protein

In my busy world, I also appreciate energy-packed foods that are easy to make and keep on hand for when I'm on the run but don't want a prepackaged energy bar; in fact, I'm not an energy bar lover. They generally taste too "vitamin-ish" to me and I find the textures dense, gummy, and overly sweet.

These power-packed, chock-full-of-health treats (that are also gluten free and dairy free) hit that sweet spot in your mouth, are made only of simple natural ingredients, and are energy filled rather than just sugary. They are superfast to make (like 10 minutes) and can be prepared from pretty much any dried fruit, nut, and nut butter combination that pleases you and your family and that you can easily keep stocked in your pantry.

1 cup of almonds, walnuts, or other nuts (you can use one type or a combination)
½ cup of raisins, dried apricots, dates, or prunes (any of these or a combination)
2 tbsp. almond or other nut butter
¼ cup dried coconut flakes, plus 2 tbsp. extra for rolling the balls in at the end
4 tbsp. ground flaxseeds
Optional for the chocolate version: ¼ cup unsweetened cacao powder

Put the nuts into your food processor and grind until they are close to finely ground. Add in the dried fruit and grind to form a thicker mess of stuff in your processor. Add in the nut butter and mix until a dough forms. Sometimes you might have to add a little extra to get the dough to form. Add in the ¼ cup of coconut flakes and flaxseeds (and add the cacao powder if making a chocolate version). Remove your blade from your food processor, then form round balls using about 2 tbsp. of "dough" per ball. Roll these in your hands, then roll in the extra coconut flakes (or you can roll in some extra walnuts, almonds, or cacao powder) and place on a platter or into a glass storage container for later enjoyment. These can be eaten straightaway or kept in the fridge and enjoyed over the next 3 to 4 days. They can be taken anywhere in a small storage container.

Serving size: 1 to 3 "bites"

Chocolate Tahini Date Fudge

Provides 2 servings healthy fat, 1 nuts/seeds + protein

¾ cup pitted dates (Deglet or Medjool)
¼ cup good-quality unsweetened dark chocolate cocoa powder
⅓ cup tahini (or enough to make it into a fudgy paste)
½ tsp. vanilla extract

Line a 5" × 5" pan with parchment paper, which makes it easier to remove and serve the fudge. Put all ingredients into a food processor with the mixing blade in. Mix until it forms a fudgy dough. Press the dough into the prepared pan. Place in the fridge for an hour. Cut into squares to serve.

Makes 8 servings. This recipe can easily be doubled for a larger pan. Keeps about 5 days in the fridge in a covered glass container.

Teas, Lattes, Spritzers, and Mocktails

Simple Herbal Tea

Keep a nice supply of herbal teas on hand. Serve hot and with lemon or iced. Example: Holy Basil, Mint + Hibiscus, Chamomile-Lavender-Mint.

Ginger Lemon Tea

Steep 1 tsp. freshly grated gingerroot in boiling water for 5 minutes. Strain and add lemon. Drink hot. Great for digestion, aches and pains, cold symptoms, and a natural anti-inflammatory.

Golden Milk Chai Latte

This is my favorite coffee alternative. It's still got a wee bit of caffeine from the black tea in the chai (though you can make this with decaf chai as well) and has a rich body and flavor. It is also anti-inflammatory and great for digestion and metabolism boosting. Just be careful working with turmeric—it stains.

Blend 1 cup unsweetened nondairy milk of choice (almond or cashew milk work the best) with either 2 pitted dates or 2 tsp. raw honey; heat until it's just about to simmer.

Add 1 tsp. vanilla extract plus ½ to 1 tsp. turmeric powder to the warm milk and stir.

Fill 2 cups halfway with the hot Masala chai (I use Rishi brand and make it in a French press; or use 2 teabags per cup of boiling water), then top off with the nut milk blend.

Enjoy hot or iced. Makes 2 cups

Sleepy Time Chai

Bring 1 cup of your favorite nut milk, or water, to a simmer. Turn off heat and pour over the following in your favorite mug:

1 heaping tsp. ashwagandha powder
½ tsp. reishi mushroom powder
1 tsp. honey (honey is calming and relaxing, so this is an okay time to have it, as long as you don't have a problem with your blood sugar) OR a few drops of high-quality stevia extract to sweeten
Dash of cinnamon or cardamom powder
Dash of vanilla

Enjoy in the evening for sleep, or anytime, for a calming warm beverage *sans* caffeine.

Nourish Your Womb Tea

While we think of red raspberry leaf for toning the uterus in pregnancy to prepare for an easier birth, it's also beneficial for all women with a uterus, especially if you tend to have heavy or crampy periods. This tea is rich in magnesium, vitamin C (ascorbic acid), and other nutrients. Enjoy as a beverage anytime, or during the week before your period.

Herbal Medicine 101

Turmeric, which you'll see throughout this book, is profoundly anti-inflammatory and helps to reset cortisol, especially when elevated due to chronic stress.

Ginger is also anti-inflammatory, and both ginger and turmeric heal the gut lining and symptomatically relieve gas and bloating, and both are helpful for pain.

Cinnamon not only tastes great and also benefits digestion; it helps lower high blood sugar and improves insulin resistance.

Green tea is a powerful anti-inflammatory with compounds that improve natural detoxification while supporting healthy metabolism.

Mix ¼ ounce of each of these organic dried herbs and store them in an airtight jar as your tea stash:

Red raspberry leaf
Nettle leaf
Rose hips
Hibiscus flower (omit during pregnancy!)
Peppermint leaf

To prepare: Steep 2 tbsp. of dried herb mix in 1 quart of boiling water for 15 minutes. Strain. Enjoy 1 to 2 cups daily, plain or iced. In warm weather, place the herbs in 1 quart of cold water and steep in the sun for an hour to make "sun tea."

WomanWise (Better Than Ibuprofen) Carrot-Apple-Ginger Juice

1 organic apple
6 organic carrots
1 inch of fresh gingerroot
Optional: ¼ organic lemon with the peel

Run all the ingredients through your juicer and drink fresh, 1 cup daily for preventing or reversing cramps or pelvic pain—or just because it's delicious, anti-inflammatory, great for your gut, and healthful.

Reishi "Hot Cocoa" Latte

When I was a kid, hot cocoa was my and my little brother's favorite "after snow play" warmer-upper. My mom would make us steaming cups of Swiss Miss with mini marshmallows. This is a healthier grown-up version that not only has the mood-boosting brain benefits of dark chocolate, but also adds in a healthy dose of reishi mushroom to reduce stress and support your immune health. If you're craving a comforting beverage premenstrually—or any time—this one will hit the spot.

2 cups organic nut milk, blended thoroughly with 4 pitted dates
4 tbsp. organic dark chocolate cocoa powder
2 tbsp. Dagoba (or similar) xocolatl chili hot chocolate powder if you like it spicy, or 6 tbsp. of the plain dark chocolate powder
1 to 2 tsp. reishi mushroom powder per cup
2 cinnamon sticks
Pink or sea salt
1 tbsp. shaved dark chocolate

Whisk together the date-sweetened nut milk, cocoa powder, chocolate powder, and reishi mushroom powder (or you can mix in a blender, instead). Heat in a saucepan on low-medium heat until just about to simmer. While heating, place a cinnamon stick into each mug. Pour the hot cocoa over the cinnamon sticks and sprinkle salt and shaved chocolate on top.

Makes 2 cups.

Sweet Dreams Adaptogen Latte

1 tsp. ashwagandha powder
½ tsp. reishi powder
⅛ tsp. cardamom seed powder
⅛ tsp. cinnamon powder
1 cup unsweetened almond milk or coconut milk
¼ tsp. vanilla extract
Optional (but recommended!): 2 pitted dates or 1 tsp. of raw honey (honey can help you sleep, too!)

Add all ingredients to blender and blend until smooth. Bring to the gentlest simmer. Pour into your favorite mug, dust with a pinch of cinnamon, and enjoy this anti-inflammatory, mind- and mood-soothing, cortisol-balancing drink before bed, or anytime.

Ginger Lemon Spritzer

Squeeze the juice of 1 tbsp. freshly grated ginger and ¼ of a fresh lemon into sparkling water. Stir and serve as is or with ice.

Love Your Liver Bitters and Tonic

Use the Love Your Liver Bitters Tonic mix on page 234 or Angostura bitters in ¼ cup of sparkling water, plain or on the rocks, for a liver detox tonic and after-dinner digestive.

Pomegranate Spritzer

Combine 2 ounces pomegranate concentrate in 6 ounces sparkling water. Antioxidant boosting.

Clean Green Mojito

Muddle 1 tbsp. fresh mint leaves in 8 ounces sparkling water. Add the juice of ¼ fresh lime. Serve over ice.

Lemon-Raspberry (or Cucumber)-Basil Cooler

Muddle several fresh basil leaves and 4 fresh or frozen red raspberries leaves in sparkling water and add a squeeze of lemon. Serve over ice. If you'd like a cucumber cooler instead, whiz ¼ of a cucumber in ¼ cup of water, strain, and add the liquid to the sparkling water with basil and lemon.

BOTANICAL AND SUPPLEMENT QUICK REFERENCE GUIDE

Herbs and nutrients can have tremendous health benefits; however, natural isn't synonymous with safe, and more isn't always better. Therefore, before you start taking the supplements discussed in this book, here are some basic safety rules:

- Please **follow all precautions** and **discuss herb and supplement use with your medical provider** before starting any new treatments, particularly if you have a medical condition or are on medications.

- **Do not exceed the recommended doses**, including being aware of ingredient redundancies if you're on more than one product.

- As this book is not intended for guidance once you become pregnant, assume that these are **not to be used in pregnancy** unless otherwise specified for fertility treatment, in which case unless otherwise stated, discontinue when you conceive. Overall, the herbs and supplements in this book are safe for use during breastfeeding.

Herb or Supplement	Uses	Dose	Notes & Precautions
5-HTP	Menstrual migraines Sleep support	100–300 mg 3x/day	Avoid combining with SSRIs, MAOIs, and tramadol.
Alpha lipoic acid (ALA)	Blood sugar balance Fertility PCOS	600 mg/day	—
Artichoke leaf	Detoxification	320–640 mg 3x/day	—
Ashwagandha (an adaptogen)	Endometriosis Low libido Perimenopause PCOS PMS-mood, cravings Sleep support Stress/adrenal support Thyroid support	Powder, capsule, tablet: 500 mg 3x/day, but up to 6 gm a day is safe and can help to optimize results. Tincture: 40–60 drops 3x/day	Safe with Hashimoto's, but can occasionally cause flares in some autoimmune conditions; discuss with your medical provider and start at the lowest dose, discontinuing if you notice any symptom exacerbation. It is a nightshade though not usually troublesome for those avoiding nightshades; use at your discretion.
Berberine	Blood sugar balance	400 mg 3x/day for 4 months	Avoid if you have liver disease.
Bitters	Constipation Detoxification Gas, bloating	2 droppers of tincture in a half glass of still or sparkling water before or after evening meal	—
Black cohosh	Hot flashes PCOS Uterine fibroids	40 mg/day	Remifemin, a commonly available product, can be taken to achieve this /daily dose.
Broccoli extracts (DIM, indole-3-carbinol [I3C])	Cyclic breast pain Detoxification Endometriosis Elevated estrogen PMS Uterine fibroids	I3C: 250–600 mg/day DIM: 100–200 mg/day	—
Butterbur	Menstrual migraines	75 mg 2x/day	Purchase the "PA-free" type only.
Calcium	Menstrual cramps PMS Sleep support	800 mg For special menstrual pain dosing see page 133.	Discuss use with your doctor if you've been told you have a high "coronary artery calcium score."
California poppy	Sleep support	Tincture: 20–40 drops before bed, repeat one time if needed	Can make you sleepy; do not take before driving.
Cannabis (CBD)	Endometriosis Low libido Menstrual cramps PMS-anxiety Sleep support	A product containing 15 mg 1–2x/day	Can be taken during the day, but take before bed for sleep.

Herb or Supplement	Uses	Dose	Notes & Precautions
Chamomile (extract)	Cyclic breast pain Leaky gut, digestion PMS-depression, anxiety Sleep support	Tincture: 40–60 drops in water 1–2x/day Tea: 1–2 cups/day	—
Choline	Fertility	400 mg/day	—
Cinnamon	Blood sugar balance Heavy periods Menstrual cramps, nausea	420 mg/day	Do not exceed this dose; use products intended as supplements (vs. kitchen spice).
Cinnamon & Poria Formula (traditional Chinese medicine product)	Uterine fibroids	Use as directed on package.	Avoid products imported from China due to possible contamination with heavy metals and herbicides.
Coenzyme Q10 (ubiquinone)	Menstrual migraines Mitochondrial support Ovulation support PCOS	150–200 mg/day	—
Cramp bark	Menstrual cramps	¼ tsp. in water as directed on page 259. If you use capsules, follow the dosing directions on the product you purchase.	—
Cranberry/D-mannose	Urinary tract infection (UTI)	500 mg 2x/day for prevention; up to 2 g/day for early symptoms	This is for prevention and mild symptoms only; always consult your medical provider for urinary tract infections.
Curcumin/Turmeric	Detoxification Endometriosis Leaky gut PMS Stress/adrenal support Uterine fibroids	Curcumin: dose depends on formulation, so take as directed on the package Turmeric: 2–10 g/day in food	Curcumin: look for Meriva on the package or a product formulated with piperine from black pepper or lecithin to improve absorption. Avoid if you have gallstones or gallbladder disease.
DGL licorice	Leaky gut	1–3 chewable tablets or capsules	Take between meals or before bed; discuss use with your doctor if you have high blood pressure.
DHEA	Perimenopause	25 mg/day	Do not exceed this dose; avoid if you've had hormone positive cancer.
FertilityBlend	Fertility	Take as directed on the package.	—
Feverfew	Menstrual migraines	25 mg/day	Do not take if on blood thinners.

Herb or Supplement	Uses	Dose	Notes & Precautions
Ginger	Endometriosis Heavy periods Leaky gut / IBS Menstrual cramps, nausea Menstrual migraines PMS-bloating	500 mg of ginger powder in capsules 3x/day, up to 3,000 mg/day, is considered safe.	Tea and tincture can also be used but aren't as effective for pain.
Ginkgo	Cyclic breast pain	80–160 mg standardized extract (24% ginkgo flavonglycosides) 2x/day	Avoid if you are on blood thinners.
Glycine	Blood sugar Detoxification Sleep support	3–5 g/day in capsule or powder form in foods	Take one hour before sleep.
Green tea extract (decaffeinated)	Detoxification support Endometriosis PCOS hair loss Uterine fibroids	800 mg of green tea extract (standardized to 45% EGCG, 95% polyphenols)	Do not exceed 200 mg of green tea catechins/day (will specify amount on package).
Guggul	Hormonal acne Thyroid support	500 mg/day	May cause nausea or GI upset so take with food.
Holy basil (an adaptogen)	Low energy Stress/adrenal support	2–3 mL (40–60 drops) tincture in water 3x/day	—
Hops	Hot flashes Perimenopause Sleep support Vaginal dryness	Tincture: 30 drops 1 hour before bed, repeat one time immediately before going to sleep	Before sleep only, do not drive. Do not drink alcohol while using. Avoid if you suffer from moderate to severe depression or have a history of estrogen receptor positive cancer.
Inositol	Insulin resistance PCOS Thyroid support	600 mg/day Sensitol or Ovasitol	—
Iodine	Cyclic breast pain Elevated estrogen Fertility Heavy periods Irregular periods Ovulation PCOS Thyroid support	Take as part of your prenatal or multivitamin.	—
Iron chelate	Anemia Hair loss Heavy menstrual flow Iron deficiency	30–60 mg/day	Take with 500 mg vitamin C (ascorbic acid) for absorption.

Herb or Supplement	Uses	Dose	Notes & Precautions
Kava kava	Anxiety Depression Perimenopause mood	100 mg for up to 6 months	Do not use if you have history of liver disease; check with your primary care provider before combining with other medications.
Krill oil	Cyclic breast pain PMS	1 g 2x/day	18% EPA and 12% DHA
L-arginine	Mitochondrial support Ovulation support	3 g/day	Discuss with your doctor before use if you're on any heart medications or have high or low blood pressure.
L-carnitine	Fertility support Mitochondrial support	3 g/day	—
L-glutamine	Leaky gut	5–10 g powder 2x/day	Take for 1–3 months.
Lavender	Anxiety Menstrual migraines PMS Sleep support	Essential oil (Lavela): 81 mg in capsule / day Aromatherapy oil: 2–3 drops applied to your temples, or 5–7 drops in a bath Tea: 1 cup/day Tincture: 20–40 drops/day	Avoid if you have a history of estrogen receptor positive cancer.
Lemon balm	Sleep support	80 mg/day or, if using tinctures, use 40–60 drops	—
Licorice	PCOS ovulation	150–300 mg; if using DGL up to 1,800 mg daily for 4 weeks	Avoid if you have high blood pressure or are on cortisol, and check with your medical provider before using if you are on other medications.
Krill oil	PMS	2 g of krill oil (1 g twice a day; 18% EPA and 12% DHA) for 8 days each month before your period is due	Expect results in about 8 weeks.
Maca (an adaptogen)	Fertility Low libido Perimenopause anxiety, depression Stress/adrenal support	600–900 mg of standardized maca in capsules (it will say this on the label) or 2–3 g/day in powder (mix into hot water, nut milk, or a smoothie) 75–100 mg/day 3 g/day for low libido	The Quechua people of Peru consider maca a food that promotes mental acuity, physical vitality, endurance, and stamina. Maca reduces anxiety and depression and is rich in essential amino acids, iodine, iron, and magnesium, as well as sterols that may possess a wide range of activities that support adrenal and hormone function. Maca comes in a few varieties, each with its own color—white, yellow, red, or black. There's no evidence, despite any company saying there's proof otherwise, that any one variety is more effective than the other.

Herb or Supplement	Uses	Dose	Notes & Precautions
Magnesium (citrate or glycinate)	Blood sugar / insulin resistance Constipation (use magnesium citrate Detoxification Menstrual cramps Menstrual migraines PCOS PMS-anxiety, bloating "Post-Pill" Sleep support Stress/adrenal support	200–600 mg/day For period pain up to 600–800 mg/day (see page 127)	If on blood pressure medication, discuss with your doctor before use as magnesium can lower BP.
Maitake mushroom	Blood sugar balance Ovulation support	50 mg/day of extract	Discuss with your doctor if you have an autoimmune condition.
Marshmallow root	Heals the gut lining	Infusion: 1–2 cups/day or 2 capsules 2x/day	To prevent interference with other medications, take >1 hour after medications you take orally.
Melatonin	Endometriosis Fertility support Hot flashes Leaky gut Menstrual migraines Ovarian health PCOS Primary ovarian insufficiency Sleep support	Sleep: 0.3–3 mg/day before bed Ovarian support: 1–3 mg/day	Allow 2 hours after eating before taking; do not exceed 3 mg/day when trying to conceive as higher doses can suppress fertility.
Methylfolate	Detoxification Fertility Menstrual cycle regularity Ovulation PMS	400–800 mcg/day	Take separately or as part of your multi- or prenatal vitamin.
Milk thistle	Detoxification Hormonal acne	200 mg 3x/day of a product standardized to 80% silymarin	—
Motherwort	Menstrual cramps Perimenopause PMS-mood	Tincture: ¼ tsp. up to 4 times daily or as directed on a capsule/tablet product	—
N-acetylcysteine (NAC)	Detoxification Endometriosis Fertility Ovarian health PCOS	600 mg 3x/day	—

Herb or Supplement	Uses	Dose	Notes & Precautions
Nettles	Hormonal hair loss	Infusion 2 cups/day (see page 369)	—
Omega-3 fatty acids (EPA/DHA—fish or algae derived)	Endometriosis Fertility Gut health Menstrual cramps PCOS PMS	850 EPA / 200 DHA 1–2x/day (or as directed in your Advanced Protocol, which may be a higher dose)	Use products from companies that have low heavy metal contamination.
Passionflower	PMS-anxiety Sleep support	Tincture: 30–60 drops Capsule/tablet: 320 mg up to 3x/day	Take before bed (see page 192).
Peppermint (oil)	Menstrual cramps Nausea	3 capsules containing about 187 mg of peppermint oil per capsule, once per day during the first 3 days of your period	Avoid if you have gastric reflux.
Phosphatydil serine (PS)	Stress response	100 mg 3x/day	—
Probiotic	Endometriosis Fertility Gut health (leaky gut, dysbiosis, IBS) Hormonal acne Nervous system support PCOS PMS-depression, anxiety Stress/adrenal support UTI Vaginal health	1–2 capsules/day, with a minimum of 10 billion CFUs (colony forming units)	Strains may include *Lactobacillus* and *Bifidobacterium* species, specifically *Bifidobacterium infantis* and *B. longum*.
Pueraria mirifica	Perimenopause Vaginal dryness	25–100 mg/day; take for at least 6 months	—
Pycnogenol	Detoxification Endometriosis Hot flashes Insulin sensitivity	25–200 mg/day	—
Red ginseng	Low libido	1 g/day	—
Reishi (an adaptogen)	PCOS hair loss Perimenopause Sleep support Stress/adrenal support	3–9 g dried mushrooms in capsules or tablets / day or 2–4 mL tincture in water 2–3x/day	Possibly avoid if you have a true mushroom allergy.

Herb or Supplement	Uses	Dose	Notes & Precautions
Relora	Sleep support	500 mg/day at bedtime	Proprietary combination of the traditional Chinese herbs magnolia and phellodendron
Rhodiola	Anxiety Inflammation Mood support Sleep support Stress/adrenal support	200–400 mg in capsules or tablets daily or 2–3 mL (40–60 drops) of tincture, in water 2–3 times daily	Avoid in bipolar affective disorder.
Rhubarb (Chinese or Siberian)	Hot flashes	Dosing is complex so I use a proprietary product called Estrovera, following the dosing on the package.	Avoid with a history of estrogen receptor positive cancer.
Saffron	PMS-depression	5–15 mg 2x/day	Take with food to avoid nausea. Do not exceed the upper dose.
Selenium	Blood sugar balance Detoxification Endometriosis Fertility Hormonal acne Ovarian health Ovulation PCOS "Post-Pill" support Thyroid support	200 mcg/day	Do not exceed this dose. Safe during pregnancy and while breastfeeding.
Senna	Constipation	1 cup of senna and mint tea before bed	—
Shatavari (an adaptogen)	Perimenopause-mood PMS-mood Stress/adrenal support	2–4 mL (40–80 drops) of tincture in water 2–3x/day	Avoid if you have a history of estrogen-receptor-positive cancer.
Shepherd's purse	Heavy periods	Tincture: 30–40 drops in water 2–3x/day	Avoid if you are on medications for blood coagulation or have a blood clotting disorder.
Spearmint	PCOS ovulation	Tea, 1–3 cups daily	—
St. John's wort	Detoxification PMS/PMDD-anxiety, depression	300 mg 3x/day	Use with black cohosh.
Tea tree oil	Hormonal acne	5% solution of the oil diluted in a carrier oil (i.e., about 2 drops of the essential oil in 1 tsp. of another oil such as coconut, avocado, jojoba or grapeseed oil), can be applied as a spot treatment.	For topical and suppository use only; use diluted only.
Thiamine (vitamin B1)	Severe menstrual cramps	100 mg/day for 3 months	—

Herb or Supplement	Uses	Dose	Notes & Precautions
Triphala (herbal blend)	Constipation	Take as directed on package.	—
Uva ursi	UTI	Tea, or take as directed for a packaged product.	Avoid if you have kidney disease.
Valerian	Hot flashes Menstrual cramps Sleep support	255–500 mg 3x/day	Do not take before driving.
Vitamin B2 (riboflavin)	Menstrual migraines Mitochondrial support Ovulation support	400 mg/day	—
Vitamin B6	Detoxification Fertility Hormonal acne Ovulation PCOS Period problems PMS "Post-Pill" Skipped periods Sleep support	25–100 mg/day	Do not exceed this dose so cross-check your supplements for your total intake.
Vitamin B12	Detoxification Sleep support	400–1,000 mcg/day	I recommend taking it before noon as some find it too stimulating in the evening.
Vitamin C (ascorbic acid)	Detoxification Endometriosis Fertility Ovarian support Skipped periods Stress/adrenal support	500–1,000 mg/day	—
Vitamin D3	Blood sugar balance / insulin resistance Endometriosis Fertility Menstrual cramps PCOS PMS "Post-Pill" Thyroid support Uterine fibroids	To replenish, take up to 4,000 IU/day for 3 months. For maintenance, take 2,000 IU/day.	To optimize your vitamin D levels, have your medical provider check your blood levels; however for most people, these dosing instructions are appropriate.

Herb or Supplement	Uses	Dose	Notes & Precautions
Vitamin E	Endometriosis Menstrual cramps Vaginal dryness	500 IU/day	Do not exceed this dose; do not supplement if you are currently a smoker.
Vitex (chaste tree)	Cyclic breast pain Fertility Heavy periods Hot flashes Low progesterone Menstrual migraines Ovulation Perimenopause PCOS PMS Skipped periods	Capsules 180–200 mg 1–2x/day Tincture: 5 mL/day (~1 measured tsp.) in water	May rarely exacerbate depression; if you notice this symptom, discontinue.
White peony	Fertility Ovulation PCOS	As directed for white peony and licorice combination products	Avoid the licorice if you have high blood pressure.
Yarrow	Heavy periods	1–2 cups of infusion/day during heavy flow days	—
Zinc (citrate, picolinate, or sulfate)	Endometriosis Fertility Hormonal acne Menstrual cramps PCOS hair loss PMS-depression Stress/adrenal support Thyroid support	15–45 mg/day	Take with meals to prevent nausea.
Zinc carnosine	Leaky gut	75–150 mg/day	Take with meals to prevent nausea.

ACKNOWLEDGMENTS

They say it takes a village to raise a child. I couldn't agree more. As an author, one could say the same about a book. The village that supported me with this book includes:

My publishing team: Gideon Weil, for honoring the importance of this book from day one and for letting it become a very big book; and Sydney Rogers, for keeping it "true to me."

Jeff Jump, MD, my BFAM, and Robin Gellman, LAc, who read first drafts and told me to keep going because women need this.

Michelle Collins, MD, my bestie, without whom this book would not be here, because sometimes I wanted to quit, and she gave me permission to, which meant everything.

My daughter Yemima, for invaluable edits that shaped the first draft and who said, "Mom, your readers are looking for answers they can trust—and you have those." My daughters Forest and Naomi, whose insights helped make this book relevant to women of any age.

My life partner—Tracy Romm, EdD, for breakfasts, dinners, tea, walks, for editing, listening to my doubts (even at four in the morning), coming up with some truly helpful insights when I hit roadblocks, and for being in on this journey every step of the way—and I hope, every step to come.

And all of the women who have trusted me with their health.

I am ever grateful.

ON HER TERMS

Amenorrhea: The absence of a menstrual period in a woman of reproductive age.

Androgens: Hormones typically defined as leading to male characteristics, also important in women's reproductive and gynecologic health. The principle androgens are testosterone and androstenedione, which are produced in the ovaries, adrenal glands, and fat cells.

Anovulation: Lack of ovulation; not ovulating.

Cervix: The lower end of the uterus, shaped like the narrow end of a balloon, has an opening for sperm to enter from the vagina and babies and menstrual blood to exit.

Clitoris: Sitting at the top of your vulva like a little head with a hood on it, this sensation powerhouse runs below the surface of your vulva and has over fifteen thousand nerve endings. Cool fact: this is the only body part whose sole job is providing pleasure.

Dysmenorrhea: Period pain.

Ecosystem: A complex, interconnected network, the interaction of an organism and its physical environment.

Endometrium: The interior lining of the uterus; it thickens during the menstrual cycle in preparation for possible implantation of an embryo and is shed during menstruation.

Entrainment: The process that includes harmonization between the functions of the organ systems with the circadian rhythm.

Environment: The internal and external factors that can affect health, including the totality of living and working conditions as well as physical, biological, social, and cultural responses to these conditions.

Exposome: The sum total of factors you're exposed to that interact with your own genetic predispositions or that independently influence health or disease.

Fallopian tubes: The structures attached to the horns of the uterus that receive the egg from the ovaries at ovulation; this is where conception usually occurs if egg meets sperm.

Hypothalamus: This "conducting gland" in your brain links the nervous system to the endocrine system via the pituitary gland. It stimulates the release of hormones that activate the thyroid, adrenal glands, and ovaries, regulating sleep, hunger, metabolism, circadian rhythm, and even emotional bonding.

Menopause: The cessation of menstrual cycles, usually occurring after age 45 and by age 54.

Ovaries: These organs are your estrogen-, progesterone-, and testosterone-producing powerhouses, and where you mature and release an *ovum* (fancy word for egg) from ovarian follicles (fluid-filled sacs that nourish the ova) when you ovulate.

Perimenopause: The period of time, which can be as long as eight years, leading up to menopause.

Pituitary gland: This tiny organ the size of a pea, below the hypothalamus in the brain, produces many hormones that travel throughout the body, directing numerous processes and stimulating other glands to produce other hormones.

Uterus: The powerful muscular organ lined with a layer called the *endometrium*; this is the site of action for menstruation, pregnancy, and powerful contractions that occur with orgasm and childbirth.

Vagina: A seemingly miraculous muscular tube, about four to seven inches long, where tampons go into, menstrual blood and babies come out of, and you (hopefully) experience pleasure, which can also stretch to accommodate a baby's head when it's serving as the birth canal. It includes the G-spot, responsible for a deeper orgasm sensation than clitoral stimulation alone, though very few women orgasm without clitoral stimulation.

Vulva: What you see when you're standing naked in front of the mirror, or have a look at what's going on between your legs, is your external genitalia, collectively called the vulva. It includes the mons pubis (mountain of Venus), the fleshy pad about six inches south of your navel, the labia majora (outer lips), labia minora (inner lips), nerves, glands, and then some.

REFERENCES

Over fifteen hundred scientific papers were reviewed in the development of this manuscript; however, space limitations allow me to provide only a fraction of these. You can find the complete references, by chapter, at my website, avivaromm.com/hormone-intelligence-resources.

ACOG Committee on Adolescent Health Care. ACOG Committee Opinion No. 349, November 2006: Menstruation in girls and adolescents: using the menstrual cycle as a vital sign. *Obstet Gynecol* 108, no. 5 (Nov. 2006): 1323–28.

Agarwal, A., et al. The role of oxidative stress in female reproduction: a review. *Reprod Biol Endrocrinol* 10 (2012): 1–32.

Akbari, M., et al. The effects of vitamin D supplementation on biomarkers of inflammation and oxidative stress among women with polycystic ovary syndrome: a systematic review and meta-analysis of randomized controlled trials. *Horm Metab Res* 50, no. 4 (Apr. 2018): 271–79.

Allen, J. M., et al. Exercise alters gut microbiota composition and function in lean and obese humans. *Med Sci Sports Exerc* 50, no. 4 (Apr. 2018): 747–57.

American College of Obstetricians and Gynecologists. Adult manifestations of childhood sexual abuse. Committee Opinion No. 498. *Obstet Gynecol* 118 (2011): 392–95.

American College of Obstetricians and Gynecologists. Alternatives to hysterectomy in the management of leiomyomas. ACOG Practice Bulletin. *Obstet Gynecol* 112 (2008): 387–400.

Armour, M., et al. Self-management strategies amongst Australian women with endometriosis: a national online survey. *BMC Complem Altern Med* 19 (2019): 17.

Ata, B., et al. The endobiota study: comparison of vaginal, cervical and gut microbiota between women with stage 3/4 endometriosis and healthy controls. *Sci Rep* 9, no. 2204 (2019).

Bailey, M. T., and C. L. Coe. Endometriosis is associated with an altered profile of intestinal microflora in female rhesus monkeys. *Hum Reprod* 17, no. 7 (July 2002): 1704–8.

Baker, F. C., and H. S. Driver. Circadian rhythms, sleep, and the menstrual cycle. *Sleep Med* 8, no. 6 (Sept. 2007): 613–22.

Baker, J. M., et al. Estrogen-gut microbiome axis: physiological and clinical implications. *Maturitas* 103 (Sept. 2017): 45–53.

Balachandran, K., et al. Increased risk of obstructive sleep apnoea in women with polycystic ovary syndrome: a population-based cohort study. *Eur J Endocrinol* Feb. 13, 2019. doi: 10.1530/EJE-18-0693.

Ballard, K., et al. What's the delay? A qualitative study of women's experiences of reaching a diagnosis of endometriosis. *Fertil Steril* 86 (2006): 1296–301.

Belkaid, Y., and T. Hand. Role of the microbiota in immunity and inflammation. *Cell* 157, no. 1 (Mar. 27, 2014): 121–41.

Brown, S. L., et al. Social closeness increases salivary progesterone in humans. *Horm Behav* 56, no. 1 (June 2009): 108–11.

Bruner-Tran, K., et al. Medical management of endometriosis: emerging evidence linking inflammation to disease pathophysiology. *Minerva Ginecol* 65, no. 2 (Apr. 2013): 199–213.

Buck, L. G., et al. Bisphenol A and phthalates and endometriosis, the ENDO study. *Fertil Steril* 100, no. 1 (July 2013): 162–69.e2.

Buck, L. G., et al. Persistent environmental pollutants and couple fecundity: the LIFE study. *Environ Health Perspect* 121, no. 2 (Feb. 2013): 231–36.

Carignan, C. C., et al. Urinary concentrations of organophosphate flame retardant metabolites and pregnancy outcomes among women undergoing in vitro fertilization. *Environ Health Perspect* 125, no. 8 (Aug. 2017).

Cedars, M., et al. The sixth vital sign: what reproduction tells us about overall health. Proceedings from a NICHD/CDC workshop. *Hum Reprod Open* 2017, no. 2 (July 12, 2017).

Chocano-Bedoya, P. O., et al. Intake of selected minerals and risk of premenstrual syndrome. *Am J Epidemiol* 177, no. 10 (May 15, 2013): 1118–27.

Cobey, K., J. Havlicek, K. Klapilova, and S. C. Roberts. Hormonal contraceptive use during relationship formation and sexual desire during pregnancy. *Arch Sex Behav* 45 (2016): 2117–22.

Cooney, L. G., et al. High prevalence of moderate and severe depressive and anxiety symptoms in polycystic ovary syndrome: a systematic review and meta-analysis. *Hum Reprod* 32, no. 5 (May 1, 2017): 1075–91.

Copp, T., et al. Are expanding disease definitions unnecessarily labelling women with polycystic ovary syndrome? *BMJ* 358 (2017): j3694.

Corona, L. E., et al. Use of other treatments before hysterectomy for benign conditions in a statewide hospital collaborative. *Am J Obstet Gynecol* 212 (Mar. 2015): 304.e1.

Crain, D. A., et al. Female reproductive disorders: the roles of endocrine-disrupting compounds and developmental timing. *Fertil Steril* 90, no. 4 (Oct. 2008): 911–40.

Daily, J. W., et al. Efficacy of ginger for alleviating the symptoms of primary dysmenorrhea: a systematic review and meta-analysis of randomized clinical trials. *Pain Med* 16, no. 12 (Dec. 2015): 2243–55.

de Melo, A. S., et al. Pathogenesis of polycystic ovary syndrome: multifactorial assessment from the foetal stage to menopause. *Reproduction* 150, no. 1 (July 2015): R11–24.

Diamanti-Kandarakis, E., et al. Endocrine-disrupting chemicals: an Endocrine Society scientific statement. *Endocr Rev* 30, no. 4 (June 2009): 293–342.

Diaz, A., et al. Menstruation in girls and adolescents: using the menstrual cycle as a vital sign. American Academy of Pediatrics Committee on Adolescence; American College of Obstetricians and Gynecologists Committee on Adolescent Health Care. *Pediatrics* 118, no. 5 (Nov. 2006): 2245–50.

Dokras, A., et al. Androgen Excess-Polycystic Ovary Syndrome Society: position statement on depression, anxiety, quality of life, and eating disorders in polycystic ovary syndrome. *Fertil Steril* 109, no. 5 (May 2018): 888–99.

Donga, E., et al. A single night of partial sleep deprivation induces insulin resistance in multiple metabolic pathways in healthy subjects. *J Clin Endocrinol Metab* 95, no. 6 (June 2010): 2963–68.

Doufas, A., and G. Mastorakos. The hypothalamic-pituitary-thyroid axis and the female reproductive system. *Ann NY Acad Sci* 900 (2000): 65–76.

Dunson, D. B., et al. Increased infertility with age in men and women. *Obstet Gynecol* 103, no. 1 (Jan. 2004): 51–56.

Facchinetti, F., et al. Results from the International Consensus Conference on myo-inositol and d-chiro-inositol in obstetrics and gynecology: the link between metabolic syndrome and PCOS. *Eur J Obstet Gynecol Reprod Biol* 195 (Dec. 2015): 72–76.

Fahs, B. Demystifying menstrual synchrony: women's subjective beliefs about bleeding in tandem with other women. *Women's Reprod Health* 3, no. 1 (2016): 1–15.

Fernando, S., and L. Rombauts. Melatonin: shedding light on infertility? *J Ovarian Res* 7 (2014): 98.

Fisher, M., and E. Eugster. What is in our environment that effects puberty? *Reprod Toxicol* 44 (Apr. 2014): 7–14.

Fjerbaek, A., and U. B. Knudsen. Endometriosis, dysmenorrhea and diet—what is the evidence? *Eur J Obstet Gynecol Reprod Biol* 132, no. 2 (2007): 140–47.

Forsyth, C. B., et al. Circadian rhythms, alcohol and gut interactions. *Alcohol* 49, no. 4 (June 2015): 389–98.

Gabriel, B., and J. Zierath. Circadian rhythms and exercise—re-setting the clock in metabolic disease. *Nat Rev Endocrinol* 15, no. 4 (Apr. 2019): 197–206.

Gaskins, A. J., and J. E. Chavarro. Diet and fertility: a review. *Am J Obstet Gynecol* 218, no. 4 (Apr. 2018): 379–89.

Gildersleeve, K., et al. Do women's mate preferences change across the ovulatory cycle? A meta-analytic review. *Psychol Bull* 5 (2014): 1205–59.

Girman, A., et al. An integrative medicine approach to premenstrual syndrome. *Am J Obstet Gynecol* 188, no. 5 (2003): 56–65.

Goldstein, C. A., and Y. R. Smith. Sleep, circadian rhythms, and fertility. *Curr Sleep Med Rep* 2 (2016): 206–17.

Gollenberg, A., et al. Perceived stress and severity of perimenstrual symptoms: the biocycle study. *J Womens Health (Larchmt)* 19, no. 5 (May 2010): 959–67.

González, F. Inflammation in polycystic ovary syndrome: underpinning of insulin resistance and ovarian dysfunction. *Steroids* 77, no. 4 (Mar. 10, 2012): 300–5.

Grindler, N., et al. Persistent organic pollutants and early menopause in U.S. women. *PLOS ONE* 10, no. 1 (Jan. 28, 2015): e0116057.

Guo, Y., et al. Association between polycystic ovary syndrome and gut microbiota. *PLOS ONE* 11, no. 4 (Apr. 19, 2016): e0153196.

Hanson, S. O., and L. B. Kundsen. Endometriosis, dysmenorrhea, and diet. *Eur J Obstet Gynecol Reprod Biol* 169, no. 2 (July 2013): 162–71.

Harlev, A., et al. Targeting oxidative stress to treat endometriosis. *Expert Opin Ther Targets* 19, no. 11 (2015): 1447–64.

Hennig, B., et al. Nutrition can modulate the toxicity of environmental pollutants: implications in risk assessment and human health. *Environ Health Perspect* 120, no. 6 (2012): 771–74.

Herington, J. L., et al. Dietary fish oil supplementation inhibits formation of endometriosis-associated adhesions in a chimeric mouse model. *Fertil Steril* 99 (2013): 543–50.

Hoffmann, D., and A. Tarzian. The girl who cried pain: a bias against women in the treatment of pain. *J Law Med Ethics* 29 (2001): 13–27.

Houghton, S. C., et al. Intake of dietary fat and fat subtypes and risk of premenstrual syndrome in the Nurses' Health Study II. *Br J Nutr* 118, no. 10 (Nov. 2017): 849–57.

Hunt, P., et al. Female reproductive disorders, diseases, and costs of exposure to endocrine disrupting chemicals in the European Union. *J Clin Endocrinol Metab* 101, no. 4 (Apr. 2016): 1562–70.

Husby, G. K., et al. Diagnostic delay in women with pain and endometriosis. *Acta Obstet Gynecol Scand* 82 (2003): 649–53.

Irani, M., and A. Merhi. Role of vitamin D in ovarian physiology and its implication in reproduction: a systematic review. *Fertil Steril* 102, no. 2 (Aug. 2014): 460–68.

Johnson, P. A., et al. Sex-specific medical research: why women's health can't wait. A Report of the Mary Horrigan Connors Center for Women's Health & Gender Biology at Brigham and Women's Hospital. 2014.

Kamel, H. H. Role of phytoestrogens in ovulation induction in women with polycystic ovarian syndrome. *Eur J Obstet Gynecol Reprod Biol* 168, no. 1 (May 2013): 60–63.

Kashefi, F., et al. Effect of ginger on heavy menstrual bleeding: a placebo-controlled randomized clinical trial. *Phytother Res* 29 (2015): 114–19.

Kennaway, D., M. Boden, and T. Varcoe. Circadian rhythms and fertility. *Mol Cell Endocrinol* 349, no. 1 (Feb. 5, 2012): 56–61.

Khan, K. N., et al. Escherichia coli contamination of menstrual blood and effect of bacterial endotoxin on endometriosis. *Fertil Steril* 94, no. 7 (Dec. 2010): 2860–63. e1–3.

Kloss, J. D., et al. Sleep, sleep disturbance and fertility in women. *Sleep Med Rev* 22 (Aug. 2015): 78–87.

Kuang, B., et al. O-55: Fertility and infertility: What do students at an Ivy League college really know? *Fertil Steril* 86, no. 3, Supplement (Sept. 2006): S24.

Labyak, S., et al. Effects of shiftwork on sleep and menstrual function in nurses, *Health Care Women Int* 23, no. 6–7 (2002): 703–14.

Lamvu, G., et al. Patterns of prescription opioid use in women with endometriosis: evaluating prolonged use, daily use, and concomitant use with benzodiazepines. *Obstet Gynecol* 133, no. 6 (June 2019): 1120–30.

Laschke, M. W., and M. D. Menger. The gut microbiota: a puppet master in the pathogenesis of endometriosis? *Am J Obstet Gynecol* 215, no. 1 (July 2016): 68.e1–4.

Lin, T. Y., et al. Risk of developing obstructive sleep apnea among women with polycystic ovarian syndrome: a nationwide longitudinal follow-up study. *Sleep Med* 36 (Aug. 2017): 165–69.

Lin, W. C., et al. Increased risk of endometriosis in patients with lower genital tract infection: a nationwide cohort study. *Medicine* (Baltimore) 95, no. 10 (Mar. 2016): e2773.

Lindheim, L., et al. Alterations in gut microbiome composition and barrier function are associated with reproductive and metabolic defects in women with polycystic ovary syndrome (PCOS): a pilot study. *PLOS ONE* 12, no. 1 (Mar. 2017).

Liu, R., et al. Dysbiosis of gut microbiota associated with clinical parameters in polycystic ovary syndrome. *Front Microbiol* 8 (2017): 324.

Louis, G. M., et al. Environmental PCB exposure and risk of endometriosis. *Hum Reprod* 20 (2005): 279–85.

Ma, B., et al. The vaginal microbiome: rethinking health and diseases. *Annu Rev Microbiol* 66 (2012): 371–89.

Marziali, M., et al. Gluten-free diet: a new strategy for management of painful endometriosis related symptoms? *Minerva Chir* 67, no. 7 (2012): 499–504.

Marziali, M., and T. Capozzolo. Role of gluten-free diet in the management of chronic pelvic pain of deep infiltrating endometriosis. *J Minim Invasive Gynecol* 22, no. 6S (Nov.–Dec. 2015): S51–52.

Mendonça, L., et al. Non-steroidal anti-inflammatory drugs as a possible cause for reversible infertility. *Rheumatology* 39, no. 8 (Aug. 1, 2000): 880–82.

Merhi, I. M. Role of vitamin D in ovarian physiology and its implication in reproduction: a systematic review. *Fertil Steril* 102, no. 2 (Aug. 2014): 460–68.

Mesen, T., and S. Young. Progesterone and the luteal phase: a requisite to reproduction. *Obstet Gynecol Clin North Am* 42, no. 1 (Mar. 2015): 135–51.

Messerlian, et al. The Environment and Reproductive Health (EARTH) study: a prospective preconception cohort. *Hum Reprod Open* 2018, no. 2 (Feb. 2018).

Michels, K. A., J. Wactawski-Wende, and J. L. Mills. Folate, homocysteine and the ovarian cycle among healthy regularly menstruating women. *Hum Reprod* 32, no. 8 (Aug. 1, 2017): 1743–50.

Mier-Cabrera, J., et al. Women with endometriosis improved their peripheral antioxidant markers after the application of a high antioxidant diet. *Biol Endocrinol* 7, (2009): 54.

Missmer, S. A., et al. A prospective study of dietary fat consumption and endometriosis risk. *Hum Reprod* 25, no. 6 (June 2010): 1528–35.

Moore, J. S., et al. Endometriosis in patients with irritable bowel syndrome: specific symptomatic and demographic profile, and response to the low FODMAP diet. *Aust N Z J Obstet Gynaecol* 57, no. 2 (Apr. 2017): 201–5.

Moran, L. J., et al. Sleep disturbances in a community-based sample of women with polycystic ovary syndrome. *Hum Reprod* 30, no. 2 (Feb. 2015): 466–72.

Mumford, S., et al. Dietary fat intake and reproductive hormone concentrations and ovulation in regularly menstruating women. *Am J Clin Nutr* 103 (2016): 868–77.

Mumford, S. L., et al. Serum antioxidants are associated with serum reproductive hormones and ovulation among healthy women. *J Nutr* 146, no. 1 (Jan. 2016): 98–106.

Murri, M., et al. Circulating markers of oxidative stress and polycystic ovary syndrome (PCOS): a systematic review and meta-analysis. *Hum Reprod Update* 19, no. 3 (May–June 2013): 268–88.

Netsu, S., et al. Oral eicosapentaenoic acid supplementation as possible therapy for endometriosis. *Fertil Steril* 90 (2008): 1496–502.

Neuman, H., et al. Microbial endocrinology: the interplay between the microbiota and the endocrine system. *FEMS Microbiol Rev* 39, no. 4 (July 2015): 509–21.

Parazzini, F., et al. Dietary components and uterine leiomyomas: a review of published data. *Nutr Cancer* 67, no. 4 (2015): 569–79.

Parazzini, F., P. Viganò, M. Candiani, and L. Fedele. Diet and endometriosis risk: a literature review. *Reprod Biomed Online* 26, no. 4 (Apr. 2013): 323–36.

Patel, S., et al. Effects of endocrine-disrupting chemicals on the ovary. *Biol Reprod* 93, no. 1 (2015): 20.

Pearcea, K., and K. Tremellena. Influence of nutrition on the decline of ovarian reserve and subsequent onset of natural menopause. *Hum Fertil* 19, no. 3 (2016): 173–79.

Purdue-Smithe, A., et al. Vitamin D and calcium intake and risk of early menopause. *Am J Clin Nutr* 105, no. 6 (June 2017): 1493–501.

Rattan, S., et al. Exposure to endocrine disruptors during adulthood: consequences for female fertility. *J Endocrinol* 233, no. 3 (June 2017): R109–29.

Robinson, O., and M. Vrijheid. The pregnancy exposome. *Curr Environ Health Rep* 2, no. 2 (June 2015): 204–13.

Roca, C., et al. Differential menstrual cycle regulation of hypothalamic-pituitary-adrenal axis in women with premenstrual syndrome and controls. *J Clin Endocrinol Metab* 88, no. 7 (2003): 3057–63.

Roshdy, E., et al. Treatment of symptomatic uterine fibroids with green tea extract: a pilot randomized controlled clinical study. *Int J Womens Health* 5 (Aug. 7, 2013): 477–86.

Saeed, S. A., et al. Depression and anxiety disorders: benefits of exercise, yoga, and meditation. *Am Fam Physician* 99, no. 10 (May 15, 2019): 620–27.

Schecter, A., and D. Boivin. Sleep, hormones, and circadian rhythms throughout the menstrual cycle in healthy women and women with premenstrual dysphoric disorder. *Int J Endocrinol* 2010 (2010): 259345.

Schliep, K. C., et al. Perceived stress, reproductive hormones, and ovulatory function: a prospective cohort study. *Epidemiology* 26, no. 2 (2015): 177–84.

Schliep, K. C., et al. Sexual and physical abuse and gynecologic disorders. *Hum Reprod* 31, no. 8 (Aug. 2016): 1904–12.

Sen, A., and M. T. Sellix. The circadian timing system and environmental circadian disruption: from follicles to fertility. *Endocrinology* 157, no. 9 (Sept. 2016): 3366–73.

Sesti, F., et al. Dietary therapy: a new strategy for management of chronic pelvic pain. *Nutr Res Rev* 24, no. 1 (June 2011): 318.

Sinaii, N., et al. High rates of autoimmune and endocrine disorders, fibromyalgia, chronic fatigue syndrome and atopic diseases among women with endometriosis: a survey analysis. *Hum Reprod* 17, no. 10 (Oct. 2002): 2715–24.

Siobán, D., et al. The ReSTAGE Collaboration: defining optimal bleeding criteria for onset of early menopausal transition. *Fertil Steril* 89, no. 1 (Jan. 2008): 129–40.

Skovlund, C. W., et al. Association of hormonal contraception with depression. *JAMA Psychiatry* 73, no. 11 (Nov. 2016): 1154–62.

Sood, R., et al. Paced breathing compared with usual breathing for hot flashes. *Menopause* 20, no. 2 (Feb. 2013): 179–84.

Tersigni, C., et al. Celiac disease and reproductive disorders: meta-analysis of epidemiologic associations and potential pathogenic mechanisms. *Hum Reprod Update* 20, no. 4 (July 2014): 582–93.

The NAMS 2017 Hormone Therapy Position Statement Advisory Panel. The 2017 hormone therapy position statement of the North American Menopause Society. *Menopause* 24, no. 7 (2017): 728–53.

Thompson, M., and K. Boekelheide. Multiple environmental chemical exposures to lead, mercury and polychlorinated biphenyls among childbearing-aged women (NHANES 1999–2004): body burden and risk factors. *Environ Res* 121 (Feb. 2013): 23–30.

Toledo, E., et al. Dietary patterns and difficulty conceiving: a nested case–control study. *Fertil Steril* 96, no. 5 (Nov. 2011): 1149–53.

Torres, P. J., et al. Gut microbial diversity in women with polycystic ovary syndrome correlates with hyperandrogenism. *J Clin Endocrinol Metab* 103, no. 4 (Apr. 1, 2018): 1502–11.

Trabert, B., et al. Diet and risk of endometriosis in a population-based case-control study. *Br J Nutr* 105, no. 3 (Feb. 2011): 459–67.

Treloar, S. A., et al. Early menstrual characteristics associated with subsequent diagnosis of endometriosis. *AJOG* 202 (2010): 534.e1–6.

Upson, K., et al. Organochlorine pesticides and risk of endometriosis: findings from a population-based case-control study. *Environ Health Perspect* 121 (2013): 1319–24.

Valdes, A. M., and J. Walter. Role of the gut microbiota in nutrition and health. *BMJ* 361 (2018): k2179.

van der Zandenm, M., and A. W. Nap. Knowledge of, and treatment strategies for, endometriosis among general practitioners. *Reprod Biomed Online* 32, no. 5 (May 2016): 527–31.

Vujic, G., et al. Efficacy of orally applied probiotic capsules for bacterial vaginosis and other vaginal infections: a double-blind, randomized, placebo-controlled study. *Eur J Obstet Gynecol Reprod Biol* 168, no. 1 (2013): 75–79.

Walter, J., et al. Better reporting needed for cosmetics and women's health. *AJOG* 218, no. 2 (Feb. 2018): 265–66.

Wang, YY., et al. Menstrual cycle regularity and length across the reproductive lifespan and risk of premature mortality: prospective cohort study. *BMJ* 371 (2020): m3464.

Weiss, G., et al. Inflammation in reproductive disorders. *Reprod Sci* 16, no. 2 (Feb. 2009): 216–29.

Werner, A., and K. Malterud. It is hard work behaving as a credible patient: encounters between women with chronic pain and their doctors. *Soc Sci Med* 57 (2003): 1409–19.

Wise, L. A., et al. Intake of fruit, vegetables, and carotenoids in relation to risk of uterine leiomyomata. *Am J Clin Nutr* 94, no. 6 (Dec. 2011): 1620–31.

Wise, L. A., et al. A prospective study of dairy intake and risk of uterine leiomyomata. *Am J Epidemiol* 171 (2010): 221.

Woosley, J. A., and K. L. Lichstein. Dysmenorrhea, the menstrual cycle, and sleep. *Behav Med* 40, no. 1 (2014).

Yang, H., et al. Pleiotropic roles of melatonin in endometriosis, recurrent spontaneous abortion, and polycystic ovary syndrome. *Am J Reprod Immunol* 80, no. 1 (July 2018): e12839.

Zarei, S., et al. Effects of calcium—vitamin D and calcium—alone on pain intensity and menstrual blood loss in women with primary dysmenorrhea: a randomized controlled trial. *Pain Med* 18, no. 1 (2017): 3–13.

Zee, P. C., and F. W. Turek. Sleep and health: everywhere and in both directions. *Arch Intern Med* 166 (2006): 1686–88.

Zelieann, R., et al. Endocrine-disrupting chemicals in ovarian function: effects on steroidogenesis, metabolism and nuclear receptor signaling. *Reproduction* 142 (2011): 633–46.

Zota, A. R., and B. Shamasunder. The environmental injustice of beauty: framing chemical exposures from beauty products as a health disparities concern. *Am J Obstet Gynecol* 217, no. 4 (Oct. 2017): 418.e1–6.